HEALTHCARE TECHNOLOGIES SERIES 17

Patient-Centered Digital Healthcare Technology

Other volumes in this series

Volume 1	**Nanobiosensors for Personalized and Onsite Biomedical Diagnosis** P. Chandra (Editor)
Volume 2	**Machine Learning for Healthcare Technologies** D.A. Clifton (Editor)
Volume 3	**Portable Biosensors and Point-of-Care Systems** S.E. Kintzios (Editor)
Volume 4	**Biomedical Nanomaterials: From design to implementation** T.J. Webster and H. Yazici (Editors)
Volume 6	**Active and Assisted Living: Technologies and applications** F. Florez-Revuelta and A.A. Chaaraoui (Editors)
Volume 7	**Semiconductor Lasers and Diode-Based Light Sources for Biophotonics** P.E. Andersen and P.M. Petersen (Editors)
Volume 9	**Human Monitoring, Smart Health and Assisted Living: Techniques and technologies** S. Longhi, A. Monteriù and A. Freddi (Editors)
Volume 13	**Handbook of Speckle Filtering and Tracking in Cardiovascular Ultrasound Imaging and Video** C.P. Loizou, C.S. Pattichis and J. D'hooge (Editors)
Volume 14	**Soft Robots for Healthcare Applications: Design, modelling, and control** S. Xie, M. Zhang and W. Meng
Volume 16	**EEG Signal Processing: Feature extraction, selection and classification methods** W. Leong
Volume 19	**Neurotechnology: Methods, advances and applications** V. de Albuquerque, A. Athanasiou and S. Ribeiro (Editors)
Volume 20	**Security and Privacy of Electronic Healthcare Records: Concepts, paradigms and solutions** S. Tanwar, S. Tyagi and N. Kumar (Editors)
Volume 23	**Advances in Telemedicine for Health Monitoring: Technologies, design and applications** T.A. Rashid, C. Chakraborty and K. Fraser
Volume 24	**Mobile Technologies for Delivering Healthcare in Remote, Rural or Developing Regions** P. Ray, N. Nakashima, A. Ahmed, S. Ro and Y. Soshino (Editors)
Volume 26	**Wireless Medical Sensor Networks for IoT-based eHealth** F. Al-Turjman (Editor)
Volume 29	**Blockchain and Machine Learning for e-Healthcare Systems** B. Balusamy, N. Chilamkurti, L.A. Beena and T. Poongodi (Editors)

Patient-Centered Digital Healthcare Technology

Novel applications for next generation healthcare systems

Edited by
Leonard Goldschmidt, M.D., Ph.D. and Rona Margaret Relova, M.D.

The Institution of Engineering and Technology

Published by The Institution of Engineering and Technology, London, United Kingdom

The Institution of Engineering and Technology is registered as a Charity in England & Wales (no. 211014) and Scotland (no. SC038698).

First published 2020

The Institution of Engineering and Technology
Michael Faraday House
Six Hills Way, Stevenage
Herts, SG1 2AY, United Kingdom

www.theiet.org

British Library Cataloguing in Publication Data
A catalogue record for this product is available from the British Library

ISBN 978-1-78561-565-8 (hardback)
ISBN 978-1-78561-566-5 (PDF)

Typeset in India by MPS Limited

To my wife and daughter, who have always provided inspiration and support.

– L. Goldschmidt

To Rogelio & Nancy Relova, and Lolita Patacsil, who inculcated that disrupting the status quo is not necessarily a bad thing. The influence of your fearless out-of-the-box thinking lives on.

– R. Relova

Contents

Preface

Patient-Centered Digital Healthcare Technology: Novel Applications for Next Generation Healthcare Systems
Featuring the Game Changers of Emerging Technologies in Medicine and Public Health

Leonard Goldschmidt, M.D., Ph.D. and Rona Margaret Relova, M.D.

The past decade has seen the introduction of new information technologies for healthcare, ranging from systematic to the more subtle. Whether approaching a whole ecosystem of a health process such as computerized medical records, or the granular patient needs addressed in mobile apps, or the new industry of wellness, innovators are addressing the gaps of healthcare systems and their patients. This book explores several themes of current and near-future healthcare information technology by presenting innovations and approaches to solving peoples' medical and mental health needs.

This book of digital health technologies (DHTs) features novel and emerging applications and system modifications that intersect with healthcare. The authors' contributions often challenge the existing healthcare systems in ways that aim to transform healthcare, with the single overarching objective of improving clinical outcomes and advocating wellness. The concept of encountering or treating a medical condition when it has already become disturbingly manifest is being replaced by earlier awareness, diagnosis, and proactive intervention.

Dr. Young and Dr. Klein introduce us to the topic of what makes information systems successful and the components of designing such systems. This chapter should be recommended reading for someone beginning to think about the human interface to information, and the process needed to achieve a measurable end.

The collaboration of Dr. Lesselroth, Dr. Mastarone, K. Adams, S. Tallett, Dr. Kushniruk, and Dr. Borycki further outline the methods of evaluating health information technology in their contribution. Their chapter explores pragmatic techniques of assessing technologies in the real-world operational setting.

The wealth of information that can be acquired with today's substantial health information systems, so-called "big data," is tackled by Dr. Luxton and C. Poulin. They investigate the potential use of big data analytics to advance public health issues such as contact tracing during an infectious outbreak as well as concomitant ethical implications.

Moving from the more theoretical to the practical side of health technologies, Dr. Kleinman, Dr. Orr, Dr. Heier, G. Benyamini, J. Johnson, and Dr. Rapp demonstrate an information-technology-based intervention for age-related macular degeneration. The home-monitoring device is a model of telemedicine device and clinical process improving clinical outcomes in macular degeneration (a condition caused by deterioration of the central portion of the retina).

Not only patients with physical impairments, but also those with mental health conditions have been shown to be amenable to the influence of ubiquitous mobile health technology applications, as exemplified by Dr. Crooks, S. Mack, J. Nguyen, and Dr. Kaslow. They examine the behavioral health landscape with a prototype application, which may lead to the prompt detection of condition exacerbations, improved clinical outcomes, and enhanced quality of life for patients who use them.

Further illustrating mental health support for children and adolescents in clinical applications, R. Anthony and Dr. Reilly discuss how health gaming platforms can provide a supportive space for end users. The goal is to develop validated programs that integrate playful learning with reinforcement of behavioral coping strategies, which may be consequential in patients' mental health.

Another contribution to this book illustrates remote access to care for one of the most common chronic diseases, diabetes, through a mobile health platform. Dr. Perry and Dr. Cross scrutinize specific complications of the disease and underscore how the application, which is linked to specialty diagnostic and interpretive algorithms, may be cost-effective in care delivery by encouraging patient compliance.

The team of U. Feldman, C. Larsen, E. Paramonova, and D. Theobald offer up the future of robotics in medical care as they document the strengths and limitations of current design and construction of intelligent machines. This subject matter is invaluable to readers who wish to understand the various uses of robotics in telepresence for continuity of patient care or in supply chain distribution.

Dr. Barad and Dr. McCaney probe how immersive simulation technology can radically reshape the next generation of medical education and surgical training. A virtual reality or augmented reality platform may improve patient outcomes, increase the adoption of higher value medical technologies, and ameliorate the scarcity of quality medical training and education around the globe.

The book further offers the contribution of R. Urwongse and K. Culver, who thoroughly explore how blockchain technology could remold the healthcare information management. Blockchain technology has the potential to play a significant role in supporting the digitization of medication supply chains or transmission of medical records or health providers' credentials with increased transparency and efficiency.

K. Lyman aptly illustrates the use of artificial intelligence and machine learning to advance medical diagnostics, specifically looking through the lens of the radiologist. The decision support platform integrates seamlessly into various stages of radiological workflow.

The succeeding chapter by E. Kiruluta, B. Stade, and Dr. Relova delineates the new technology that allows rapid, actionable genomic testing, thereby paving the way to customized care. Precision medicine will require a new generation of clinicians and medical informaticians who are well versed in digital literacies and the nuances of validating critical genomic insights and translating these findings to clinical care.

Change is the engine of progress. Taken altogether, all the contributors (better yet, the pioneering "disruptors") articulate how their work and creative thinking may revolutionize medical progress. By precipitating change, these novel and emerging technologies may represent the future potential of healthcare in industrialized countries.

Indeed, DHT elicits an epochal shift in healthcare; from an absolute dependence on clinician's skills and intellect in medical diagnostics and therapeutics to one where interventions are derived partly from software-based data analyses and proprietary algorithms. Another motivating vision is healthcare administration, and information systems will also be fundamentally altered as interoperable, meaningful solutions intended to optimize workflow. Ultimately, enhanced patient engagement and empowerment may be enabled by diverse impact-driven DHTs, as they involve end users to be partners in their care. People pursuing a healthier way to live would have effortless access to their personal health records for self-improvement and self-monitoring. This may perhaps lead to yet the most gratifying consequence of all, the transformative democratization of healthcare.

The chapters collectively appraise the existing landscape and gaps, highlight the evolving current approaches, detail groundbreaking pragmatic frameworks, and convey the current limitations in the healthcare industry. Some more mature solutions elucidate paths toward implementation and outline early trends. We, the editors, hope you remain intrigued to learn what is taking place around you. May you also be inspired to proactively contribute and engage commensurate with your skills and interests.

About the Editors

Dr. Leonard Goldschmidt is a Clinical Associate Professor (Affiliated) of Ophthalmology at Stanford University, School of Medicine and leads the Eye Clinic at the Livermore Division of VA Palo Alto Health Care System, Livermore, CA, USA. For many years, he was the Director for Telehealth and Medical Informatics at the latter facility, one of the five largest hospitals in the U.S. Department of Veterans Affairs. He has been working to improve patient health care using information technology tools for more than twenty years. Among his accomplishments that utilized telehealth and medical informatics are projects involving remote video consultation for patients with spinal cord injury, home telehealth using personal messaging and other tools, patient health education portals including web-enabled kiosks, web portals for triage and education of selected clinical conditions, and teleretinal imaging or diabetic retinopathy screening. He has been the Ophthalmology lead for the U.S. Department of Veterans Affairs Teleretinal Diabetic Screening Program since its inception in 2006, and the program has screened more than 1.8 million diabetics in primary care and eye clinics in VA medical centers. He has also developed innovative multimedia patient education health kiosks, which have been used within the U.S. Department of Veterans Affairs and community clinics in California.

Dr. Rona Margaret Relova serves as a Research Health Scientist at VA Palo Alto Health Care System, Palo Alto, CA, USA. Her principal research interest is in creating a successful roadmap for translating evidence into practice, policy and public health. She directs numerous multidisciplinary, patient-centered projects that demonstrate the full spectrum of translational research facilitating practice guideline development, implementation of innovative health care interventions, and conducting clinical drug trials to evaluate the comparative effectiveness. She provides oversight for Medical Informatics projects that create kiosk/tablet applications for health screening with mindful designs, i.e. demonstrating universal accessibility for end-users. She launched a proof-of-concept study evaluating a measurement-based care (MBC) platform that utilizes Artificial Intelligence. After completion of the health assessments, the application provides real-time feedback to providers, with flags for at-risk conditions. After the MBC tool is validated, the next phase is integration in clinical workflow. Overall, her investigator-initiated projects focus in novel ways to improve patient accessibility and care coordination, underscoring strategies that achieve triple aim of delivering of quality care, achieving measurable health outcomes, and demonstrating cost effectiveness of interventions. She holds leadership roles in National Institutes of Health (NIH) Precision Medicine Initiative (https://allofus.nih.gov/) and VA Genomic Medicine Program (https://www.research.va.gov/mvp/). These programs share the foundational mission to accelerate health research and medical breakthroughs, enabling individualized prevention, treatment, and care. She served in Advisory Committees of VA Cooperative Studies Program and Stanford School of Medicine's SPECTRUM, and as a reviewer for the Stanford Medicine X (https://medicinex.stanford.edu/), Stanford's premier initiative that explores how emerging technologies can advance the practice of medicine. She is a regular speaker at the Association of Clinical Research Professionals (https://acrpnet.org/) and Society for Brain Mapping and Therapeutics (https://www.worldbrainmapping.org/). She currently sits on the Advisory Board of Health, Wellness & Society International Research Network (https://healthandsociety.com/).

Chapter 1

Information systems in health: what do you need and how will you get it?

Terry Young, Ph.D.[1,2] *and*
Jonathan H. Klein, M.Sc., Ph.D.[3]

1.1 Introduction

Healthcare information systems are interesting, intellectually compelling and challenging in equal measure: interesting because they lie between people and technology and, at their best, facilitate remarkable activity; intellectually compelling because information technology has faced serious problems in healthcare, requiring investigation and reflection. The field is challenging for similar reasons: it crosses the boundaries of the technical and the human, and so there are rich corpuses of literatures in social science, from the information systems and informatics communities, by computer scientists and engineers, and as part of the wider academic pursuit of systems in health, not to mention the clinical corpuses related to specialist information systems in diverse fields such as radiology or pathology, to name but two prominent examples.

One cannot, therefore, introduce any writing on healthcare information systems with full recognition of all that has gone before and yet some context setting is necessary. At the same time, if any useful contribution is to be made for clinicians, such writing will have to step neatly from looking back and around to propose guidelines for better development of new systems or for getting better value from what exists.

In this chapter, we acknowledge that information systems in health cannot be addressed under a single disciplinary umbrella, and indeed that the variety of umbrellas that exist exhibit a degree of arbitrariness in terms of the best mix of disciplines to consider and how to combine them. We explore conceptual frameworks to address the information needs of individuals in healthcare systems, and the needs of networks of people if they are to make systems or services function

[1]Brunel University London, Uxbridge, UK
[2]Datchet Consulting Ltd, Newbury, UK
[3]Southampton Business School, University of Southampton, Southampton, UK

well. We draw these ideas together with some recommendations on critical questions to ask in evaluating systems now, or in specifying systems for the future.

1.2 Healthcare as a sociotechnical pursuit

Many authorities have commented on the complexity of healthcare, and found reasons why this should be. They have observed that healthcare systems typically span a number of domains [1], that they involve many stakeholder groups and millions of individuals, and that, in a modern society, they involve a degree of systemic complexity that may be unrivalled – elsewhere, we have characterised modern healthcare systems as uniquely *hypercomplex* [2]. This unprecedented degree of complexity carries with it very testing demands for designing and implementing information systems which will provide productive support. The healthcare field is littered with the carcasses of information systems which have been deemed failures [3–6], not forgetting that there are also a number of systems which, at one time or another, have been considered successes. Nor is it a simple binary classification: history may yet show that the UK's *Connecting for Health* project [7], generally dismissed as a failure, may, by driving the digitisation of radiological images across the United Kingdom, have delivered a lasting benefit worth much more than the cost of the programme. Success is an issue of degree, subjective [8] and multi-faceted.

In this chapter, we consider healthcare as a system of interrelated activities involving, typically, a large number of actors and stakeholders and a diverse set of technologies directed at the overall goal of improving the health of 'target' stakeholders (individuals, groups, or populations). In short, healthcare is a sociotechnical pursuit: carried out by and through people and involving various forms of technology. While much of this technology is 'front-line', used by those delivering healthcare, a growing proportion of it is concerned with the management of healthcare delivery. The latter are the information systems (IS) concerned with generating, storing, providing and using information, data and knowledge to support healthcare delivery.

While we tend to think of advanced information technology (IT) as the platform that supports healthcare information systems, a great deal of information management in healthcare is not based in sophisticated technology. Healthcare is a people-centred activity – involving patients, medical personnel, healthcare managers and others (including carers) – and the interactions between people are central to most healthcare provision. Much of this activity is face-to-face or mediated by fairly standard and ubiquitous commodified technology (such as the telephone). Realistically, this is likely to remain so for the foreseeable future. However, this in no way reduces the challenging complexity of the healthcare management problem – quite the reverse, in fact.

Given the complexity of healthcare systems, how can we characterise the healthcare environment in a way which is conducive to providing appropriate IS solutions? Many authorities advocate an explicitly multi-perspective view when addressing complex sociotechnical problems. Mingers and Brocklesby [9], for example, advocate a 'three-world' approach to problems: problems need to be addressed not only in the material world (physical and objective) but also in the subjective worlds of the stakeholders (the understandings, beliefs and needs of individuals) and in the social world in which the problems are immersed (the constraints and opportunities latent in the collective cultural environment which prevails). Problems must be addressed in all three worlds, they argue, or solutions will not work, although they note the attention needed in each of the three worlds (loosely, the need for change within each world) may differ substantially from problem to problem. In each world, four phases of an intervention need to be carried out: appreciation (of the problem); analysis (of the causal structure of the problem); assessment (of alternatives); and action (for change).

We concur with this, but would suggest that within the domain of healthcare, a tighter focus can be realised by further directing attention specifically to three Es (Figure 1.1): engineering (the physical world, including information); ethnography (individual and collective perceptions and needs); and economics (resource allocation). These are not natural bedfellows, but it would be very difficult to have confidence that a system is robust and sustainable and works for all involved without eventually applying methods from each of the three disciplines to a formal evaluation. Engineering, particularly systems engineering, focuses on capturing requirements from users, characterising their needs, and designing systems that can be tested and shown to meet those needs. The perspective of ethnography (and, more generally, social science) considers the experiences, cultures and practices of people within the system. Attention to economics acknowledges that, as health budgets are increasingly stretched, it is not simply a case of finding any solutions, but of finding affordable and cost-effective solutions: economic evaluation can no longer be ignored. While the concept of utility has served well in developing the field of health economics, enabling different interventions and drugs to be

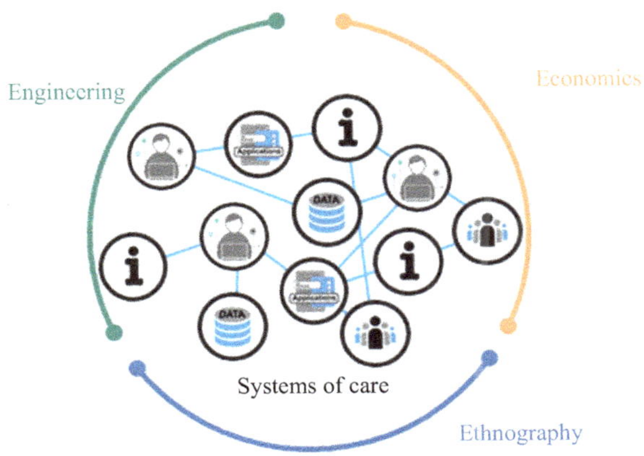

Figure 1.1 A combination of disciplines for a multi-world evaluation of IS in the delivery of healthcare

compared with one another, applying this thinking to health information systems is not straightforward: in an early attempt, for example, to determine the cost-effectiveness of a picturing archiving and communications system (PACS), benefits were identified but not the cost savings anticipated and so the case for adoption was not clear cut, but nonetheless, and presciently, there was confidence that 'in the hospital of the future, PACS will be seen as standard' [10].

In order to provide a framework to guide the practical introduction of information systems solutions to healthcare problems, we adapt Mingers and Brocklesby's three-world framework with our own 3E conceptualisation. We limit the focus of our attention to the first three of Mingers and Brocklesby's four intervention phases: appreciation, analysis and assessment. Within each of the resulting nine cells of the adapted three-world framework, we direct explicit consideration towards engineering, ethnographic and economic aspects. Thus, within each cell, three sets of concerns arise (see Table 1.1). These concerns, in turn, give rise to questions that can be asked of the situation (Table 1.2).

1.3 A simple model of what information someone in healthcare needs

In this section, we consider the needs of individuals within healthcare systems. No matter how complicated the world is, we recognise that people are able to live in such a world and routinely make decisions. Our next step, then, is to focus upon the individual seeking to make a decision and therefore seeking information upon which to base that decision. Since we are exploring the world of healthcare, we will call this person the *health information seeker*.

Thus, we centre our thinking on information seeking, rather than a particular clinical or social role. The *health information seeker* may be, for example, a patient who has recently received a diagnosis and is trying to find out more about what it means and what needs to be done; a carer, trying to arrange an appointment at a wheelchair clinic; a hospital nurse wanting to know whether it is time for a patient to have another dose of medicine; or a doctor reading a radiologist's report to see if the X-ray taken last week has revealed signs of cancer. The term is deliberately general. Moreover, the health quest may be for clinical information, economic information or relate more widely to the person's private life or social setting.

Thus, while we put a person at the centre of the enquiry, we are not doctrinaire about what sort of person it is. We simply recognise that people make decisions about their own health or the health of others, and that to do so, they need information. Figure 1.2 illustrates how a *health information seeker* will typically have a choice of sources to consult. Clearly, the options open to the *health information seeker* and the choice selected will vary: patients and carers, for instance, would tend to have fewer, and less formal, sources than clinicians and health managers, who might also have access to deeper professional knowledge and information. The ease of consulting various sources (in terms of time, cost and effort) may also vary. Further, the seeker may not be aware of the full range of available sources, and the

Table 1.1 A framework for healthcare system development

		Appreciation: assimilate the richness of the content (structure and processes) of the world	**Analysis: understand (conceptualise and model) underlying mechanisms**	**Assessment: formulate and evaluate alternative solutions or ways forward**
Material	Engineering: information technology	Material and physical processes and arrangements	Underlying causal structures: nature of decisions	Alternative physical and structural arrangements: alternative information sources, decision processes
	Ethnography: decision processes	Information: its availability, how it is transmitted, stored, used, changed…	How information contributes to the decision	Alternative ways of generating and using information
	Economics: resources; costs	Costs and benefits of IS/IT	Sources of costs of providing data and information	Costs and benefits of alternatives
Individual	Engineering: human–computer interaction (HCI) considerations	Individual needs and capabilities	How individuals seek, use and conceptualise information	Alternative ways of using and interacting with systems
	Ethnography: beliefs and attitudes about IS/IT and decision processes	information skills, perceptions of information environment	Understand belief systems of individuals	Alternative individual understandings
	Economics: individual utilities	Value of resources used and outputs generated to individuals	Understand underlying value systems of individuals	Alternative value systems of individuals
Social	Engineering: role of IS/IT within society; societal constraints	Social practices regarding IS/IT	How social practices manifest in behaviour and conflicts of interest	Alternative social practices
	Ethnography: cultural aspects of IS/IT	Cultural beliefs about healthcare systems	Why people believe what they do	Alternative social understandings
	Economics: societal utilities	Social values	Understand social value systems	Alternative social values

Table 1.2 Information systems questions

Material: engineering: information technology	Appreciation: • What physical processes are encompassed by the system, and how might they be informed by data and information flows? • What, in material terms, does the system do, and by what data and information is it informed? Analysis: • What are the underlying causal mechanisms that explain the physical processes within the system, and the way in which they are informed by data and information? Assessment: • What alternative configurations for the physical processes and data and information flows can be devised? • How do these alternatives function in terms of the effectiveness of the system? • How might a chosen alternative be developed?
Material: ethnography: decision processes	Appreciation: • What decision processes are encompassed by the system? • By whom are the decisions made? • How do they access the data and information which inform their decisions? • Is full use made of the available data and information? Analysis: • How do decision-makers make use of the data and information they obtain in order to make their decisions?

	Assessment: • How might decisions be configured differently within the system? • How effective might alternative configurations be? • How might a chosen alternative be developed?
Material: economics: resources; costs	Appreciation: • What are the costs and benefits of different information sources? Analysis: • How do information sources add value to decisions? Assessment: • Which alternative offers the best cost-benefit profile? • How might a chosen alternative be developed?
Individual: engineering: HCI considerations	Appreciation: • Who are the stakeholders in the system? • How do the stakeholders interact with system? Analysis: • Why do the stakeholders interact with the system as they do? Assessment: • What alternative ways of interaction with the system are possible? • How might a chosen alternative way of interacting with the system be developed?

(Continues)

Table 1.2 (Continued)

Individual: ethnography: beliefs and attitudes about IS/IT and decision processes	Appreciation: • What do stakeholders perceive the system to be? • How do stakeholders understand their own role in the system? Analysis: • Why do stakeholders hold the beliefs they do? • In what way does the system confirm their beliefs? • How do their beliefs explain their actions? Assessment: • What alternative ways of understanding the system might be available to stakeholders? • How might such alternatives impact on the way in which stakeholders interact with the system? • How might stakeholder beliefs be changed?
Individual: economics: individual utilities	Appreciation: • What are the costs and benefits of the system in terms of money, time and other criteria, to the various stakeholders? Analysis: • How are costs and benefits calculated? • What assumptions underlie such calculations? Assessment: • What alternative measures of costs and benefits might be proposed?

	• What alternative ways of assessing such costs and benefits exist? • How might an alternative set of costs and benefits be made acceptable to stakeholders?
Social: engineering: role of IS/IT within society; societal constraints	Appreciation: • What are the cultural and social constraints under which the system operates? Analysis: • How do the cultural and social constraints influence the system? Assessment: • How might different cultural and social constraints influence the system? • How might alternative cultural and social environments be created?
Social: ethnography: cultural aspects of IS/IT	Appreciation: • How do cultural and social constraints influence beliefs about the system? Analysis: • How do the cultural and social constraints operate to influence beliefs? Assessment: • How might different cultural and social constraints result in different understandings? • What actions might be taken to change the culture and consequent beliefs?

(Continues)

Table 1.2 (Continued)

Social: economics: societal utilities	Appreciation: • How does the culture value the inputs to and outputs from the system? Analysis: • Why does the culture value inputs and outputs in the way that it does? Assessment: • What alternative value systems might be introduced? • How might a culture be steered towards such alternatives?

quality of different sources may vary (and be poorly understood). A *health information seeker* may be able to modify information at source, perhaps by scribbling a note on a leaflet, by adding a comment on a website, or by making a formal entry into a record. A source may also contain information that has been generated by a machine – such as an image or a clinical laboratory test result.

There is much more detail in the upper half of this diagram, which indicates IT-mediated sources, than in the lower half, indicating sources which are generally not IT dependent. There are more apps and systems available today that support the interactions indicated in the upper half. Person-to-person happens for free in corridors, offices, and elsewhere, and more expensively in meetings and at conferences. Meanwhile, though phones and video conferencing services would be placed in the lower half of the diagram, we do not yet have systems to capture and process natural interactions routinely. Our phones, for instance, cannot yet interrogate us after a consultation to make sure we understand all that the doctor said, nor are there systems to listen to a conversation between primary and secondary care physicians and appropriately update the notes of each. Such services would align with the aspirations of care delivery, and they are starting to appear, but mature adoption is still some way away.

The utter and critical dependency of care delivery on the interpersonal dimension, we argue, sets healthcare apart from other sectors.

Figure 1.2 is not an attempt to provide a taxonomy of information sources but to illustrate the many options that are open to those seeking information. The choice could be broadened, for instance, by including sources that are encountered in a less purposeful way, such as in watching TV. We note that some social media could be placed in the bottom half of the diagram, but in its present form, it is sufficient to assess whether a given system meets the needs of existing *health information seekers*, or whether unmet needs remain.

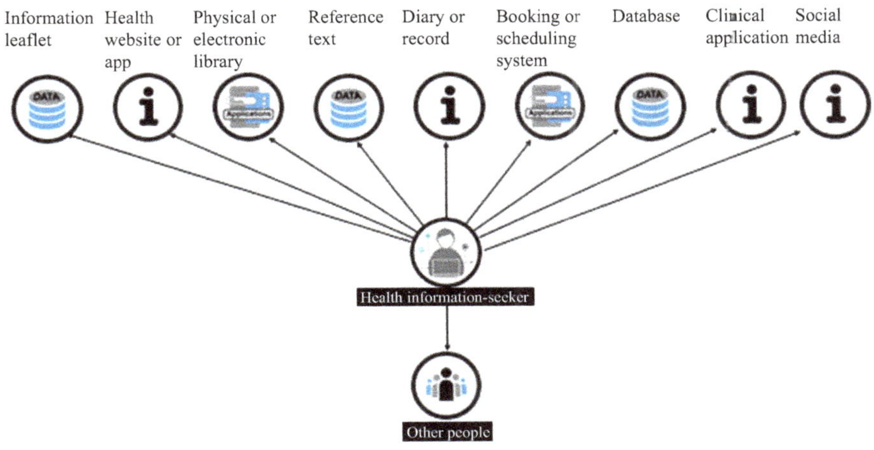

Figure 1.2 A view of information sources that a health information seeker might typically use

Our initial observation is that most health information systems connect sources and support services in the top half of the diagram: databases, clinical libraries, medical devices, hospital equipment, clinical laboratory systems, scheduling services, transaction, procurement or prescription processing and, of course, medical records. Even with phone calls and video conferences, the knowledge that is communicated tends to remain in human memories and may only make it into the top half of the diagram if the humans record it separately.

How, then, does this help to evaluate information systems or assess the benefits a new service? First, this conceptual model focuses on the match between what the stakeholders need to know, and what the system or service can provide. At its simplest, this might reveal there is information some stakeholders need but cannot get directly. It may be that the underlying data is not provided, either because it does not exist or because it is not visible to particular seekers. Perhaps, a nurse in primary care wants to know why a patient missed an anticoagulation clinic and suspects that the patient may have been admitted to hospital recently but cannot see into the hospital systems because they cannot be accessed by primary care clinicians.

Trickier is the apparent overprovision of information: where it appears that an individual has two routes to the same information. If it is genuinely the same information, that may not present a problem, but if two or more sources are poorly synchronised, appearing to contain the same data, but one being more regularly updated or generally better managed, it may create difficulties.

More broadly, we might enquire as to whether a source and a need are mutually appropriate: can the seeker get information that is sufficient to make a good decision in a timely manner? Our conceptual model, then, suggests the questions: how useful is this information, and to whom is it useful? The interest in summary records (see, for example, [11]), abridged data sets that can be shared more widely than the original records, indicates that completeness is only part of the requirement for care provision. Some information in a medical record may never be used to deliver any form of care.

Most importantly, this modelling approach enables systems designers to imagine themselves as any of a range of stakeholders who will use the system, and to work systematically through each person's needs, identifying multiple connections, inappropriate provision and, of course, disconnects. A disconnect need not be a problem if there is another route to the information. But such measures tend to add effort and the risk of mistakes to the activities they are supporting. Such workarounds [12] may be regarded positively or pejoratively (when described in terms of resistance to adoption). However, in terms of this conceptual model they are a likely outcome of any form of mismatch between the need of a stakeholder and the provision of the information system.

We must not forget the undesirable *health information seekers* – the nosey, the malicious and the hackers. The way in which information systems prevent illegitimate use will impact on the usability of the system for legitimate *health information seekers*. Passwords, even swipe cards, combined with time-consuming login and logout sequences can make a system much less attractive and convenient for the clinician to use.

A final issue – particularly when a system is being deployed – is that the architecture of the information system may mean that certain sources only become available after others are working. Hendy identified this in connection with the National Programme for IT, where the clinical systems would not work without an underlying patient administration system (PAS) [7,13]. The decision to make the PAS, with its demographic information, a foundational element was a design decision with the (unintended) consequence that doctors could not access clinical information until after the managers could access theirs.

Knowledge is not usually sought in a vacuum, and the context for healthcare information is usually to inform a decision or to enable a process. And so, the *health information seeker* is generally in search of information to make a decision or to expedite a process for themselves or for someone else. Without anticipating the dynamics of driving end-to-end processes in Section 1.4, we recognise that even a static representation such as ours has a strong sense of the passage of time:

(i) Retrospective information – a medical history or a statistical process chart – may contribute to a diagnostic decision: what is wrong with a patient or with a part of the service. There is a lot of interest in mining repositories of such data in the hope of generating new knowledge about other people with the same complaint or about the services or similar services.
(ii) Current knowledge transfer addresses the questions: how and what can I find out to help me make a decision now or how will it lessen my worry now?
(iii) What next? The key in all knowledge systems is to connect people and processes so things can happen in the future, often somewhere else. A service such as kidney dialysis at home is a complicated logistical challenge in setting up and then supplying a small chemical laboratory in a bedroom, and managing it safely. More than one stakeholder always needs to know what will and what might happen next.

We can take this one step further, by circumscribing a 'circle of knowledge' around each *health information seeker* – with an upper hemicircle that is the ***interactive*** knowledge exchange region and a lower hemicircle that is the ***interpersonal*** knowledge exchange region, as shown in Figure 1.3.

For an individual to be part of a care delivery system, as patient, carer, associated professional, clinician or manager, their circles of knowledge need to connect or overlap in some way. People need to talk to people and they need to share knowledge that provides them with a common situational awareness of what is happening and that allows them to plan together to make things happen in the future. We might visualise it as shown in Figure 1.4.

Figure 1.4 is an illustration of the idea that as an individual progresses along a pathway (supporting care, receiving care or providing care), the forward movement requires knowledge. Sometimes this knowledge may be through other people – the overlapping circles on the left indicate a shared acquaintance or colleague – or through shared access to information stored somewhere and modified or recalled by one or more parties. Sometimes the information flow will be to prepare for the future or it may be to use the past to inform the present or prepare for the future.

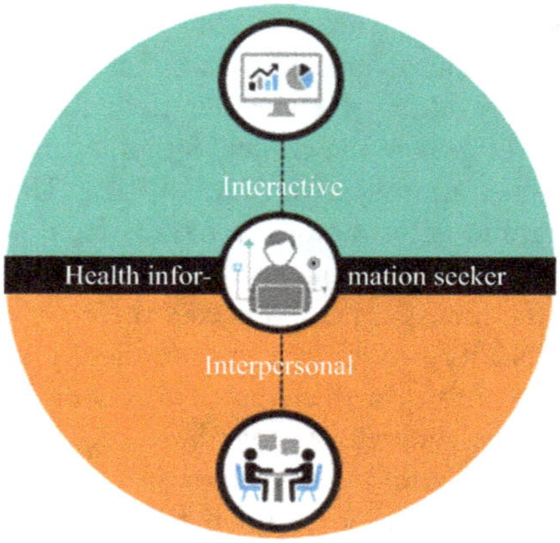

Figure 1.3 A health information seeker's circle of knowledge

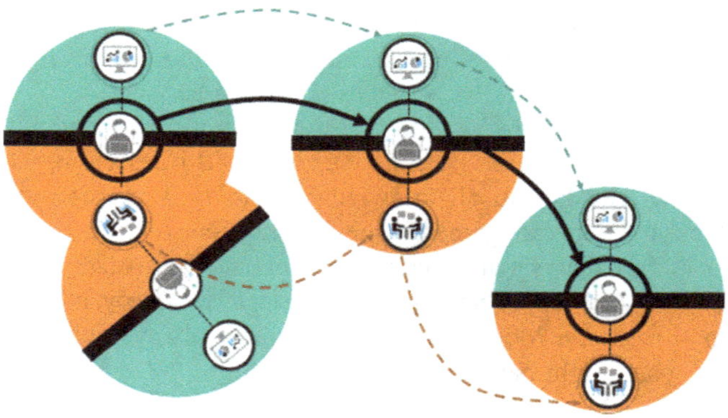

Figure 1.4 A way of visualising the sharing of interactive knowledge exchange and interpersonal knowledge exchange as a health information seeker progresses along a pathway

To summarise this section: we started by putting a person at the centre of the healthcare world and considered the knowledge that such a person would need. We have undertaken a very coarse binary classification, identifying interactive information or knowledge and interpersonal knowledge or information. We have considered the appositeness of the sources of data, information and knowledge that might constitute each type of exchange, and developed the idea of evaluative questions that will assist in troubleshooting or specifying new systems. Critically, however, we identify that health information systems simply contribute to an individual's circle of knowledge and the way in which individuals can develop, align and manage their circles of knowledge will determine the types of processes of which they can be part and to which they can contribute.

1.4 A way of thinking about the role of information in care provision

We now move on to consider the role of information in empowering process.

The literature is rich with frameworks on how to evaluate and assess information systems. Because, however, the accent here is on a pragmatic approach to making decisions about technology selection and use, we adopt a very pragmatic approach that was proposed for a small project a decade ago by one of the authors. It is certainly not the only way to structure one's thinking, and we do not claim universality, but commend it as providing (as does the conceptual model in Section 1.3) a way of thinking about information systems that should prove useful in the context of service delivery, troubleshooting or design.

This approach starts with a mnemonic, **PIQuED** (**P**rocess, **I**nformation, **Qu**ality, **E**quipment, **D**ata) that should be accessible to individuals and can be readily shared around a team.

1.4.1 Process

In healthcare, neither people nor information can be productive in isolation and the context is usually a process. Sometimes a *protocol* captures the same idea, and in the United Kingdom, the term *models of care* is gaining currency. We note that sometimes people see a new information system as the catalyst to drive better process – for instance, *Connecting for Health* was conceived as a transformation programme through technology [14] – while others see the role of IT in terms of its alignment with existing process. However, in terms of evaluation or design, it is much easier to think of information in the context of process rather than the other way around. Specific issues to focus on will include the following:

- Process maps. A process map illustrates a sequence or combination of sequences of events, with emphasis on who meets with whom or what. It has become popular to sketch out patient pathways, but every person involved has a pathway that will intersect with, or in places run alongside, the patient pathway. Simulation modelling [15,16] is a good way of capturing the complexity of these interactions, and such models allow stakeholders to explore how the interactions play out under different demand and staffing regimes or when differently configured. However developed, a set of mutually consistent sequences, governed appropriately, is essential.
- Decisions. A critical feature of process maps are the points at which someone has to make a decision, which in healthcare is usually a diagnosis or treatment decision. Decisions usually require information and communication between those involved in the decision. Understanding the timing of decisions, the availability of key stakeholders and relevant information, and having communication channels that support shared decisions where necessary, is critical to connecting a good process to an appropriate information infrastructure.
- Logistics. People have to move around: the choreography of care – ensuring that people and things (such as items of equipment, documents, samples, *etc.*)

meet up at the right time – is very complicated. The traditional way of simplifying such a problem was that patients travelled and waited, but this is less acceptable today, so coordinating care for the best experience all round requires excellent logistics.

- Management. Systems cannot run themselves and operational oversight and control is needed.
- Customers. There is no customer in health who is – as the old adage says – always right. In truth, the process will have many stakeholders, all of whom might function as a customer might in other sectors.

1.4.2 Information

Given the process, the next question is what information is needed by the people (or the equipment) in the process to make it work well. Issues such as the applicability to, or accessibility by, particular *health information seekers* will be critical to a successful design. The process outlined in Section 1.4.1 enables us to sit where each *health information seeker* sits, and, combined with a clear picture of the decision-making points, allows us to identify the two main issues.

- What needs to be known by whom (and when, and where): The dependence of effective process upon the availability of timely, accurate, appropriate and accessible information cannot be overstated.
- Who needs to communicate with whom: Again, the traditional way to manage care has been to focus on bilateral conversations, connected up with slower media, such as letters. As noted, new technologies are emerging and there may well be many more options in the future than there are today.

1.4.3 Quality

This entry is a mark of the arbitrariness of frameworks such as this, and a case could be made that quality relates to the process or that data quality is primarily a technical issue. We focus attention on it to make sure that, in designing processes and in considering the information flows needed to make them work, high quality has been designed in and poor quality has been designed out. Making it easy for *health information seekers* to do the right thing, and making it hard for them to lose situational awareness, or become confused, is about the interplay between the process and the information system supporting it. There are several dimensions to the question of quality, including the following:

- Service quality. This covers everything from governance and accreditation, to efficiency, management and user experience, and will rely upon the training, morale and performance of the staff providing the service.
- Quality of experience of all stakeholders.
- Equipment quality. This relates to the next heading, and relates not just to the technical quality, but also to ease of maintenance, calibration, configuration

management and upgrade strategy. Note that equipment must deliver appropriate information, not necessarily the most precise available, which in turn raises questions about who will interpret and make decisions based on such information.

- Quality of outcomes. Clearly, clinical outcomes are the gold standard, although linking process changes to such outcomes is not always easy.
- Information quality. As discussed above, this relates to the timeliness, accuracy, accessibility and relevance to the decision-maker. Too much information may undermine quality as much as too little.

1.4.4 Equipment

As noted above, many sources of information (and some destinations for information) are not people but computer systems or healthcare equipment (such as scanners or point of care diagnostics) with information interfaces. The role that such equipment plays in the pathway will determine whatever is appropriate, and what information is required of it. The field is huge, but some observations are helpful.

- Point of care technologies and fixed infrastructure: In many fields, from home dialysis to diagnostics, there is a marked move to bring care to the patient rather than vice versa. The technical performance of portable or decentralised equipment may be inferior to that provided in central facilities, but the access is much better. Home dialysis, for instance, may take more needle-time, but may be much more comfortable for the patient, especially when travel is taken out of the equation. The onward march of 'good enough' technologies, fuelled by a desire for portability, is a key theme of The Innovator's Dilemma [17] and its subsequent application to health [18,19].
- Configuration management: Knowing how equipment has been set up and whether it is sufficiently well calibrated is a task more easily performed in a central facility, and issues around such management need to be considered when designing new services.
- Interfaces: Again, there is a vast literature on equipment read-outs and the potential for error around the human-computer interface [20]. Here, we simply note the nature of displays and direct-to-human transfer of data needs to be a factor in evaluating equipment. Similarly, the compatibility of the information that interfaces to a network with other equipment supporting the same processes needs to be considered.

1.4.5 Data

It is easy to focus on the data at an early stage. While we acknowledge much good has come from coding systems and standards, there are two aspects of a strong data focus that are not helpful. The first is that the quest to standardise can obscure the purpose for wanting the data in the first place. It is easy to get caught up in lengthy discussions over exactly what will and will not be allowed – and indeed, the quest for coding standards has taken decades – and to lose sight of why it is needed. A second observation is that data is too often used for audit rather than operational delivery [7,13]. We contend that the first priority of an information system in healthcare is to facilitate better delivery of healthcare and audit for policy or financial purposes should not shape the systems architecture.

For these reasons, and perhaps a little idiosyncratically, we have put data at the bottom of the list of what to address. Once everything else is clear, the data sets you need should be relatively straightforward to identify and specify.

1.5 Knowledge and process in care delivery

Finally, we present one other very simple conceptual model about knowledge and process. Healthcare service provision is perhaps the most knowledge-intensive sector in the world. Because of the number of variables and people, and the scale and complexity of the interactions between them, it is also one that requires an enormous capability to deploy and manage processes effectively. However, the knowledge piece and the process piece are not separate issues.

In other sectors, such as logistics and supply chain or manufacturing, the really successful players have managed to use knowledge and process in the sort of virtuous circle that is shown in Figure 1.5.

It is easy to be cynical about on-line vendors, who track your purchases in order to predict what you will require and to sell you more, but the information systems and process controls behind such service are really quite spectacular. At its best, it has managed to wrap the customer and the service delivery system in processes that collect information, which can be turned into knowledge, and vendors use the knowledge to be even smarter with their processes.

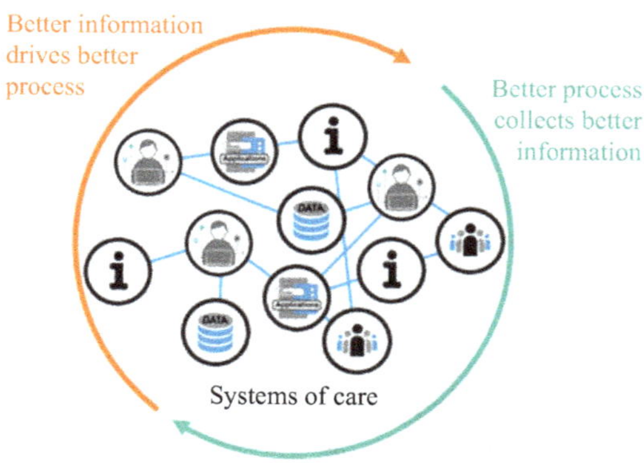

Figure 1.5 A simple view of the potentially reinforcing role of knowledge and process in care delivery

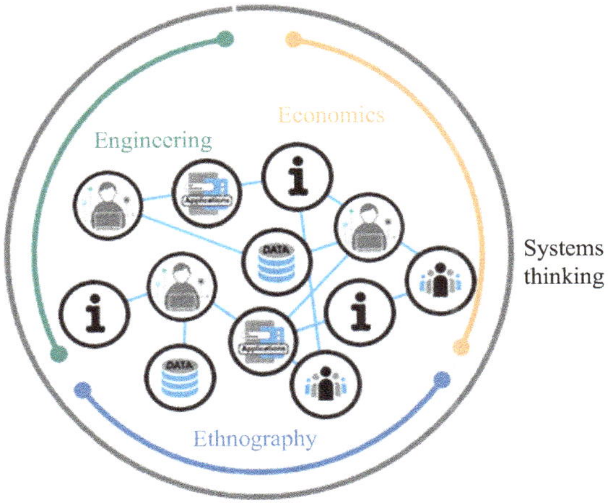

Figure 1.6 The 3E model for analysing the delivery of healthcare

Very simply, this is the ideal to which all information systems in healthcare should aspire, in order to facilitate a continuously improving experience for all concerned and a generally increasing freedom from fear and worry.

It is clear we have not explored a complete set of methods to be able to answer the questions posed in the title of this chapter: what do you need and how will you get it? We add, therefore, the ideas of knowledge drivers and process drivers to propose a connected model for continuous improvement in one more conceptual model – shown in Figure 1.6. This concept was developed as part of a proposal in 2016 and is used here to emphasise that thinking about systems is not just an engineering pursuit, but a service such as healthcare is a system with people and one that consumes resources and delivers value.

1.6 Conclusion and critical design questions

In this paper we have sought, using a framework and a set of conceptual models, to cut through the complexity of what is currently available in healthcare information services, systems and apps. Our aim has been to provide help for clinicians involved in evaluating or specifying services and their supporting information systems, so that they may have a fruitful dialogue with all stakeholders, including those who are providing the information systems. To do this, we have adapted the Mingers and Brocklesby framework by appealing to disciplinary backdrops in engineering, ethnography and economics. From there, we considered the individual's quest for information by imagining a *health information seeker*. In doing so, we have been able to highlight the information such a person would want to have in order to make effective decisions, and we have partitioned that information into what we have termed either *interactive* – information that is stored somewhere, updated and may be interacted with by the *health information seeker* – or *interpersonal* – communication-based exchange of information in natural language involving shared decisions, mutual learning, accommodation and consensus.

We moved on to see that information and communication systems need to support both *interactive* and *interpersonal* exchanges of data, information and knowledge, and the ease with which the most appropriate connections may be made will influence the effectiveness of the processes of care.

From here, we went on to provide a framework comprising process mapping, identification of key decision points, specifying the information flows needed, the quality of the overall service, the equipment and finally, the data sets needed. Clearly, many of these components will already be fixed by the existing infrastructure or purchasing decisions made by others, but the approach allows the choices at each stage to be formally assessed.

And finally, we returned to the question of how better knowledge can drive the design of better process which in turn can lead to the gathering of better knowledge.

We contend that healthcare professionals could get a lot more out of existing systems, and could have more impact on the development of new systems, if they could use these thinking tools to ask better questions at whatever stage they encounter the system. Our hope is the debate around healthcare information systems can return to the basics of who needs what, while setting the business of agreeing standards and formats on a firmer basis in which specific types of user are always in view.

There may be other pieces of information system design theory that would help – use cases, for instance, are a way to stimulate the dialogue between information system users and designers by drawing pictures that describe how each user expects to encounter and engage with the system. If you have not seen the use-case diagrams for the system you are expected to use, you might have a fruitful conversation by asking for them. But, that is a subject for consideration elsewhere.

We contend although the health information technology scene exhibits a bewildering range of products and services, information management is relatively straightforward at heart and has remained so since the late 1960s. New technologies and apps introduce new ways of addressing what are essentially old questions. The key issue is to keep returning to the old questions in new ways.

To end with, we present a series of possible questions that might be asked when evaluating an existing system or considering a new one. (These questions can be viewed as an informal summary of the questions appearing in Table 1.2.)

- **What is the problem I am reviewing?** What is the physical system and the social challenge? Who are the individuals?
- **Who are the main information seekers in this process?** Can I work through what they want using the *health information seeker* model?
- **How do the information and the process that I am reviewing interact?** What are the stakeholders in the process trying to do and how does the timing and availability of information affect their decisions? What are the engineering challenges of providing this information in a timely way and what are the costs and benefits of doing so?

- **What formal and informal sources of knowledge and information are the individual stakeholders using already and how will a new service or system change this?** How would they like it to be changed? What are the reasons that individuals may or may not want to use the system in the way that the designers have planned that it be used?
- **What are the constraints that limit me?** Is it the engineered solution – can it simply not do what needs to be done? Would it cost too much to get it to do what is really needed? If so, have I fully costed the impact of it not doing what it really needs to do? Does the way individuals will have to use it present a barrier to its effectiveness?
- **If this is a proposed solution, how will I evaluate it:**
  - With and against alternatives before it is implemented?
  - After it has been implemented?

Good luck!

Acknowledgements

The 3E expression of the critical disciplines helpful for analysing healthcare systems was developed while Professor Terry Young was putting a proposal together. We acknowledge contributions from Davina Allen (Cardiff), Claire Donovan, Susan Jobling, and Subhash Pokrel and Teresa Waller (Brunel). We also thank a number of informal reviewers.

References

[1] Dawson S. 'Managing, organising and performing in health care: what do we know and how can we learn?' in Mark A.L, and S. Dopson (eds.) *Organisational Behaviour in Health Care: The Research Agenda*. 1999; Basingstoke: Palgrave Macmillan.

[2] Klein J. H., and Young T. P. 'Health care: a case of hypercomplexity?' *Health Systems*. 2015;4:104–110.

[3] Detmer D. 'Information technology for quality health care: a summary of United Kingdom and United States experiences'. *Quality in Health Care*. 2000;9(3):181–189.

[4] Benson T. 'Why general practitioners use computers and hospital doctors donot – Part 1: incentives'. *BMJ* 2002;325(7372):1086–1089.

[5] Benson T. 'Why general practitioners use compute\rs and hospital doctors do not – Part 2: scalability'. *BMJ* 2002;325(7372):1090–1093.

[6] Heeks R., Mundy D., and Salazar A. 'Why health care information systems succeed or fail' in Armoni A. (ed.) *Health Care Information Systems: Challenges for the New Millennium*. Hershey, PA: Idea Group Publishing; 1999.

[7] Hendy J., Reeves B. C., Fulop N., Hutchings A., and Masseria C. 'Challenges to implementing the national programme for information technology (NPfIT): a qualitative study'. *BMJ* 2005;331:331–336

[8] Wilson M., and Howcroft, D. 'Re-conceptualising failure: social shaping meets IS research'. *European Journal of Information Systems.* 2002;11 (4):236–250.

[9] Mingers J, and Brocklesby J. 'Multimethodology: towards a framework for mixing methodologies'. *Omega.* 1997;25;489–509.

[10] Bryan S., Weatherburn G., Buxton M, Watkins J., Keen J., and Muris N. 'Evaluation of a hospital picture archiving and communication system'. *Journal of Health Services Research & Policy*. 1999;4(4):204–209.

[11] Anderson R. 'Do summary care records have the potential to do more harm than good? Yes'. *BMJ* 2010;340:c3020

[12] Alter S. 'Theory of workarounds'. *Communications of the Association for Information Systems*. 2014;34:1041–1066.

[13] Connell N. A. D, and Young T. P. 'Evaluating healthcare information systems through an 'enterprise' perspective'. *Information and Management.* 2007;44(4):433–444.

[14] Protti, D. 'The benefits of computer technology can only be realised when systems of work are changed'. UK: Connecting for Health NHS; 2005.

[15] Brailsford S. C., Harper P., Patel B., and Pitt M. 'An analysis of the academic literature on simulation and modelling in health care'. *Journal of Simulation.* 2009;3(3):130–140.

[16] Jahangirian M., Naseer, A., Stergioulas, L., *et. al.* 'Simulation in health-care: lessons from other sectors'. *International Journal of Operational Research.* 2012;12(1):45–55.

[17] Christensen C. M. *The Innovator's Dilemma* 2003; New York: Harper Collins.

[18] Christensen C. M., Bohmer R., and Kenagy J. 'Will disruptive innovations cure health care?' *Harvard Business Review*. 2000;78:102–112.

[19] Christensen C. M., and Grossman J. H., and Hwang J. *The Innovator's Prescription: A Disruptive Solution for Health Care*. New York: McGraw-Hill; 2009.

[20] Thimbleby, H. 'Safer user interfaces: a case study in improving number entry'. *IEEE Transactions on Software Engineering*. 2015;41:711–729.

Chapter 2

Hybrid usability methods: practical techniques for evaluating health information technology in an operational setting

Blake J. Lesselroth, M.D., MBI, FACP, FAMIA, UXC[1], Ginnifer L. Mastarone, Ph.D, M.S., UXC[2], Kathleen Adams, M.P.H., FAMIA, UXC[3], Stephanie Tallett[3], Andre Kushniruk, Ph.D., M.S., FACMI[4] and Elizabeth Borycki, Ph.D., RN, MN, FACMI[4]

2.1 Introduction

2.1.1 Problem statement

The considered application of human factors engineering principles to system design can improve user satisfaction, accelerate innovation adoption, and promote skilful technology use [1,2]. For professionals across disciplines, proficiency with technology is a critical prerequisite for successful performance. Technology developers understand this and recognize that system usability can be an important determinant of user satisfaction and marketplace dominance [3,4]. Industries outside of healthcare including nuclear engineering, aviation, and online retail have traced technical and economic catastrophes to usability missteps and responded by investing heavily in usability evaluation throughout the product design lifecycle [5–10].

By contrast, healthcare has lagged behind other industries [11,12]. Health information technologies (HIT) including electronic health records (EHRs), biomedical device interfaces, and a broad array of clinical software applications suffer from usability flaws that impact patient safety, clinician efficiency, and health outcomes [13–21]. In response, informaticians, systems engineers, and human factors experts have hard fought to raise awareness among stakeholders including

[1]Department of Medical Informatics, University of Oklahoma-Tulsa (OU-TU) School of Community Medicine, Tulsa, OK, USA
[2]Department of Communication, College of Liberal Arts & Sciences, Portland State University, Portland, OR, USA
[3]Office of Human Factors Engineering, Department of Veterans' Health Affairs, Portland, OR, USA
[4]School of Health Information Science, University of Victoria, Victoria, BC, Canada

clinicians, health administrators, policy makers – and, of course, technology vendors. The healthcare landscape has seen some progress as evidenced by the increase in published human factors research, a burgeoning demand for human factors specialists, the appearance of better-designed technologies, and public policies such as Safety-Enhanced Design – a requirement for "meaningful use" certification of health records in the United States [10,13,22,23]. Nevertheless, a variety of mediators – including business market forces, testing cost, competing executive agendas, and limited methodological expertise – have slowed integration of usability evaluation into HIT design [24–26].

Although there are many well-documented examples of usability engineering activities improving product safety and reducing downstream cost, clinical stakeholders struggle with practical issues that can undermine commitment [10,13,27]. Competitive market forces and cost considerations may temper enthusiasm for investing in lengthy testing protocols [24,25]. Instead, software engineers and product owners frequently forego usability evaluation to quickly innovate [28].

This phenomenon is by no means isolated to commercial EHR vendors. Healthcare administrators and government agencies – embattled by competing institutional priorities, fiscal concerns, and public or political scrutiny – are also pressured to compress development and deployment timelines. Measuring the return on investment (ROI) associated with human factors evaluation can be challenging. Cost savings from increased usability may not be immediately visible upon deployment, particularly if the ROI is measured by non-events (e.g., "near-misses" or potential errors avoided) [20,28].

Even organizations boasting a relatively mature user experience (UX) culture grapple with methodological and logistic issues that confound usability evaluation. First, methods developed in other industries can be difficult to adapt to healthcare – particularly, when measuring dimensions such as safety, error tolerance, and data reliability [9,29]. For example, usability specialists tend to rank usability based upon the UX or frequency of occurrence [3]. However, infrequent or unnoticed errors can have catastrophic consequences to downstream patient outcomes – particularly, when few recovery systems exist [20,21,30]. New measurement instruments are needed to assess products supporting decision-making, clinical triage, or distributed cognition (as in the case of team-based cardiopulmonary resuscitation). As the discipline matures, it will be crucial leverage lessons learned from the related disciplines of health informatics and patient safety to develop valid algorithms or prediction models that suitably measure the risk and prioritize mitigation strategies.

Second, the perceived rigor required for healthcare evaluations may discourage novice usability practitioners, operational staff, or executive sponsors [28]. Techniques described in the peer-reviewed literature often require dedicated funding, protected time, specialized technologies, and highly trained personnel with years of research experience [9,11,24,31,32]. Understandably, implementers may quickly become frustrated with the resource demands or overwhelmed by the complexity of the data analysis. Similarly, healthcare executives may be disinclined to sponsor such an investment when an ambitious testing protocol promises to slow a highly anticipated product implementation.

The stakes are often higher in healthcare and products can benefit from carefully designed, quantitative, and scientific evaluation. However, when such rigorous protocols are not feasible, some testing is almost always better than no testing [28]. Therefore, many usability professionals have advocated for "discount usability testing" [12,24,28,33,34]. Discount usability testing is an approach that promotes frequent, small tests to rapidly debug a design and inform iterative development. There are many well-documented reports from other industries demonstrating that discount usability testing can improve design and maximize ROI [12,34–37]. It follows then, that clinical stakeholders need descriptive reports of usability techniques that are simple, efficient, and evaluate as many usability dimensions concurrently as possible.

In many cases, "hybrid" techniques represent a practical way to increase the speed of evaluation. Hybrid usability techniques combine two or more usability measurement strategies into a single test protocol. By combining protocols, it is possible to measure several related or orthogonal dimensions concurrently. This, in turn, increases the validity of findings, improves the explanatory power of conclusions, and helps meet the needs of multiple stakeholders. In our own work, we typically combine methodologies (e.g., simulations with surveys) either concurrently or in rapid succession to quickly identify usability concerns, forecast training needs, and develop new technology requirements.

2.1.2 Aims and goals

The purpose of this chapter is to provide clinical leaders, informaticians, and novice usability specialists with practical approaches to usability testing when stakeholders need to answer multiple research questions on a tight timeline. As the title implies, we emphasize the mechanics of combining several methods, using real-world examples to illustrate the instrumentation and analytic processes. There are many possible ways to combine methods, and each project may demand a slightly different approach.

We begin Section 2.1.3 of this chapter by introducing two frameworks to approach HIT usability evaluation: the cognitive-socio-technical framework and a framework organized by evaluation focus. The cognitive-socio-technical framework organizes usability activities into distinct levels of analysis and articulates the effect technology has on user perception, workflow, and team collaboration. The UX Evaluation Focus framework organizes usability dimensions in relation to the level of analysis: the interface, processes, or environment [38]. In Section 2.1.3 of the chapter, we inventory and briefly describe common techniques that provide the "building blocks" for hybrid techniques and several of the most common combinations. Finally, we conclude the chapter with two case studies that illustrate use of hybrid protocols in sufficient detail to permit replication and adaption.

After reading this chapter, the audience will be able to (1) understand how combining two or more methods in a single protocol can improve testing sensitivity and explanatory power; (2) describe combinations that can accelerate data collection; (3) purposefully select testing combinations that best measure usability dimensions of interest for a specific technology; and (4) leverage the included examples to design hybrid testing protocols.

2.1.3 Background and principles

2.1.3.1 Approaching usability evaluations

Usability assessments in clinical environments are often driven by one of three needs: (1) the need to design a technological solution to a problem; (2) the need to improve HIT to reach a performance target; or (3) the need to assess ROI following HIT implementation. Informaticians often use systems thinking to evaluate HIT effectiveness. This approach examines the interaction between clinical actors, technology, and the organizational context. Unfortunately, a systems-based evaluation is often challenging to operationalize; it can be daunting to gather and analyse a large mixed-methods data set in an operational environment. In response, we have found that applying a theoretical framework during the planning and implementation stages of usability assessments simplifies data management. Theory provides a framework to scope projects and identify key relationships between system components, evaluative dimensions, or research findings. In this section, we present two frameworks that we regularly use for operational projects. The cognitive-socio-technical framework provides a vocabulary to articulate the purpose, evaluative method, and types of findings that can be expected as a function of the product development-deployment lifecycle [39]. The UX Evaluation Focus framework operates on a more micro-level by proving informaticians heuristics to link evaluation focus and usability dimensions.

2.1.3.2 Cognitive-socio-technical framework

Cognitive studies that focused on analysing the interaction of individual users with systems typically drew from cognitive models, such as the Human Information Processor model of human-computer interaction (HCI), whereby a focus is on detailing the steps taken by both humans and machines in carrying out a task. In the healthcare domain, this might involve analysing how an individual physician interacts with an EHR system to enter patient data into the record. The methods most associated with this level of interaction (referred to in the Borycki and Kushniruk model as Level 1 in Figure 2.1) include basic usability testing [39]. Basic ("classic") usability testing has become a popular way of assessing the usability of systems in terms of their effectiveness, efficiency, learnability, enjoyability, and safety. The approach typically involves observing and recording a user interacting with a system to carry out a task while the user is asked to "think aloud" or verbalize their thoughts while using the system [40]. This approach may also include a cued recall, whereby users are asked to comment on the recordings of their interactions upon completion of the task (e.g., interacting with a decision support tool or an EHR to carry out a health-related task). Cued recall may be more practical for tasks where it may not be natural for the user to be thinking aloud while using the system under study. The data from this cognitive level (i.e., screen recording, video recordings, and audio recordings of think-aloud data) can be analysed at a fine-grained and micro-level to identify specific usability problems, user interface flaws, and problems in a system's interaction in terms of its impact on clinician reasoning and decision-making [40,41].

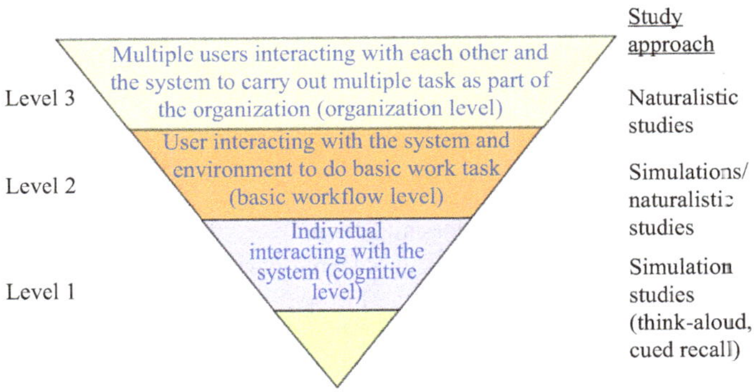

Figure 2.1 The 3 layers of the cognitive-socio-technical framework proposed by Borycki and Kushniruk

Despite the importance of understanding HCI at Level 1, to assess a system's usability in terms of how well a system works when users are carrying out real tasks in complex settings (typically involving multiple "players" or users, e.g., a medical team) other methods are needed. Furthermore, it has become apparent that ensuring a system works at Level 1 (i.e., that it satisfies testing goals when an individual user interacts with an individual system in isolation of real-world work contexts) does not guarantee it will work well when released and put to work in real clinical settings, involving multiple health professionals, patients, and complex organization goals and objectives. Therefore, the cognitive-socio-technical framework in Figure 2.1 was expanded to include a Level 2 (see Figure 2.1) where further evaluation of a system requires the analysis of users interacting with a system to carry out basic work tasks (e.g., using an EHR system to guide an interview with a patient and to support note taking during the interview). The methods required for this level can be based on and expand the approaches taken from Level 1 but do require a consideration of social factors that come into play when a system is being used for real tasks in a healthcare setting. This is a level where one can begin to see the impact of system on workflow. Methods used at this level include clinical simulations, which extend classic usability testing by ensuring the testing is conducted in real or highly realistic simulation environments that consider interactions involved in carrying out more complex work processes than at the purely cognitive level – i.e., those interactions that involve both technical aspects of user interface/system design and social aspects. Clinical simulation extends usability testing (which is conducted using representative users doing representative tasks) to include a third dimension – representative or real contexts and environments [42]. Examples of work at this level include evaluation of doctor-patient-computer interaction, where the 3-way interaction between doctors, patients, and computers (e.g., EHR systems) has been video recorded, analysed, and iteratively improved based on this analysis [40]. Furthermore, studies of use of system in real naturalistic settings can be introduced at Level 2 that may involve use of methods such as observational ethnographic data collection, shadowing key participants (where an observer follows a health professional around taking notes and observations), and an approach to data collection known as contextual inquiry. Contextual inquiry involves "getting as close as possible to the real work" when observing human-system interactions, and may involve shadowing or following health professionals as they interact with systems, asking the participant(s) questions where further delineation of goals and actions taken is needed to understand their interactions with systems [43].

At Level 3 of Borycki and Kushniruk's framework (see Figure 2.1), the focus on evaluating extends to multiple user interacting with each other (e.g., a clinical team) to carry out multiple tasks as part of the organization's higher-level goals. This level extends from Level 2 in terms of number of participants and task complexity. As this level is the least constrained, it is depicted in Figure 2.1 as being at the broad end of the upside-down triangle. Methods used at the level typically involve observational methods, including tracking multiple user interactions (from multiple users) over time (e.g., using software tracking), ethnographic observational methods, and more extensive application of contextual enquiry and clinical simulation [44].

In response to the complexity of studying health information system interactions with human, Borycki and Kushniruk's (2010) cognitive-socio-technical framework posits that the cognitive and socio-technical aspects of the modern clinical environment must be examined concurrently. That is, to ensure systems have been tested effectively more than one level from the framework needs to be considered. The cognitive-socio-technical framework initially grew from applied work and consulting in health informatics where we found that multiple levels of evaluation were needed to ensure that health information systems were useful and usable in multiple contexts. Specifically, we found that testing systems at the level of the individual user (i.e., Level 1) was essential to identify and rectify basic surface level usability problems. However, we needed additional approaches (i.e., Level 2 and Level 3) to evaluate how a health information system would affect clinical workflow, and ultimately, complex social interactions. Indeed, what Borycki and Kushniruk propose is what they have applied in numerous studies that involve evaluating and improving systems at Level 1 and Level 2 at a minimum. For example, a round of basic usability testing may detect issues with a system at Level 1 that may be corrected along with other issues that arise from testing at Level 2 or 3. Along these lines, a multi-level, multi-method approach to applying usability engineering is argued for due to the complexity of application and interactions in the healthcare field [39].

2.1.3.3 Evaluation focus and usability dimensions

With the proliferation of web-based interfaces, the ways in which we approach and think about usability have evolved. Table 2.1 reflects the range of published usability definitions and the dimensions used to operationalize measurement.

For novice usability practitioners, a challenge with these dimensions is that, depending on the source, the underlying construct is conceptualized differently. For example, "efficiency" in some models refers to how quickly the system responds to

Table 2.1 Commonly cited definitions for usability and the associated dimensions of analysis

Usability Definition	Factors (Dimensions)	Theorist or Organization
"A quality attribute that assesses how easy user interfaces are to use"	Easy to Learn Efficient Memorable Satisfying Error Tolerant	Nielsen Schneiderman
Responsive and easy to use	Easy to Use Accessible Intuitive Architecture	U.S. Department of Health and Human Services
"the quality or characteristic of a usable product"	Effective Efficient Engaging Error Tolerant Easy to Learn	Quesenbery
A system that is useful, usable, and satisfying	Useful Usable Functional Satisfying	Zhang and Walji

the user [45,46]. In this case, the technology is the primary focus. In others, efficiency addresses all aspects of the user's environment, including the time required to execute a complex series of actions of which the technology is only one aspect [47]. Another elusive, yet critical usability dimension is "satisfaction". In many models, satisfaction is defined as "the user liked using the system" or the system was "pleasing" [3,46,48]. In others, satisfaction is conceptualized as user engagement and measured in terms of emotional experience [47,49]. Zhang and Walji' conceptualization of usability reminds us that a system can be useful even when it is not implemented well [48]. The context dictates what is useful at any given moment.

Mapping out usability factors allows the usability researcher to clarify the strategic goals associated with a given project. For example, when considering new user requirements or evaluation of an early HIT prototype, it may be reasonable to begin identifying what is functional and useful (e.g., Zhang & Walji's framework). However, a conceptually straightforward inquiry may not be fruitful since stakeholders often struggle to communicate a prioritized list of crucial usability factors and may not know which dimensions address their clinical goals. Therefore, to draft an evaluation protocol, we begin by identifying the focus of the evaluation (Figure 2.2). Broadly, these include process and procedure, context and environment, and the interface. We then trace the usability dimensions that explore the selected focus.

Practical use of the UX Evaluation Focus map is best demonstrated through example. Consider the challenge of developing an interface that permits medical scheduling assistants (MSAs) to identify, track, and schedule electronic specialty

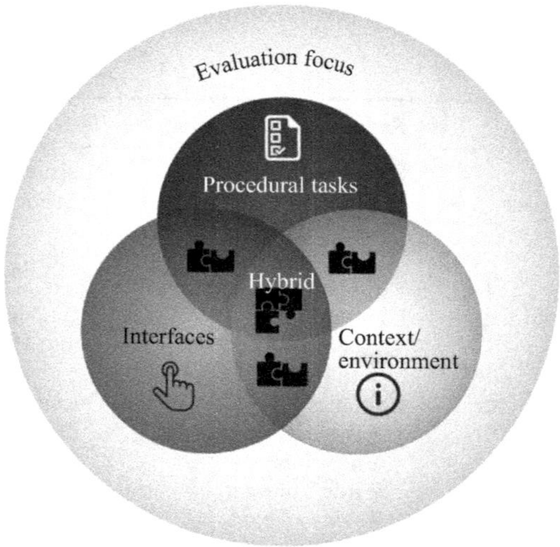

Figure 2.2 Evaluation focus

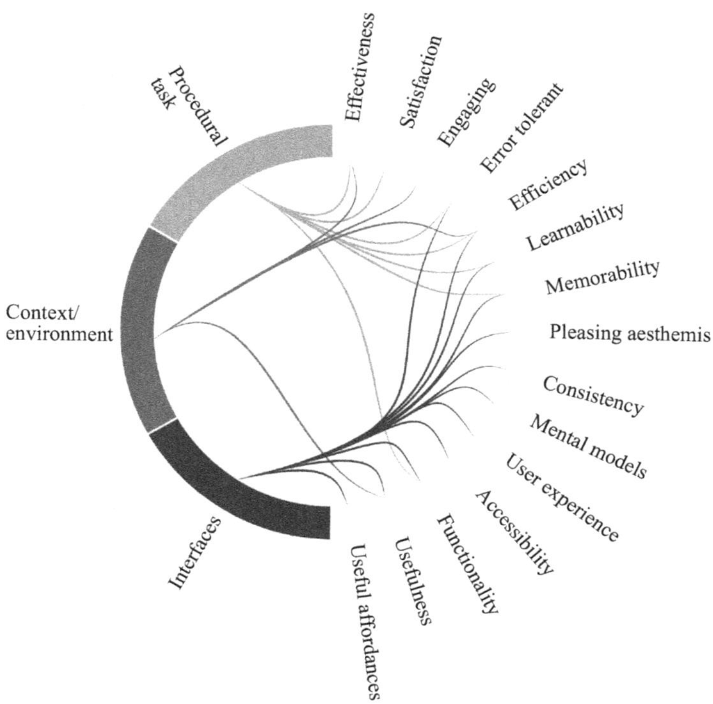

Figure 2.3 UX Evaluation Focus map of usability dimensions by evaluation focus

consult requests across multiple clinics. Clinic managers were clear they wanted an innovation to display specialty consults in relation to status (e.g., active, pending). What they did not realize was the clerks did not use a standardized workflow or set of heuristics; processes varied between specialties. In our experience, this situation is not unique to this project. Operational stakeholders are often focused on process; they know the clinical work that they want a new technology to improve; however, they are often less clear on the environmental factors that impact the clinical environment. We discovered this difference through our examination of HIT consistency and effectiveness for clinical workflow (e.g., on the context/environment dimension above).

2.2 Commonly used methods

2.2.1 Heuristic evaluation

Heuristic evaluation is one of the most commonly used usability techniques [11,34,35]. A usability specialist – often a usability researcher with additional domain-specific subject matter expertise – conducts a systematic evaluation of the interface to search for design issues [3,41,50]. The specialist uses a set of heuristics, or usability "rules of thumb", to organize a step-through, document usability findings, and summarize violations of usability principles (i.e., best practices).

Typically, a single expert evaluator evaluates a target application. However, Nielsen recommends that several evaluators – ideally five – evaluate the interface independently and pool findings [34]. While a single evaluator will identify 35–40% of the usability problems, three evaluators will typically identify 60–70% of the usability problems (with some overlap) and five evaluators will identify 75–85% of the usability problems [33–35]. The number of evaluators depends upon the project, the content domain, the estimated level of risk, and a cost-benefit analysis [33,34]. The team can then compile the violations into a single document, organized by heuristic or theme, along with their severity scores and design recommendations.

Several standardized heuristic lists are available, the most widely cited developed by Nielsen and Molich (i.e., Nielsen's 10 Usability Heuristics) [50–52]. Other popular heuristic lists include Shneiderman's Eight Golden Rules and Tognazzini's Nineteen Principles of Interaction Design [53]. Notably, Zhang, and colleagues at the University of Texas at Houston combined and expanded the lists originally developed by Nielsen and Shneiderman to create the Nielsen-Shneiderman heuristics. This is a list of 14 heuristics adapted for the healthcare domain and EHR evaluations (Table 2.2).

Table 2.2 Nielsen-Shneiderman heuristics described by Zhang and colleagues

Principle	Definition
Consistency and standards	Words, functions, display appearance should remain consistent across a product, interface, or workflow
Visibility of system state	Users should be aware of system preferences, processes, and state through feedback and messaging
Match between system and world	Image and behaviour of a system should match users' mental models
Minimalist	The interface design should be free of extraneous content
Minimize memory load	Users should not be expected to hold information in working memory to complete tasks
Feedback	Users should receive prompt and informative feedback
Flexibility and efficiency	Give users tools to streamline workflow and accelerate processes
Good error messages	Error messages should help users understand, learn, and recover from errors
Prevent errors	The interface should minimize the opportunity for error
Reversible actions	The interface should have tools that enable the user to recover from an error easily
Use users' language	Interface language should be in terms understandable to the user
Users in control	Do not give users the impression that they are controlled by the system
Help and documentation	Always provide clear help and resources at the point-of-service

Considerations

Because heuristic evaluations can be quickly conducted by a small number of specialists, they remain a vital tool for usability testing. The strengths of heuristic evaluation include (1) the relative ease of administration, (2) the low cost, and (3) the ability to perform on virtually any phase of the design life-cycle, including paper prototypes. If the purpose of an evaluation is to examine the overall design in terms of standout usability problems, a reasonable approach is to use established heuristics to identify elements such as figure-ground contrast, useful error messages, information architecture, or standardize design across organizational innovations. Heuristic evaluations take much less time to complete in comparison to simulations, hierarchical task analysis (HTA), or even cognitive walkthroughs. Heuristic evaluation can be performed at any stage of the development cycle.

A limitation of heuristic evaluations is that they cannot provide any information about product performance, efficiency, or user perceptions. This is because heuristic evaluations don't typically involve direct user observation; experts might not experience interfaces in the same way as actual users. Experts might have high sensitivity to relatively trivial design flaws. Heuristic evaluations require that the evaluation team be knowledgeable and comfortable with the given heuristic. Initially, time must be expended for team members to learn and practice applying the heuristic. Omitting this training might introduce concerns about inter-rater reliability into evaluations.

2.2.2 *Cognitive walkthroughs*

A cognitive walkthrough can be a powerful technique for identifying procedural barriers to usability [54]. It was originally designed to evaluate how well users without prior training can learn and interact with consumer technologies such as self-service kiosks. However, cognitive walkthroughs have since been adapted to understand how new or occasional users experience more complex software systems. Participants attempt to complete a predetermined set of tasks and then flag any issues that arise. Walking through a process in this way explores whether its expected behaviours are intuitive to the user.

By their very nature, cognitive walkthroughs are a practical, cost-effective way to assess usability. They can be performed at any stage in development and normally involve just a small group of stakeholders or members of the design team, rather than target users [53]. A shared understanding of how users are expected to interact with the technology serves as a starting point. It is then essential to determine the tasks that the user is expected to perform while using the technology (including any task variations). Moving through the process can provide valuable feedback to designers as they ensure that their design concept matches user expectations. Though a cognitive walkthrough may be performed by an individual, an evaluation team is recommended [50].

Because the evaluation team may be interacting with their own product design, it is essential to determine a set of ground rules that focus on capturing any insights or issues rather than any discussions about design solutions. For each user task, the team attempts to answer the questions developed by Wharton *et al.* [55]: (1) *Will the user try to achieve the right effect?;* (2) *Will the user notice that the correct action is available?;* (3) *Will the user associate the correct action with the effect that the user is trying to achieve?; and* (4) *If the correct action is performed, will the user see that progress is being made toward the solution of the task?* The use of a standard form is helpful when documenting any issues that arise, any ideas to improve design, any successes or failures, any insights about the users, and any comments about the tasks themselves. This facilitates the evaluation team to (1) arrive at a consensus when identifying overall strengths/weaknesses and (2) discuss solutions to any problems identified in the design.

Considerations

This technique is a straightforward way to test learnability. It is a scalable process that can accommodate designs that are more robust at any stage of development. Moreover, it can be used to detect serious problems as well as providing an assessment of the "walk up and use" nature of the design. One should note, however, that cognitive walkthroughs do require very careful planning and are best conducted by experienced facilitators. Training the evaluation team is a prudent first step. Since cognitive walkthroughs can sometimes provide a relatively limited analysis of affordances and identified issues, a hybrid approach might better serve the evaluation team.

2.2.3 Goals, operators, methods, and selection (GOMS) rules

GOMS borrows from HCI concepts to better understand user performance. Each task is broken down into discrete actions to discern interaction and flow. This method helps to identify redundancies so they can either be eliminated or redesigned to produce a more efficient critical path (interactions that are required to achieve the task goal). In GOMS, the task ***goal*** is typically a user-defined end state. Any actions taken to accomplish the task goal are defined as ***operators***. The series of operators needed to carry out the task goal are categorized under the ***method***. If there are competing methods to consider, ***selection rules*** determine the order in which they are executed [56].

Advantages to using GOMS include: an engineer's perspective to protocol design, an estimate of cost savings associated with improved user interaction, a detailed account of the specific actions and time required to achieve user goals, and a well-documented method for comparing competing designs. GOMS is one of the few HCI models based on strong, empiric research [57]. It is best suited to products that have a clearly defined critical path.

Variants [58,59]

- Keystroke-Level Model (KLM) – Estimates execution time; limited to a specified sequence of actions and keystroke-level operators
- Card, Moran, and Newell GOMS (CMN-GOMS) – Predicts execution time and operator sequence; can be modified to include a qualitative dimension
- Natural GOMS Language (NGOMSL) – Predicts operator sequences, execution time, and time to learn; incorporates high-level goals

- Cognitive-Perceptual-Motor GOMS (CPM-GOMS) – Assumes that the operators of cognitive, perceptual, and motor processors can work in alignment; because CPM-GOMS models overlapping actions, it is able to predict skilled behaviour
- Touch Level Model (TLM) – Adapted from the KLM to include touchscreen devices; better able to predict user performance due to adding several operators, but requires proper criteria

Considerations

Due to its detailed methodology, GOMS requires formal training. It is time-consuming, and its focus tends to be so narrow that it does not consider overall context. Consequently, GOMS may not be suitable for open-ended tasks, multiple user types or settings. However, GOMS has been adapted to include multiple variants. When evaluating complex adaptive systems (e.g., healthcare), a modified version might better align with user goals.

2.2.4 Hierarchical task analysis

HTA is one of the most widely accepted and frequently used techniques for breaking down complex activities into smaller units [60,61]. First described by Annett and Duncan in 1967 as a training application to model and teach complex procedures, the approach has undergone multiple revisions and extensions over the last 50 years [62]. By studying individuals interacting with tools in the work environment, practitioners can gain a deeper understanding of physical and cognitive work from the user's perspective. This knowledge, in turn, can be used as a problem-solving approach for a range of human factors, quality improvement, and systems engineering applications.

Since its introduction, practitioners have recognized the inherent flexibility of HTA, using core techniques in a variety of contexts and for a broad range of investigations [63]. For example, HTA can be used to study HCIs such as EHR use, complex adaptive environments such as intensive care units, team-based tasks such as cardiopulmonary resuscitation, and error-prediction across a range of process from hospital drug administration to endoscopic surgery [5–7,60,63]. Other application areas include development of personnel training curriculum and manuals, workload assessment, and error analysis [61,63,64]. Similarly, HTA outputs can satisfy a variety of goals depending upon the intended audience. For example, deliverables for software design teams can be in the form of technical requirements whereas reports for quality specialists or hospital executives can be in the form of team performance assessments, failure mode mitigation plans, or training protocols.

In an HTA, the usability practitioner decomposes work into a detailed list of goals and tasks. To accomplish this, it is critical to first gather a detailed description of the work from the user's perspective by asking four main questions: (1) How is the work performed?, (2) What was required to perform the work?, (3) What is the high-level goal of the work?, and (4) Why is each step performed in this way? [63].

Structuring the inquiry in this way enables the practitioner to understand both observable physical tasks and the motivating cognitive processes [63].

Stanton outlined the accepted heuristics for executing the HTA: (1) define the problem statement and purpose; (2) clarify the boundaries of the target system; (3) use mixed methods to gather information about the system; (4) describe system goals, sub-goals, and tasks; (5) keep the sub-goals to a small number (i.e., between 3 and 10); (6) organize the goals into a hierarchy; (7) establish the logic and conditions under which sub-goals are triggered; and (8) validate the analysis either through member checking or iterative ethnography [65]. These heuristics only provide a general framework; specifics can be tailored to the purpose so long as the output lends insight into cognition and planned behaviour [66,67].

Task analysis findings are typically documented in a task specification document, which may include task lists, narrative details, workflow diagrams, hierarchical diagrams, and tables organized according to the study purpose (e.g., cognitive needs for a requirements document or error types for a risk analysis). In the hierarchical diagram (i.e., task analysis diagram), the highest-level goal defines the objective of the system or behaviour in practical and realistic terms such as "deliver medications to patient" [9,68]. The goal is then broken down into sub-operations defined by sub-goals (e.g., check record for medication orders), which can be measured in terms of performance standards. The sub-goals can be further decomposed into progressively more atomic units depending upon the level of granularity required. Practitioners denote task sequencing using a numbering scheme, and an associated decision taxonomy (e.g., procedure-based, chain sequencing, time-sharing). This fact notwithstanding, tasks can happen concurrently, iteratively, or in a series of nested feedback loops [63]. Hence, HTA convention tends to organize the work by goal, emphasizing purpose over a normative flow [69]. The analysis is complete when the sub-goals are sufficiently clear to the subject matter expert and the analyst [70].

Ultimately, this top-down systems approach to analysis enables the usability specialist or systems engineer to identify and manage factors that have the largest effect upon process performance, variance, outputs, defects, and errors [67]. External representations (e.g., using software or communicating with colleagues) are then catalogued in sequence. In summary, the usability specialist describes how a user establishes mental goals and selects actions to execute these goals.

Considerations

The key considerations to keep in mind are to gather as much detail as possible, document through the lens of the user, and avoid developer contrivances (e.g., artificial sequencing, organization by interface or functionality, and applying developer language).

2.2.5 Surveys

Survey questionnaires are a systematic way to gather demographic data during usability evaluations. While some informaticians might be hesitant to collect user demographic information, we have found that position, time in position, and participant age provide more data to contextualize usability findings. For example, if we observe that MSAs with less than 5 years of experience on the job have a difficult time learning to use the interface in comparison to those with more time on the job, we would suggest that this group receive more at-the-elbow educational support post-implementation. Collecting demographic information is also useful when practitioners must validate to stakeholders that they tested the correct user group during evaluations.

Questionnaires are an ideal way to gather attitudinal perceptions of an interface, including satisfaction, ease of use, perceived system usability, aesthetic appeal, and the level of cognitive effort required. A strength of such instrumentation is that the questionnaires are standardized, quick to administer and quantifiable. There are several well-established and validated survey questionnaires that we regularly use in our evaluations. They can be divided into two types: overall usability and satisfaction. These include the System Usability Scale (SUS), the abbreviated Usability Metric for User Experience questionnaire (UMX-Lite), the Computer System Usability Questionnaire (CSUQ), the Questionnaire for User Interface Satisfaction (QUIS), and the Software Usability Measurement Inventory (SUMI) [71–75].

While most usability scales have been validated and used in a variety of settings, they were not specifically designed to assess healthcare technologies. Several, however, have been used extensively in healthcare and are endorsed by the Certification Commission for Healthcare Information Technology (CCHIT), an accreditation body for the Office of the National Coordinator (ONC) [76]. These include the SUS and the After-Scenario Questionnaire (ASQ) [77]. Also, Columbia University researchers have published a customizable questionnaire designed to evaluate HIT – the Customizable Health IT Usability Evaluation Scale (Health-ITUES) [78]. The instrument addresses four factors thought to be central to technology adoption: (1) quality of work life; (2) perceived usefulness of technology; (3) perceived ease of use of technology; and (4) degree of user control.

A benefit of surveys is they are relatively easy to administer when staff have adequate training. This ease of administration allows for even novice members of the human factors team to reliably collect data. Additionally, self-administered surveys save time during usability evaluations because they can be sent to participants ahead of time. This might drastically reduce time spent in the laboratory while still acquiring important data (e.g., demographics). When cost and time is a consideration, practitioners might consider administering the entire usability assessment by survey (e.g., the SUS). In this case, internet survey packages and remote usability testing applications might be used to reach as many clinical staff as possible within the data-collection phase.

Considerations

There are limitations and drawbacks to the use of surveys. First, questionnaire items are predetermined and do not enable investigators to explore emergent issues encountered during simulation testing [41]. Second, user responses about use might diverge from observations of actual use [79,80]. Prior research suggests that users overestimate their competency when asked to estimate their ability. Certain responses might also be influenced by social desirability bias, or the user's desire to respond to testing in a way they believe the evaluator or stakeholders would approve [81]. This fact notwithstanding, it is important to note that some usability dimensions, such as satisfaction, can only be gathered via self-report. Accordingly, the usability practitioner should be careful interpreting survey findings and reconciling apparent disconnects between the qualitative (e.g., observation) and quantitative data through triangulation.

Third, validated instruments might not completely meet the needs of a given project. There might be questions that are not applicable or the instrument might not include the specificity needed to answer an operational question. In this case, practitioners have three choices: (1) they might ask all the questions; or (2) modify the instrument to meet the needs of their project; or (3) create their own instrumentation. When using a standardized scale, findings can be compared over time (i.e., within subject comparisons) as a product evolves or to other products within a content domain (i.e., between subject comparisons). Such comparisons might help the development team benchmark products and track performance or value over development sprints. In contrast, a consideration when editing validated questionnaires is that it is inappropriate to compare these findings to other evaluations that used the validated version. Therefore, we take this approach when comparison between other similar innovations is not a key factor for our stakeholders. A limitation of creating a new, contextualized survey instrument is that the practitioner should pre-test items (e.g., cognitive interviewing) in addition to piloting the instrumentation. Clearly, this approach requires more time and cost.

Fourth, questionnaires that are particularly long, redundant, or abstract can quickly exhaust the time and patience of busy clinicians and medical staff. In this case, the practitioner must weigh the implications of longer evaluations vs. specific needs.

2.2.6 Semi-structured interviews and probes

Semi-structured interviewing is often used to collect qualitative data during usability studies [82–84]. The strength of qualitative techniques such as interviewing is that usability specialists can gather deep data and insights into the UX. Quotes or specific user feedback can be captured during simulations, at the end of tasks, or at the conclusion of the evaluation session. In this section, we describe two interviewing techniques: probing and semi-structured interviews.

Probing consists of asking clarifying statements during usability tasks or think-aloud protocols [41]. Examples include: "Can you describe what you meant by..." or "You seem to be focusing on something – can you tell me what you are thinking?" The benefit of probing is that it is quick and flexible. However, human factors staff should be careful that the flexibility of probing does not detract from capturing a projects' key indicators. For example, if time on task is a key indicator, introducing probes during the task does not give an accurate representation of time on task. Additionally, facilitators should be mindful of how much time probing is taking up during evaluation, so they do not run out of time-subsequent usability tasks. Another limitation of probing is that it does not yield the same data point for each user; not all users may get the same probe. As usability evaluations tend to involve small sample sizes, the research team will have to determine if this is an acceptable limitation given the objectives of their project.

Semi-structured interviews have a set number of questions. When using this approach, the assessment team develops a guide that covers the key indicators of the project, such as quality of use (e.g., effectiveness dimension). The interviewer has the flexibility to rephrase questions for participants or explore a given answer in more depth. For example, each user might answer a relative advantage question, such as "how is scheduling patients using the software better or worse than your current process?" The interviewer could then dynamically ask another question to explore themes or key indicators of interest that were not anticipated when the interview guide was developed.

Considerations

Investigators should use two primary strategies to ensure qualitative data integrity. The first is to reduce facilitator bias through the training of staff and systematic execution of a protocol. This is critical for teams that divide interviewing activities among their staff members. Facilitators must be comfortable with silence and resist influencing participant answers; the goal of interviewing is to acquire user feedback, insights, and solutions in their own words.

The second strategy is to align on an evaluation method. There are several systematic ways to evaluate qualitative data. A common approach is to create themes or "buckets" within the data – often via an affinity mapping exercise [85]. Another process is conventional content analysis using a codebook to link constructs with that data. These units might reflect usability dimensions or some a priori theoretical framework. Content analysis is costlier in comparison to affinity mapping because it requires software and takes more time. For this reason, some practitioners agree on themes in their data during debriefing sessions via "consensus".

Practitioners should also be aware that interview data is unstructured, highly interpretive, and unwieldy in comparison to surveys. These attributes of the method sometimes make it difficult to justify design insights and recommendations to stakeholders who might be conditioned to quantitative data. To mitigate this, we are careful to not only summarize and synthesize data, but also to acquire verbatim quotes from users that we incorporate into our reports.

2.2.7 Simulations

Although usability testing encompasses a wide array of techniques that can be used before, during, and after the development of a product, most people consider simulation testing the quintessential method [7,35,86]. This is likely because observing a user interacting with a product is a foundational technique for understanding user perceptions and surfacing design flaws [34]. Important usability problems, though easy to find, can remain invisible to developers because they are too familiar with the design, lack domain expertise, or spend little time watching people use their products [33]. Hence, simulations offer deep insight into usability issues and design possibilities. Although there are other data-collection techniques that can help understand user behaviours in context – including ethnographic observation, time-motion, and work sampling – only simulations enable practitioners to test ideas, dissect specific activities, or isolate device features [7]. For this reason, simulations have been used to model complex clinical tasks including endoscopic surgery, cardiopulmonary bypass surgery, emergency resuscitation, and medical decision-making [41,87–89].

Stated simply, simulation-testing entails creating task-based scenarios and observing representative users working through scenarios. The observer avoids interacting with the user to provide a naturalistic and unbiased testing environment. Users are often encouraged to think aloud while using the device.

The "Think-Aloud" protocol (i.e., verbal protocol analysis) has been heralded as one of the most valuable techniques to collect user perceptions and understand user behaviours [11,34,35]. Initially developed as a research method in cognitive psychology to understand subject behaviours (i.e., cognitive interviewing), it has been effectively adapted for human factors engineering and software evaluation. In software testing, the observer asks the user to think aloud while using the application; meanwhile, the observer records field-notes. The observer keeps dialog to a minimum, but gently prompts the user to share their thoughts aloud while using the system and probes for more information when the user is either stuck or ceases to think aloud (e.g., "What are you thinking now?" and "What do you think this device does?") [11,35].

Throughout testing, the observer documents observations about the simulation [11]. The observer may collect qualitative data (e.g., observed behaviours or quotes), quantitative data (e.g., time to complete tasks or number of errors), or a combination of quantitative and qualitative data by collecting qualitative notes and direct quotes, the testing team can capture rich information about users' experiences, lending insight into how a product can be improved. By collecting quantitative data, the testing team can (1) compare competing designs, (2) measure improvement between iterations, (3) isolate important dimensions of usability – e.g., efficiency, safety, and (4) prioritize design efforts. Common measurements include the time to complete a task (efficiency), the number of errors observed (learnability; error tolerance), the ratio of successful interactions to errors (effectiveness), the number of features used (utility; engaging), and the proportion of positive statements versus critical statements (satisfying). More complicated techniques also involve collecting video, audio, on-screen, or eye-movement data for later coding and analysis [11,41].

Like heuristic evaluation, a common point of debate is how many participants are needed for each round of testing. Although there is no consensus on how many participants is "best", it has been suggested that small studies involving three to five users can identify 80–85% of findings from a test [90,91]. Although it may be tempting to test more users when evaluating a high-stakes health technology, adding more testers can be costly and often yields diminishing returns [34]. On average, three users identify 70% of findings, whereas five users identify 85% of findings. Hence, small studies uncover most findings for a *test* (the same may not be true for an *entire product* with multiple features) [35]. This means it can be more fruitful to complete more rounds of testing with a revised product and revised instruments than to wring everything out of each round.

These arguments notwithstanding, the risks associated with usability errors in healthcare can be dire [16]. Depending upon the technology purpose or context (e.g., administration of high-risk medications or data integration in ER and ICU settings), it may be necessary to test more users on one feature or design use-cases to explore high-risk "edge cases". For this reason, some healthcare investigators propose testing 25 or more users [13,92].

Considerations

When incorporating simulations into an evaluation plan, informaticians should be aware of the substantial investment in time, resources, and personnel that this method requires. A given evaluation can range from 15 to 40 minutes, depending on the critical tasks to be examined and the pace of the user. Often, clinical user time comes at a premium; careful planning is required when users are clinicians or hospital staff.

Simulations often require laboratory resources, such as computers, cameras, usability-specific software, two rooms, and staff presence. Staff must be trained to administer simulation protocols in a way that seems relaxed and natural. Therefore, protocols may need to account for the time required for investigators to achieve mastery. Staff training might be accomplished using an apprenticeship model (e.g., shadowing a senior laboratory member) or role-playing among staff. For these reasons, we consider simulations one of the most difficult techniques to engage in.

2.2.8 Severity ratings

Not every usability problem is the same and rarely can all issues be addressed concurrently. Instead, fixed resources (e.g., developer time, content expert availability, finances) and product dependencies (e.g., software components, interface standards) typically dictate the nature and timing of solutions [93]. Therefore, investigators must often prioritize findings according to a severity score.

The premise of severity scoring is conceptually straightforward. The investigator either rates the findings according to the impact upon the UX (i.e., one-dimensional system) or a composite score computed from several orthogonal scales (i.e., multi-dimensional system). Nielsen describes a method that combines user impact with the frequency and an issue is encountered [3]. The overall score is calculated from a 2 × 2 table. Alternatively, Tullis and Albert describe a system that combines four three-point scales measuring the UX, the frequency of occurrence, the impact on business goals, and the implementation costs [93]. By adding all dimensions, the overall severity score can be measured on an ordinal scale from 0 to 8.

There are several strengths and limitations to severity scales. Strengths include: (1) the ability to standardize communication across stakeholders; (2) the ability to prioritize remediation plans based upon fixed resources; and (3) the ability to make comparisons across sequential studies or between competing designs. However, critics have argued that severity scores are fundamentally subjective. Hence, limitations include: (1) poor demonstrated inter-rater reliability between usability experts [3,94]; and (2) the challenge of finding usability raters with deep content expertise (i.e., only end-users familiar with the domain or use-case may be qualified to rate the relative priority of a finding) [93].

We have found these challenges critical to our own work. Frequently, a usability finding can cause downstream patient harm even if unrecognized or rarely encountered by the end-user. For example, consider a medication order entry system that allows a physician to select an unsafe medication dose or a non-formulary item. The verifying pharmacist may be the individual responsible for identifying and correcting the error, leaving the ordering physician out of the feedback loop. An error not caught by the system can result in patient injury or death. This sort of usability finding may not trigger action by many of the most commonly used scales [93]. Given the need to operationalize predicted health outcome risks, we have adapted a scoring system developed by the VA National Patient Safety (NCPS) – the Safety Assessment Code (SAC) score [95].

The VA NCPS adopted the SAC scoring matrix to score and prioritize predicted healthcare system hazards identified during process analysis and reengineering efforts. It is like Nielsen's algorithm in that it combines two orthogonal scales: (1) the impact upon patients and patient care; and (2) the frequency or probability of occurrence. The impact dimension is a four-item scale ranging from minor (e.g., no injury) to catastrophic (e.g., death). The probability dimension is a four-item scale that ranges from remote (i.e., may happen once in 5–30 years) to frequent (i.e., may happen several times a year). The investigator then calculates the product of the two scores and uses a decision tree to determine the priority of action based upon (1) criticality; (2) absence of control measures or effective workarounds; and (3) lack of detectability. The SAC score can be used alone or combined with other scales, using the approach described by Tullis and Albert.

Considerations

Informatics staff expertise should be considered when using severity scales; teams might need to consult clinical staff to assess the impact of findings upon patient outcomes. Also, team members must be trained on how to use the assessments. They must feel comfortable explaining the severity ratings to stakeholders more accustomed to severity scales prioritizing the frequency of occurrence.

2.3 Hybrid techniques

In this section, we explain how to combine two or more of the previously described methods in novel ways. Although few texts explicitly describe combination methods or hybrid protocols, most usability specialists will either intuitively or purposefully integrate several methods to keep pace with the rapid pace of health information technology development [34]. There are many different combinations and each project will likely require a slightly different approach.

Combining methods confers several advantages. First, combining methods and complementary data-collection techniques enables testing teams to capitalize upon limited resources (or limited user availability) and gather more information about device usability. Second, combining methods permits the team to measure multiple usability dimensions concurrently. This is often critical when stakeholders and business owners have competing agendas or performance expectations. Third, gathering and "triangulating" complementary data can help explain puzzling or apparently conflicting findings. Fourth, the ability to mix and match methods depending upon the testing goals increases the agility and flexibility of the design team in the face of changing deadlines or fixed costs.

Of course, there are some disadvantages to combining methods that should be kept in mind when developing a protocol. Invariably, the protocol requires a larger investment of work including time spent on design, set-up, data collection, and analysis. Accordingly, there is an additional up-front project management cost. Similarly, there is a back-end cost required to analyse two or more sets of data. Although combined methods may not be feasible in highly resource-constrained settings, the usability specialist should be encouraged to at least design a "collapsible" protocol that can be expanded or revised as logistics dictate.

2.3.1 Simulation combined with heuristic checklist

One of the most common strategies used by specialists is to combine a heuristic checklist with a simulation. In one variant, the simulation is completed first and the observer records qualitative data during the simulation. The testing team can then organize, categorize, and report the data according to a set of usability heuristics. The testing team may elect to use only the data collected from the simulations or combine with expert findings gathered during a design step-through. For example, in a study of a medication history documentation tool, representative patients completed a series of simulated tasks while using a Think-Aloud protocol. The testing team collected screen recordings as well as hand-written field-notes on a paper collection form with printed screen shots. Screenshots were included on the field-notes collection form, making it easier to quickly mark-up design problems and potential solutions. The data was then entered in a spreadsheet and distributed to a panel of usability specialists for coding. Codes were assigned independently and discrepancies were resolved through discussion.

In a second protocol variant, the testing team completes the heuristic evaluation first to identify obvious usability problems and "clean up" the interface before recruiting users for simulation [51]. The development team updates the interface based upon the initial evaluation results. Then, users participate in a simulation using the Think-Aloud protocol to validate design revisions and sweep for remaining usability problems not originally identified. In circumstances where there is no time to change the interface before simulation testing, the expert review can be used to help clarify testing goals, narrow the scope of testing, or guide the development of the simulation tasks [35].

There are several reasons for combining simulation with heuristic evaluation. First, starting with a heuristic evaluation helps to identify obvious usability flaws without "wasting representative end-users" that might be difficult to recruit [51]. Second, the two techniques have been shown to identify different usability issues – the two techniques do not have a high degree of overlapping findings [96,97]. Third, coding findings according to heuristics can help organize results for the development team and forecast potential remediation strategies [98]. Finally, heuristics can provide a "voice" to the finding when end-users are unable to articulate why they are struggling with an interface component.

2.3.2 Simulations combined with interviews

Combining simulations with a debriefing exercise is a common and practical way to revisit an observational finding and understand the user perspective. Interviews permit the usability specialist to unpack an observation or emergent theme – even with little advance preparation. What did the user think when encountering a new interface interaction? What decision rules or heuristics did the user apply to navigate the tools or negotiate a challenge? What design modifications or new affordances would make the interface easier to use or more valuable in daily work? Combining direct observations with interview responses is a rapid technique for understanding the root causes of usability issues and tracing root causes (i.e., archetypal usability challenges) to evidence-based or best-practice solutions. Ultimately, the nature of the questions will be dictated in part by the study goals and in part by the UX.

Including interviews in a simulation confers several advantages. First, interviews guide exploratory phases of an evaluation when requirements or design problems are still unknown [3]. Second, interviews provide the opportunity to "chase down" and understand unexpected observations. Third, interviews can inform other UX efforts and deliverables including empathy maps, journey maps, needs statements, and personas. Fourth, interviews can establish the association or correlation between user perceptions and user behaviours [3,41]. By quickly establishing the relationship – or lack thereof – between user reports and technology use, it is possible to contextualize future feedback and prioritize design backlog. Finally, it can be possible to address user fears or worst-case scenarios that may not occur frequently, if ever, during simulations, but that can impede user adoption or expose the organization to risk [3].

Although it is certainly possible to extemporaneously conduct an interview driven entirely by the findings of the simulation, most researchers will assemble a general script with important themes, topics, and probes. The usability specialist can then conduct a semi-structured interview, that in equal measures, helps guide the inquiry based upon the overarching goals and provides enough flexibility to capitalize upon unanticipated findings. Depending upon where a product is in the development lifecycle, the research or development team can use an exit interview to (1) identify new requirements; (2) empathize and map the UX; (3) explore new design idea; (4) prioritize development backlog; and (5) evaluate existing designs or chart long-term optimizations.

While there are clearly many benefits to integrating an exit interview into a simulation exercise, there are challenges and risks that should be recognized. First, interviews require additional usability staff time and more participant time. This can be particularly problematic in operational settings that are resource constrained or in circumstances that pull clinicians from busy patient-care posts. Second, as stated earlier, interviews are fundamentally subjective, and prone to recall bias and social desirability bias [3,81]. It is, therefore, crucial to avoid explaining system functions, offering testing rationale, agree or disagreeing with user statements, or asking questions that favour a certain valence. Third, it can be challenging to reconcile findings when user reports and observations seem orthogonal to each other. Invariable, the research team must develop validated protocols for handling these findings.

2.3.3 Simulation combined with surveys

Adding surveys to a simulation protocol, much like combining simulations with interviews, enables the evaluation team to quickly gather user opinions about an interface. Surveys, on their own, provide only an indirect method for gathering usability data. However, when combined with direct observations, surveys lend additional explanatory power to the conclusions drawn from direct observations. Also, surveys can help link the qualitative observations associated with a simulation to quantitative statistics typically required by product owners, clinical managers, and executive sponsors.

Surveys can be an important part of a mixed-methods protocol for several reasons. First, surveys are a validated method for measuring user satisfaction. As noted in the foundational methods section, there are several instruments that have been tested across industries (e.g., SUS) and that have been developed for healthcare (e.g., Health-ITUES) [74,78]. Second, it is possible to design an instrument that rapidly assesses multiple usability dimensions or determinants of adoption (e.g., compatibility with user values, usefulness, aesthetic appeal, etc.) [99]. This is particularly useful when applying a theoretical framework or model such as Davis' Technology Acceptance Model (TAM), Venkatesh's Unified Theory of Acceptance and Use of Technology model (UTAUT), or Holahan's Effective Technology Use Model (ETUM) [2,100,101]. Finally, surveys can help operationalize a quantitative appraisal of product utility or effectiveness – even during the formative evaluation stage of the design lifecycle. Although, not always methodologically ideal, this can be a practical necessity in high stakes, fast paced, or low UX maturity operational environments.

Practically speaking, there are several common strategies to combine surveys with simulations. If it is critical to understand the interaction between user attributes, system usability, and implementation success, the usability team may elect to open a testing session with a brief demographic survey. In addition to the common attributes typically collected in any usability test (e.g., user age, occupational title, work location), the researcher may also elect to measure more specific attribute that can influence medical outcomes or patient safety (e.g., years of training in a clinical domain, functional health literacy, functional technology literacy, relationship to organizational leadership, degree of practice autonomy). If the goal is to measure satisfaction or impressions of an interface, it may be reasonable to conclude a simulation session with a short survey. Instruments that are well suited to this task are the SUS and the QUIS [74,75]. If time is limited, the UMUX-Lite is an extremely concise and validated instrument that compares favourably with longer questionnaires [73].

In our own experience, we often simply include these questionnaires at the back of our testing script and administer a paper copy after all test scripts. However, some usability experts have argued it is possible to gather more precise user estimates of ease of use by administering a subset of questions after the *user completes each task* [102]. For example, Sauro found that the Single Ease Question (SEQ) – a Likert item asking the user to rate the relative difficulty of a task – administered immediately after task completion, performed as well as more complex task difficulty measures such as the ASQ, the Subjective Mental Effort Question (SMEQ), and the Usability Magnitude Estimation (UME) [103].

2.3.4 Agile task analysis: A combination of simulation and hierarchical task analysis

Agile task analysis (ATA) is a method developed and described by Lesselroth and colleagues that combines HTA with simulation to test interface prototypes [104]. The application of HTA for interface evaluation is well-established; Annett and Stanton's ergonomics text offers a series of monographs describing modified HTAs to simulate interface operations, capture data flows between humans and artefacts, and inform iterative software engineering campaigns [67]. These HTA extensions offer the flexibility and expressivity to capture nuanced design requirements or emergent behaviours in high-stakes settings. The ATA builds upon this work by providing a prescriptive framework for organizing use-case simulations and enforcing a tabular format that matches images of representative artefacts (e.g., software interfaces, data entry forms) with tasks and findings (see **Case Study 1** for figure examples). This tabular format enables investigators to gather a variety of data types concurrently including qualitative notes, task completion rates, prototype mark-ups, and user feedback.

ATA is suited to evaluating HIT designed for a narrow set of tasks or that enforces a standardized workflow. For example, software designed to guide a clinician through a medication history might first retrieve a medication list and require review of each medication with a patient. In this case, the software is designed to solve a specific problem and expects a protocolized sequence. The ATA enables the usability practitioner to map out each step of the medication history workflow, permitting collection of usability findings at a very granular level. The investigator can then quickly organize findings by clinical task, functional unit, or interface affordance.

The integration of HTA into a traditional simulation protocol helps address some of the challenges inherent with a traditional HTA. First, the software function or clinical workflow defines the decomposition exercise, thus helping the investigator recognize “the bottom” of a hierarchy chart. Second, combining simulation with a task analysis makes it possible to anticipate and catalogue even rare errors. Finally, Think-Aloud protocols enable immediate member checking and ecological validation of the hierarchy.

To develop an ATA protocol, the testing team must first define the use-case and high-level goals for the interface. Then, investigators can break down the behavioural and cognitive steps required to complete each goal. In the tradition of HTA, a “top-down” approach is typically used where a series of larger and more complex steps are first identified that move the user through the interface to complete a goal. Once these steps are identified, they are broken down into progressively smaller sub-tasks until they cannot be decomposed any further. Once all the steps are outlined for each goal, an instrument can be assembled that lists each step in the workflow along with a representative screenshot. The design strategy is like the wireframing and storyboarding exercises that accompany Agile software engineering. The instrument is then used as a script for an eventual simulation study.

The testing team should create a script for each major software feature or use-case. The steps are listed numerically along with clear descriptions for successful task completion. While the purpose of the test is not “pass” or “fail” a participant, it is crucial to mark which screens, signals, or affordances force an error. If a user completes the task easily without assistance, the proctor marks that step as “passing”. If the user can complete the task but with some difficulty, the proctor marks that step as “marginal”. If the user cannot complete the task or the proctor needs to assist the user to advance to the next step in the scenario, the proctor marks that step as “failing”. Because the instrument includes illustrations of artefacts or screenshots of software, the proctor can quickly capture qualitative observations, record user quotes, or identify problematic areas. The testing team can then qualitatively describe the pain points in a workflow or report the numeric scores for each task and sub-task.

2.3.5 GOMS combined with simulation

The combination of GOMS with simulation came about from our attempt to solve an implementation problem that involved process and interface considerations. We needed to replace ad hoc workflows with a technology intended to enforce a standardized workflow and reduce time on task. Therefore, we designed the protocol to measure functionality and effectiveness. Anticipating a normative workflow, we identified the clinical tasks that users needed to complete. We then divided each task into discrete steps that mapped onto the information architecture of the technology. We assigned a rating scale of no difficulty, some difficulty, and difficulty to each sub-step. To this end, we call this approach “GOMS-inspired”.

By combining GOMS with simulation, the investigator can easily evaluate the steps users take to complete a task and identify pain points for each sub-task. The evaluation team can furnish to the development team with extremely granular estimates of software performance and suggested remediation strategies. In our example, we could report the proportion of users who experienced significant difficulty, some difficulty, or no difficulty with each task. These insights informed how we prioritized (and backlogged) design recommendations. Additionally, the focus on process and functionality is useful for A/B testing approaches where one design is compared to another.

Considerations

Like the ATA, this hybrid approach provides a very granular script for the tester. However, it is best suited for tasks that have a normative workflow. Unlike the ATA, combining GOMS with simulation is better suited to capturing user behaviours when the clinical goal is well defined but the precise approach may not be known.

2.3.6 Heuristic evaluation combined with cognitive walkthrough

Kushniruk, Monkman, Tuden, Bellwood, and Borycki (2015) have described a hybrid approach to usability inspection they have applied that combines heuristic evaluation with the cognitive walkthrough approach in evaluating health information systems. The approach involves systematically analysing or "stepping through" a user interface or interaction with a system to carry out tasks (e.g., entering medications into a medication administration system) as is done using the cognitive walkthrough approach [105]. As in the cognitive walkthrough, at each step in carrying out the task the following are noted by the analyst(s) carrying out the combined method: (1) the goal or sub-goal of users at each step, (2) the action (s) the user would have to take – e.g., clicking on an icon, scrolling, etc., (3) the system's response, and (4) potential user problems. In addition, at each step along the way during the cognitive walkthrough, any potential issues encountered by the analyst are captured (using screen shots) and evaluated in terms of Nielsen's heuristics, as they are applied in heuristic evaluations [51]. The severity of each issue can also be assessed, leading to a comprehensive usability evaluation that combines the heuristic evaluation method with the cognitive walkthrough.

The advantages of the cognitive walkthrough (i.e., the ability to analyse user interactions from the perspective of end-users systematically stepping through an interface at a fine-grained cognitive level) can be combined with the advantages of heuristic evaluation (i.e., the ability to classify potential problems in terms of Nielsen's well-known set of heuristics). The approach may pair a usability expert with either a subject matter expert, clinical champion, or architect. It can be applied throughout the system development life cycle, but is well suited to early design phases when considering several prototypes (agile and spiral software design methods). Although this hybrid approach does not involve testing directly with end-users (as the analyst serves as, or "plays the role" of the end-user in carrying out the evaluation), it does provide a reasonable alternative when limited access to representative end-users. It is good for simultaneously evaluating ease of use and learnability and can lead to recommendations for fine-tuning or modification of a system's user interface that can be invaluable for improving user update and satisfaction with a healthcare information system. It is also noteworthy in that it combines the advantages of two methods – i.e., heuristic evaluation and cognitive walkthrough, that are essentially conducted together (saving time and effort in having to do both separately) and that provide reinforcing and converging evidence about usability problems and issues.

2.4 Case studies

2.4.1 Case study 1

2.4.1.1 Background and usability evaluation goals

Medication reconciliation can reduce the potential for adverse drug events by improving the situational awareness at the point-of-care. Clinicians can only make informed prescribing and management decisions when they have a complete picture of a patient's medication profile. Likewise, a patient can expect the best health outcomes when taking a medication regimen as directed. To reconcile medications, the provider must (1) collect a list of patient medications and allergies, (2) compare information to institutional documentation, (3) resolve discrepancies between lists, and (4) furnish the patient with an updated list. Gathering an accurate and complete history can be challenging because: (1) systems-based strategies can be cost prohibitive; (2) the task is cognitively and procedurally complex; and (3) patients may be incapable of furnishing an accurate history.

We were asked to evaluate a patient-facing, self-service kiosk technology intended to standardize medication history collection and documentation, thereby meeting hospital key performance metrics. The technology asks patients to answer a medication and allergy review questionnaire; they must verify the accuracy of each allergy and prescription using on-screen navigation buttons and controls. The goal of this software is to improve (1) reliability of medication and allergy review in the ambulatory clinic, (2) provider documentation efficiency, and (3) clinic quality performance. We needed to determine if patients could easily learn and use the interface with minimal assistance. We, therefore, designed a mixed-method "hybrid" protocol that included (1) a simulation with Think-Aloud protocol; (2) an ATA; and (3) an expert heuristic evaluation.

2.4.1.2 Methods and protocol design

We recruited a convenience sample of 22 patients to participate in testing. We scheduled participants for 30-minute sessions with 30 minutes in between each session for debrief and to reset systems to proper test conditions. They completed several scripted scenarios using a "Think-Aloud" protocol where subjects verbally articulated their thought processes while concurrently working through representative tasks using the technology (Figures 2.4 and 2.5). We collected data using our ATA method and completed a heuristic evaluation.

The ATA outlined discrete steps of the intended workflow, enabling tracking of design flaws, process chokepoints, and granular user feedback. Task analytics were important because they (1) allowed designers to track departures from the normative workflow and (2) enable the development team to precisely measure the performance of prototype affordances. This testing served as both a means to record current usability and to identify areas where improvements were needed.

We transcribed each use-case into a table that listed user actions and software responses. As with a traditional HTA, the ATA form articulated each user goal and the subordinate tasks required to fulfil the goal. The investigator could then easily collect any narrative observations and indicate which tasks were completed. The form also included thumbnail-sized screenshots of each screen of the interface so the test facilitator could quickly indicate any problems or suggested revisions directly on the illustration.

Each participant was invited to our usability lab and asked to complete two scenarios. The usability lab was comprised of a single room with a table, a touch screen kiosk for the participant, and a laptop computer. The facilitator provided verbal and written instructions and then protocoled the simulation. While the subject worked through the use-case, the facilitator also recorded task completion rates, obtained post-task ease of use data, and took notes on participant comments. During testing, participants were encouraged to share any questions, confusion, or feedback while completing the required tasks embedded in the scripted scenarios.

Scripted test scenario 1

Proctor notes: Test patient Sharon Rhea - SSN 000-00-0001

This scenario tests a patient with

- 2 allergies in system
- on time
- changes an allergy stored in VistA,
- adds 2 new allergies
- 1 comment

Script:

You are Mr/Ms Rhea, a 69 y Veteran seeing your medical provider. You have several allergies, some of which we know about at this facility. you believe you are **not allergic to penicillin.** You want to tell the clinic you are **allergic to oxycodone and peanuts.** You are **concerned about the mistake** that we think you are allergic to penicillin and want to tell us **you have never been allergic to penicillin.**

I will now hand you a card describing this patient for your reference. Feel free to refer to the card at any time to remind you of the task. Please remember to talk aloud as you complete the task. Is there anything that I have not made clear? Do you understand the task?

Figure 2.4 Use-case for an Agile Task Analysis of a medication reconciliation technology

Agile task analysis (ATA) - Data collection instrument

Script: 1

Test patient SSN: 000-00-0001 Sharon Rhea 1

Functional test:

StartTime______

StopTest______

StopTalk______

1. Allergies	Check task if performed	Comments
a. "Let's review the allergies listed in your chart at this facility. You have 2 allergies to review"	_ _Proceed	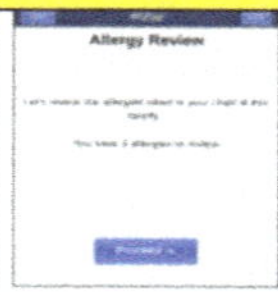
b. "Are you allergic to these items?" c. No change to aspirin d. Changes penicillin No e. "Additional allergies, reactions, or comments"	_ _Asprin: No change _Penicillin=No _Add Allergy/comment	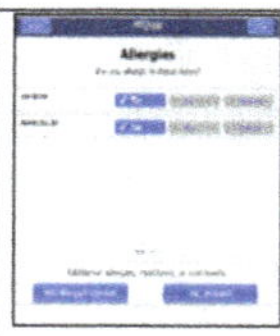
f. "Allergies/Comments: Enter your allergies and comments below" g. Adds Oxycodone h. Adds peanuts i. Enters "Not allergic to penicillin" j. Proceeds to next screen	_ _Type allergy 1 _Type allergy 2 _Type comment _Proceed	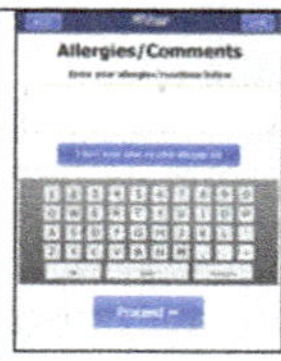
k. "Allergy review: A message is being send to your healthcare team"	_	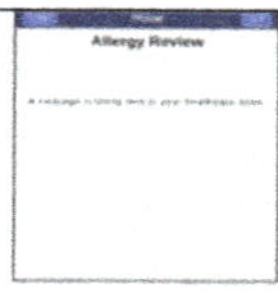

Figure 2.5 Example of the Agile Task Analysis data-collection form

The investigator captured handwritten observations on the ATA instrument; any specific graphic user interface design flaws were indicated on the thumbnail illustrations. The ATA was also used as a template to report findings (Figure 2.6).

After the session, the facilitator provided the participant with a post-test assessment that asked the participant to rate their (1) functional information technology literacy and (2) the overall software ease of use. Self-assessed functional IT literacy was rated using two Likert-type questions. Similarly, a single Likert-type question based upon a previously validated instrument was used to measure subject estimates of program ease of use. Participants' age, verbal responses, observer comments, and post-task assessment were recorded in a spreadsheet.

2.4.1.3 Data analysis

All data were analysed to identify emergent themes and to inventory design flaws. We entered handwritten notes from the ATA into a data-collection spreadsheet. Themes were identified using Grounded Theory methods. A theme was identified

Script: 1, SSN: 0001 (Sharon Rhea 1)		
Allergies	Check task if performed	Comments
a. Allergy review: "Let's review the allergies listed in your chart at this facility. You have 2 allergies to review" Observation: • While most participants read the intro page, what stood out to them was the large bolded "Allergy review", the number of allergies (e.g.2), and the proceed button • In some cases, the word "review" in the title was confusing Recommendation: • Change page title from "Allergy review" to "Allergies" • Eliminate excess wording by restating as "You have XX allergies on file at this facility"	__ __Proceed	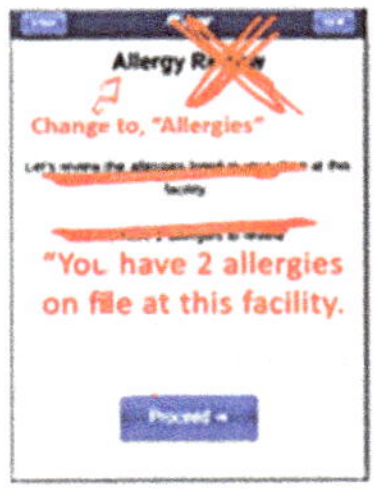
b. Allergies: "Are you allergic to these items?" (Page 1 of 1) c. No change to aspirin d. Changes penicillin No e. "Additional allergies, reactions, or comments" Observation: • On the touch screen kiosk, the "Add allergy/comment" button rendered larger than the "No, proceed" button. This worked well for discoverability and for people with large fingers who wanted to add an item. • ***Usability issue***- People were confused about the function of the "Add allergy/comment" button when the text above read "Additional allergies, reactions, or comments" • ***Usability issue***- Users consistency did not discover the blue "Back" button in the blue header	__ __Aspirin: No change __Penicillin=No __Add Allergy/comment	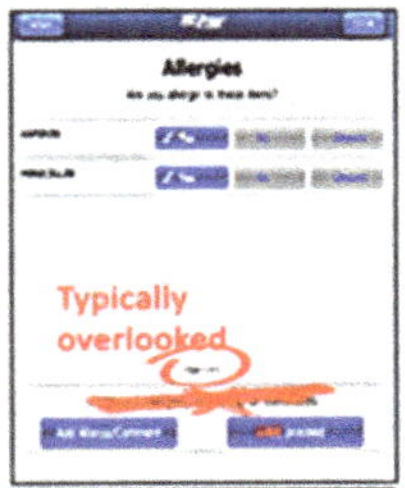 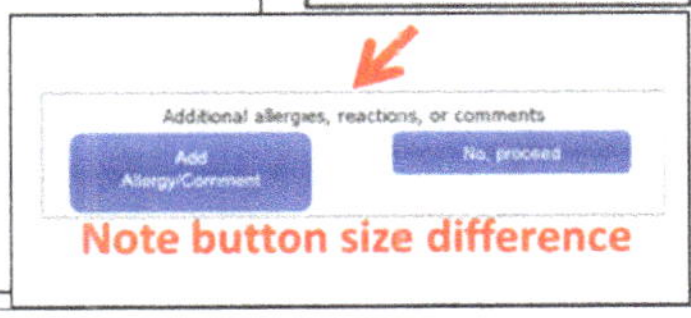

Figure 2.6 Example of the Agile Task Analysis data-collection form with recorded observations and task performance

as a barrier if (1) it affected software use or task completion, (2) was a recurrent source of confusion, and (3) contributed to user abandonment.

We then used a heuristic checklist adapted from Kushniruk and Patel [41]. Three usability specialists were given a scoring sheet with each heuristic domain listed on a 5-point Likert-type scale anchored by the labels "1 = Usability catastrophe" and "5 = Not a usability problem" with examples of strong and weak illustrations (Figure 2.7).

The experts independently completed the heuristic checklist and an average score was calculated for each dimension. We also calculated an overall average from the heuristics to provide developers with a baseline for benchmarking. Any usability dimension violation scoring less than four equated to a non-passing score for the entire application.

2.4.1.4 Results

Twenty-two subjects participated in software usability testing; 16 of the 22 completed a brief survey of self-rated IT literacy. We recorded 73 scenarios across 12

Heuristic 1: Visibility of system status

The user should be informed as to the state of the system at any given moment and should know where she or he is in terms of completing a procedure or task.

The user has difficulty determining the status of a process; the user cannot ascertain where there are in the process flow; the user cannot determine if an action is in process or if a transaction has been successful	The interface has status indicators at each point in the workflow; the interface communicates tasks in process and tasks remaining; the interface communicates when an item is processing and when a transaction has been successful

Can't judge	Usability catastrophe	Major usability problem	Minor usability problem	Cosmetic problem only	Not a usability problem
0	1	2	3	4	5

Visibility of system status–Comments:

- When comments are disabled and "Add allergy/comments" is selected, subjects are exited from the module unknowingly.
- "Add allergy" button confusing, improved with text change
- All subjects believed that the interstitial screen message indicated that data was being send to subject's primary care team and not the provider they were checking-in to see.

Figure 2.7 Heuristic checklist used to organize and score usability findings identified using Agile Task Analysis. Reprinted, with permission, from [41]

total hours of observation. Each usability session lasted approximately 30 minutes. All the survey respondents indicated they were comfortable or very comfortable using an ATA and all indicated they used a computer frequently or daily. Approximately 87.5% of subjects agreed with the statement "It was simple to use this program".

We identified several significant design flaws and heuristic violations that could influence facility implementation and user adoption. In brief, design problems tended to cluster into two categories: clarity of communication and program function. An example of a design feature that did not effectively communicate function was the button labelled "I don't know what my other allergies are". None of the participants understood the purpose of the button or how it would be effectively used in the workflow. An example of a program function issue was the on-screen "soft" keyboard lacked a conventional "return" key. Therefore, users struggled to format multiple allergies as a list.

Additional heuristic violations were identified that validated or explained a simulation finding. These violations had a significant impact upon overall module usability, task completion, and user satisfaction. Experts and participants could not track progress towards task completion and did not understand how information would reach or notify facility staff. Many on-screen affordances did not map to real-world concepts and navigation controls did not conform to design conventions for self-service kiosks. For example, participants did not discover the "Back" button in the upper left corner of the screen could not find on-screen help when they encountered novel or unexpected situations.

2.4.2 Case study 2

As an example of the application of multiple methods and approaches to address a key issue in health informatics a combination of usability methods (including human-in-the-loop simulations and computer modelling) were applied to explore the relationship between usability and patient safety. This work was motivated by the increasing reports of errors resulting from use of new health information technologies, what Borycki has referred to as "technology-induced error". Such errors may enter into a system during its design and development and are typically only detected once a system is being used in the context of the complexity of real healthcare settings and use. They may not actually be software or programming errors, but none-the-less can lead to errors ranging from minor to very serious safety hazards [39]. In considering technology-induced error, it was felt there may be a close relationship between poor usability and the occurrence of such error. To explore this, a series of complementary studies employing hybrid methods was conducted that included a full range of usability methods that involves observing end-users of systems interacting with them to carry out work tasks coupled with quantitative approaches using computer modelling [106,107].

In the initial study, participants consisting of 10 physicians were asked to perform prescription-writing tasks while using a handheld prescription-writing software application. As is done in "classic" usability testing, the screens of the device were video recorded and the participants were asked to think aloud while they entered a series of prescriptions (from a piece of paper) as accurately as possible into the application and printed them out. The approach was also extended to a more realistic context using the clinical simulation approach, with one of the investigators playing the role of the patient, and with recording of the physician participant with the "patient" recorded along with the screens being recorded of the handheld device. Initial analysis of the recorded data (consisting of video recordings of the handheld device's screens and the audio recordings) involved using methods for coding data described in detail by Kushniruk and colleagues in 2005 and more recently by Kushniruk and colleagues in 2015. The approach allows for identifying usability problems, such as display visibility problems, problems with searching and navigating for information on the screen, and printing problems. In a second (and independent) pass in analysing the same video and audio recordings, errors in the entry of the prescriptions were identified (e.g., transcription errors, wrong dosage, etc.). The statistical relation between the usability problems and technology-induced errors was then analysed. It was shown that some of the most serious usability problems were highly associated with errors in the resultant prescriptions (e.g., of the 19 coded problems related to display visibility issues, there were 16 instances of at least part of the prescription being entered with less than full accuracy, including some errors for dosage and frequency). Indeed, all the errors in entering prescriptions were associated with at least one more usability problems [106].

Although the participants were familiar with handheld mobile applications, none of them had used the application that was evaluated before. Therefore, some of the errors may have been related to lack of knowledge or lack of training on the application. To test and describe this, we also evaluated data that illustrated the learning curve of users over time. This involved following users as they improved their facility with the application over several sessions. This information was fed into a dynamic computer modelling simulation tool (Stella) model that was developed to describe and model the type of errors that emerged from the initial usability study, as well as modelling the reduction of error over time as learning occurred. The resultant computer-based simulation was then used to explore questions that arose regarding the implications of the usability errors that were identified from the initial user interactions from usability testing and simulations involving the 10 participants [107].

To carry out a computer-based simulation, parameters for a computer model (that was based on the empirical results from initial usability testing and clinical simulations) were inputted into a generalized model to explore the impact of widespread deployment of the application in terms of safety and to explore the impact of correcting and mitigating specific usability issues (i.e., by removing them from the model and by removing error rates associated with those issues). The objective was to be able to effectively extrapolate what the impact of the usability and safety errors would be when such an application was distributed on a widespread scale. This involved collecting data and estimating how often the application was being used in terms of number of physicians who used the application across the United States, integrating the learning curve data and estimations and developing cost estimates for different types of errors that the model would predict. As the application was widely used at the time of the work described above, recommendations for improving its efficacy were made and the importance of mitigating technology-induced error by applying usability-engineering methods was highlighted. The approach has been recommended as a way of integrating results from smaller scale, in-depth qualitative usability analyses (including both classic usability testing and clinical simulations) with use of quantitative computer-based simulations to extrapolate and reason about the impact of usability and safety issues on a larger scale over larger populations and regions to support decision-making about patient safety when introducing new information technologies. The approach also illustrated the potential benefits and use of combining different methods for generating and analysing usability related data [107].

2.5 Conclusions

Usability engineering studies, while critical to the design of health information technology, are often neglected or abbreviated in a misguided effort to reduce production costs, close functionality gaps, or keep pace with software development schedules. However, early shortcuts often produce frustrated users, workflow inefficiencies, and potentially catastrophic medical errors. Inevitably, usability missteps must then be revisited downstream where redesign occurs at a premium. It is, therefore, crucial that usability specialists (1) assess the UX maturity of their organization; (2) evangelize the importance of evidence-based design; (3) become conversant in a variety of usability techniques; and (4) strategically apply hybrid strategies throughout the software design lifecycle.

However, we have found that each of the recommendations above can be difficult to implement. In our own facility, we actively educate clinical stakeholders, executive leadership, and others about the value of usability testing and other human factors techniques. We do this by emphasizing discount usability methods and examining how our innovations can better meet their needs. The first step in this is operationalizing their questions and concerns (Section 2.1.3.3). This has led us to rely on relevant theoretical models that examine the complex interaction between human, technology, and clinical environment. The difficulty that stakeholders have communicating their concerns resulted in our creation of the UX Evaluation Focus Framework, which organizes usability dimensions by focus (e.g., interface, context/environment, or process).

Our endeavour to become conversant in multiple usability techniques was precipitated by the need to quickly, cheaply, and with a high level of precision address the needs of our operational stakeholders. Often, their needs required discrete methods to approach multiple research questions. However, we are unable to conduct multi-stage usability evaluations in an operational setting where developers are designing software in an agile environment. Our solution is to break a given protocol into parts, which each part using a different method to approach a research question. Key to our design process is moderating the limitations of each method. We think of these “considerations” as (1) what do we gain with each method?; (2) what do we lose with each method; and (3) what is the cost of each method in terms of personnel, expertise, time, and resources? These are detailed for the reader in Part 2 of this chapter.

Part 3 of this chapter presents combinations of methods that we typically employ. Within each section, we detail the considerations of these during triangulation. New to the reader might be ATA, which is a data instrument that we adapted from HTA to capture a granular understanding of workflow as well as any issues in the design, redundancies or problems in the process, and any qualitative feedback from users. The data gathered is organized such that it can either serve as a supplement to an executive summary to stakeholders or as a standalone agile status update to developers and the design team.

We end this chapter with two hybrid usability case studies in Part 4. The first demonstrates a cost-effective way to test multiple aspects of a complex assemblage of clinical tasks. By capturing discrete actions (ATA), cognitive context (“Think-Aloud” protocol), and qualitative feedback, we were able to identify key design flaws that may have affected both patient safety and cognitive burden. However, many more usability challenges exist at the intersection of healthcare and technology – especially outside of a controlled environment like that of our first case study. One such problem that affects the industry as it heads toward a paperless environment is ensuring that decision support tools in the electronic medical record are both safe and effective. The second case study illustrates it is possible to expand upon the largely qualitative results from comprehensive, yet small-scale usability testing and clinical simulations by way of quantitative computer-based simulations. As more hospitals implement HIT solutions to clinical processes, it is important to understand the impact of their usability across larger populations of patients and staff. Computer-based simulations help to bridge that gap.

Most of the techniques outlined in this chapter can be implemented by healthcare staff and evaluation teams who are new to usability. Combining techniques can help rapidly identify usability issues, safety risks, training needs, and system enhancements. Because a hybrid usability approach allows for measuring several dimensions at once, it is a viable option for evaluation teams that have limited time and resources. More important, it can provide comprehensive results which increase the validity of findings, help to better illustrate design decisions, and better meet the needs of stakeholders, patients, and staff.

References

[1] Holden RJ, and Karsh B-T. The Technology Acceptance Model: its past and its future in health care. Journal of Biometical Informatics. 2010;43(1): 159–72.

[2] Holahan PJ, Lesselroth BJ, Adams K, Wang K, and Church VL. Beyond technology acceptance to effective technology use: a parsimonious and actionable model. Journal of the American Medical Informatics Association. 2015;22(3):718–29.

[3] Nielsen J. Usability Engineering. San Diego: Academic Press; 1993. 362 p.

[4] Norman D. Emotional Design. New York: Basic Books; 2004.

[5] Shepherd A. Hierarchical Task Analysis. Great Britain: Taylor & Francis; 2001.

[6] Stanton N, and Young M. A Guide to Methodology in Ergonomics: Designing for Human Use. New York: Taylor & Francis; 1999.

[7] Lyons M, Adams S, Woloshynowych, and Charles V. Human reliability analysis in healthcare: a review of techniques. International Journal of Risk & Safety in Medicine. 2004; 16:223–37.

[8] Kirwan B. A Guide to Practical Human Reliability Assessment. Boca Raton, FL, USA: CRC Press 1994.

[9] Lane R, Stanton N, and Harrison D. Applying hierarchical task analysis to medication administration errors. Applied Ergonomics. 2006;37(5): 669–79.

[10] RTI International. ONC Change Package for Improving EHR Usability Washington D.C., 2018. Available from: https://www.healthit.gov/sites/default/files/playbook/pdf/usability-change-plan.pdf.

[11] Harrington L, and Harrington C. Usability Evaluation Handbook for Electronic Health Records. Chicago, IL: HIMSS; 2014 February 22, 2014. 507 p.
[12] Kushniruk A, and Borycki E, editors. Low-cost rapid usability testing: its application in both product development and system implementation. Information Technology and Communications in Healthcare (ITCH); 2017; Victoria, BC: IOS Press.
[13] Borsci S, Macredie R, Martin J, and Young T. How many testers are needed to assure the usability of medical devices? Expert Review of Medical Devices. 2014;11(5):513–25.
[14] Campbell G. FDA Guidance: "Design Considerations for Pivotal Clinical Investigations for Medical Devices". 2013.
[15] Institute of Medicine (IOM). Health IT and Patient Safety: Building Safer Systems for Better Care. Washington DC, USA: National Academies Press; 2011.
[16] Koppel R, Metlay JP, Cohen A, *et al.* Role of computerized physician order entry systems in facilitating medication errors. Journal of the American Medical Association. 2005;293(10):1197–203.
[17] Leveson N, and Turner C. An investigation of the Therac-25 accidents. Computer. 1993;26(7):18–41.
[18] Middleton B, Bloomrosen M, Dente M, *et al.* Enhancing patient safety and quality of care by improving the usability of electronic health record systems: recommendations from AMIA. Journal of the American Medical Informatics Association. 2013;20(e1):e2-e8.
[19] Ratwani R, Fairbanks T, Savage E, *et al.* Mind the gap: a systematic review to identify usability and safety challenges and practices during electronic health record implementation. Applied Clinical Informatics. 2016;07(04):1069–87.
[20] Reason J. Combating omission errors through task analysis and good reminders. Quality and Safety in Health Care. 2002;11:40–4.
[21] Reason J. Managing the Risks of Organizational Accidents. United Kingdom: Routledge; 2016.
[22] Steinbrook R. Health care and the American recovery and reinvestment act. New England Journal of Medicine. 2009;360(11):1057–60.
[23] Marcilly R, and Peute L. How to reach evidence-based usability evaluation methods. Building Capacity for Health Informatics. 2017:211–6.
[24] Lau F, Bartle-Clar J, Bliss G, Borycki E, Courtney K, and Kuo A, editors. Building capacity for health informatics in the future. Amsterdam, Netherlands: IOS Press; 2017.
[25] Beuscart-Zephir M-C, Watbled L, Carpentier A, Degroisse M, and Alao O, editors. A rapid usability assessment methodology to support the choice of clinical information systems: a case study. American Medical Informatics Association Annual Symposium; 2002; San Antonio, Texas: American Medical Informatics Association; 2002.
[26] Riskin L, Koppel R, and Riskin D. Re-examining health IT policy: what will it take to derive value from our investment? Journal of the American Medical Informatics Association. 2014;22(2):459–64.

[27] Loranger H. Effective Agile UX Product Development. 3 ed: Nielsen Norman Group. Fremont, CA, USA: NN/g Nielsen Norman Group; 2017. 113 p.

[28] Krug S. Rocket Surgery Made Easy: The Do-It Yourself Guide to Fixing Usability Problems. Davis N, editor. California: New Riders; 2010.

[29] DeRosier J, Stalhandske E, and Bagian JP. Using Health Care Failure Mode and Effect Analysis™: The VA National Center for Patient Safety's Prospective Risk Analysis System. The Joint Commission Journal on Quality and Patient Safety. 2002;28(5):248–67.

[30] Reason J. Human Error: Cambridge University Press. Cambridge, UK: Cambridge University Press; 1990.

[31] Kushniruk A, Triola M, Stein B, Borycki E, and Kannry J. The relationship of usability to medical error: an evaluation of errors associated with usability problems in the use of a handheld application for prescribing medications. Studies in Health Technology and Informatics. 2004;107 (Pt 2):1073–6.

[32] Zhang J, and Butler KA, editors. UFuRT: A Work-Centered Framework and Process for Design and Evaluation of Information Systems. Proceedings of HCI International. Berlin, Germany: Springer; 2007.

[33] Krug S. Don't Make Me Think: A Common Sense Approach To Web Usability. 2nd ed: New Riders. KG, Nordrhein-Westfalen, Germany: MITP Verlags-GmbH & Co.; 2009.

[34] Nielsen J, and Gilutz S. Usability Return on Investment. Fremont, CA, USA: NN/g Nielsen Norman Group 2003.

[35] Barnum CM. Usability Testing Essentials: Ready, Set...Test! Burlington, Massachusetts: Elsevier; 2011.

[36] Russ AL, Baker DA, Fahner WJ, *et al.*, editors. A rapid usability evaluation (RUE) method for health information technology. American Medical Informatics Association Annual Symposium; 2010 November 13, 2010; Washington D.C.: American Medical Informatics Association; 2010.

[37] Shneiderman B. Universal usability. Communications of the ACM. 2000:84–91.

[38] Mastarone GL, Adams K, Tallett S, and Lesselroth B. Hybrid Usability Methods: Practical techniques for evaluating health information technology in an operational setting. Human Factors and Ergonomics in Health Care; March 6–28; Boston, Massachusetts; 2018.

[39] Borycki EM, and Kushniruk AW. Toward an integrative cognitive-socio-technical approach in health informatics: analyzing technology-induced error involving health information systems to improve patient safety. The Open Medical Informatics Journal. 2010;4:181–87.

[40] Kushniruk AW, Borycki EM, Kuwata S, and Kannry J. Predicting changes in workflow resulting from healthcare information systems: ensuring the safety of healthcare. Healthcare Quarterly. 2006;9:114–8.

[41] Kushniruk AW, and Patel VL. Cognitive and usability engineering methods for the evaluation of clinical information systems. Journal of Biomedical Informatics. 2004;37(1):56–76.

[42] Kushniruk A, Nohr C, Jensen S, and Borycki E. From usability testing to clinical simulations: bringing context into the design and evaluation of usable and safe health information technologies. Yearbook of Medical Informatics. 2013;22(01):78–85.

[43] Holtzblatt K, and Jones S. Contextual inquiry: a participatory technique for system design. Participatory Design: Principles and Practices 1993. 177–210.

[44] Ash JS, Sittig DF, McMullen CK, Guappone KP, Dykstra RH, and Carpenter J, editors. A Rapid Assessment Process for Clinical Informatics Interventions. AMIA 2008 Symposium; 2008 November 6, 2008.

[45] Nielsen J. Usability 101: Introduction to Usability2012 April 27, 2018. Available from: https://www.nngroup.com/articles/usability-101-introduction-to-usability/.

[46] Schneiderman B. Designing the User Interface. 3rd ed. Reading, MA: Addison-Wesley; 1998.

[47] Quesenbery W. Balancing the 5Es: Usability. Cutter Business Technology Journal. 2004 February 1.

[48] Zhang J, and Walji MF. TURF: toward a unified framework of EHR usability. Journal of Biomedical Informatics. 2011;44(6):1056–67.

[49] Quesenbery W. The five dimensions of usability. In: Albers M, and Mazur MB, editors. Content and Complexity: Information Design in Technical Communication. Mahwah, NJ: Lawrence Erlbaum Associates; 2003. pp. 81–102.

[50] Nielsen J, and Molich R, editors. Heuristic evaluation of user interfaces. SIGCHI conference on Human factors in computing systems. Association for Computing Machinery, New York City, NY, USA; 1990, March 1.

[51] Nielsen J, editor. Enhancing the explanatory power of usability heuristics. SIGCHI Conference on Human Factors in Computing Systems; 1994, April 24–28; Boston, MA.

[52] Nielsen J, and Loranger H. Prioritizing Web Usability. Fremont, CA, USA: NN/g Nielsen Norman Group; 2006 April 20.

[53] Shneiderman B, Plaisant C, Cohen M, Jacobs S, Elmqvist N, and Diakopolos N. Designing the user interface: strategies for effective human-computer interaction. 2016, April 30.

[54] Wilson C. User Experience Re-mastered: Your Guide to Getting the Right Design. Burlington, MA: Morgan Kaufmann; 2010.

[55] Wharton CR, Rieman JR, Lewis C, and Polson P. The Cognitive Walkthrough Method: A Practitioners Guide. New York City, NY, USA: John Wiley & Sons, Inc; 1994.

[56] Card SK, Morgan TP, and Newell A. Computer text-editing: an information-processing analysis of a routine cognitive skill. Cognitive Psychology. 1980;12(1):32–74.

[57] Gray WD, John BE, and Atwood ME. Project Ernestine: Validating a GOMS analysis for predicting and explaining real-world task performance. Human Computer Interaction. 1993;8(3):237–309.

[58] John B. E, and Kieras D. E. The GOMS family of user interface analysis techniques: comparison and contrast. ACM Transactions on Computer-Human Interaction (TOCHI). 1996;3(4):320–51.

[59] Rice AD, and Lartigue JW, editors. Touch-level model (TLM): evolving KLM-GOMS for touchscreen and mobile devices. 2014 ACM Southeast Regional Conference; 2014, March 28–29; Kennesaw, Georgia.
[60] Dix A, Finley J, Abowd G, and Beale R. Human-computer Interaction (2nd ed.). Upper Saddle River, NJ, USA: Prentice-Hall, Inc; 1998. 639 p.
[61] Kirwan B, and Ainsworth LK. A Guide to Task Analysis. Washington D.C.: Taylor & Francis; 1992.
[62] Annett J, and Duncan KD. Task analysis and training design. Occupational Psychology. 1967;30:67–79.
[63] Stanton N. Hierarchical Task Analysis: Developments, applications, and extensions. Applied Ergonomics. 2006;37(1):55–79.
[64] Shepherd A. Hierarchical Task Analysis. London: Taylor & Francis; 2001.
[65] Stanton NA. Systematic human error reduction and prediction approach. In: Stanton N. A, Hedge A, Salas E, Hendrick H, and Brookhaus K, editors. Handbook of Human Factors and Ergonomic Methods. London: Taylor & Francis; 2005. pp. 371–8.
[66] Kirwan B, and Ainsworth L. K. A Guide to Task Analysis: The Task Analysis Working Group: CRC Press; 1992.
[67] Annett J. Hierarchical task analysis. In: Hollnagel E, editor. Handbook of Cognitive Task Design. Mahwah: Lawrence Erlbaum Associates, Inc; 2003. pp. 17–35.
[68] Annett J. Acquisition of skill. British Medical Bulletin. 1971;27:266–71.
[69] Colligan L, Anderson JE, Potts HW, and Berman J. Does the process map influence the outcome of quality improvement work? A comparison of a sequential flow diagram and a hierarchical task analysis diagram. BMC Health Services Research. 2010;10(1):7.
[70] Piso E. Task analysis for process-control tasks: The method of Annett *et al.* applied Journal of Occupational and Organizational Psychology. 1981;54 (4):247–54.
[71] Kirakowski J, and Corbett M. SUMI: the Software Usability Measurement Inventory. British Journal of Educational Technology. 1993;24(3):210–2.
[72] Lewis JR. IBM computer usability satisfaction questionnaires: psychometric evaluation and instructions for use. International Journal of Human–Computer Interaction. 1995;7(1):57–78.
[73] Lewis JR, Utesch BS, and Maher DE. UMUX-LITE: when there's no time for the SUS. Proceedings of the SIGCHI Conference on Human Factors in Computing Systems; Paris, France. 2481287: ACM; 2013. pp. 2099–102.
[74] Lewis JR, and Sauro J, editors. The Factor Structure of the System Usability Scale. Berlin, Heidelberg: Springer Berlin Heidelberg; 2009.
[75] Chin JP, Diehl VA, and Norman KL. Development of an instrument measuring user satisfaction of the human-computer interface. Proceedings of the SIGCHI Conference on Human Factors in Computing Systems; Washington D.C., USA. 57203: ACM; 1988. pp. 213–8.
[76] Technology OotNCfHI. ONC change package for improving EHR Usability. 2018.

[77] Lewis JR. Psychometric evaluation of an after-scenario questionnaire for computer usability studies: The ASQ. ACM SIGCHI Bulletin. 1991;23 (1):78–81.
[78] Yen P-Y, Wantland D, and Bakken S. Development of a Customizable Health IT Usability Evaluation Scale. AMIA Annual Symposium Proceedings. 2010. pp. 917–21.
[79] Root RW, and Draper S. Questionnaires as a software evaluation tool. Proceedings of the SIGCHI Conference on Human Factors in Computing Systems; Boston, Massachusetts, USA. 801586: ACM; 1983. pp. 83–7.
[80] Karis D, and Zeigler BL. Evaluation of Mobile Telecommunication Systems. Proceedings of the Human Factors Society Annual Meeting. 1989;33(4):205–9.
[81] Richman WL, Kiesler S, Weisband S, and Drasgow F. A meta-analytic study of social desirability distortion in computer-administered questionnaires, traditional questionnaires, and interviews. Journal of Applied Psychology. 1999;84(5):754–75.
[82] Wood LE. Semi-structured interviewing for user-centered design. Interactions. 1997;4(2):48–61.
[83] Walji MF, Kalenderian E, Piotrowski M, *et al.* Are three methods better than one? A comparative assessment of usability evaluation methods in an EHR. International Journal of Medical Informatics. 2014;83(5):361–7.
[84] Fritz F, Balhorn S, Riek M, Breil B, and Dugas M. Qualitative and quantitative evaluation of EHR-integrated mobile patient questionnaires regarding usability and cost-efficiency. International Journal of Medical Informatics. 2012;81(5):303–13.
[85] Martin B, and Hanington B. Universal Methods of Design: 100 Ways to Research Complex Problems, Develop Innovative Ideas, and Design Effective Solutions. Beverly, MA: Rockport Publishers; 2012.
[86] Dumas JS, and Redish JC. A Practical Guide to Usability Testing. 2nd ed. Portland, OR: Intellect; 1999 January 1, 1999.
[87] Cook DA, Hamstra SJ, Brydges R, *et al.* Comparative effectiveness of instructional design features in simulation-based education: systematic review and meta-analysis. Medical Teacher. 2013;35(1):e867-e98.
[88] Arriaga AF, Bader AM, Wong JM, *et al.* Simulation-based trial of surgical-crisis checklists. New England Journal of Medicine. 2013;368(3):246–53.
[89] Wright MC, Taekman JM, Barber L, Hobbs G, Newman MF, and Stafford-Smith M. The use of high-fidelity human patient simulation as an evaluative tool in the development of clinical research protocols and procedures. Contemporary Clinical Trials. 2005;26(6):646–59.
[90] Nielsen J, and Landauer T, editors. A mathematical model of the finding of usability problems. ACM INTERCHI'93 Conference; 1993 April 24–29, 1993; The Netherlands.
[91] Barnum CM, Bevan N, Cockton G, Nielsen J, Spool J, and Wixon D, editors. The "magic number 5:" is it enough for web testing. CHI 2003 Conference on Human Factors in Computing Systems; 2003, April 5–10, 2003; Ft.

Lauderdale, Florida. New York: Association for Computing Machinery; 2003.

[92] US Food and Drug Administration. National Drug Code Directory Silver Spring, MD: US Department of Health and Human Services; 2011 [updated February 4, 2016; cited 2018 January 24]. Available from: https://www.accessdata.fda.gov/scripts/cder/ndc/.

[93] Tullis T, and Albert W. Measuring the User Experience: Collecting, Analyzing, and Presenting Usability Metrics. Waltham, MA: Morgan Kaufmann; 2013.

[94] Hertzum M, and Jacobsen NE. The evaluator effect: A chilling fact about usability evaluation methods. International Journal of Human–Computer Interaction. 2001;13(4):421–43.

[95] Safety VNCfP. Safety Assessment Code (SAC) Matrix. 2015.

[96] Jeffries R, and Desurvire H. Usability testing vs. heuristic evaluation: was there a contest? SIGCHI Bull. 1992;24(4):39–41.

[97] Virzi RA, Sorce JF, and Herbert LB. A Comparison of Three Usability Evaluation Methods: Heuristic, Think-Aloud, and Performance Testing. Proceedings of the Human Factors and Ergonomics Society Annual Meeting. 1993;37(4):309–13.

[98] Li AC, Kannry JL, Kushniruk A, *et al.* Integrating usability testing and think-aloud protocol analysis with "near-live" clinical simulations in evaluating clinical decision support. International Journal of Medical Informatics. 2012;81(11):761–72.

[99] Lesselroth BJ, Holahan PJ, Adams K, *et al.* Primary care provider perceptions and use of a novel medication reconciliation technology. Informatics in Primary Care. 2011;19(2):105–18.

[100] Davis FD. Perceived usefulness, perceived ease of use, and user acceptance of information technology. Management Information Science Quarterly. 1989;13(3):319–40.

[101] Venkatesh V, Sykes TA, and Zhang X, editors. 'Just what the doctor ordered': a revised UTAUT for EMR system adoption and use by doctors. 44th Hawaii International Conference on System Sciences - 2011; IEEE; 2011.

[102] Sauro J, and Kindlund E, editors. How long should a task take? Identifying specification limits for task times in usability tests. Human Computer Interaction International Conference (HCI 2005); 2005; Las Vegas, Nevada.

[103] Sauro J, and Dumas J. S. Comparison of three one-question, post-task usability questionnaires. Proceedings of the SIGCHI Conference on Human Factors in Computing Systems; Boston, MA, USA. 1518946: ACM; 2009. pp. 1599–608.

[104] Lesselroth BJ, Adams K, Tallett S, *et al.* Design of admission medication reconciliation technology: a human factors approach to requirements and prototyping. Herd. 2013;6(3):30–48.

[105] Polson PG, Lewis C, Rieman J, and Wharton C. Cognitive walkthroughs: a method for theory-based evaluation of user interfaces. International Journal of Man-Machine Studies. 1992;36(5):741–73.

[106] Kushniruk AW, Triola MM, Borycki EM, Stein B, and Kannry JL. Technology induced error and usability: the relationship between usability problems and prescription errors when using a handheld application. International Journal of Medical Informatics. 2005;74(7):519–26.

[107] Borycki EM, Kushniruk A, Keay E, Nicoll J, Anderson J, and Anderson M. Toward an integrated simulation approach for predicting and preventing technology-induced errors in healthcare: implications for healthcare decision-makers. Healthcare Quarterly (Toronto, Ont). 2009;12 Spec No Patient:90–6.

Chapter 3

Advancing public health in the age of big data: methods, ethics, and recommendations

David D. Luxton, Ph.D., M.S.[1] and Chris Poulin[2]

The embracing of "big data" approaches is providing useful methods for public health research, surveillance, and intervention. Information is increasingly collected from traditional data sources, such as electronic health records, laboratory databases, and surveys, as well as in real time from personal mobile devices, internet use, social media, and environmental sensors – resulting in large and complex databases for analyses. Advances in technologies and data analytic techniques provide powerful ways to predict human behavior (such as health risk behaviors) or the outbreak of disease in a population. These techniques can also be used to provide helpful recommendations for risk reduction and guide clinical intervention and treatments. Importantly, the use of these modern techniques and data collection methods also raise important ethical concerns such as those associated with misuse of data, privacy, lack of transparency, and inaccurate prediction. This chapter provides an overview of "big data analytics" used in public health as well as current and emerging ethical issues and risks. Recommendations for the fields of public health and healthcare in general are provided.

3.1 Introduction

Big data is the popular term used to describe data that are too large to be processed by traditional methods [1,2]. Technological advancements such as improved computing power and data storage, artificial intelligence (AI) techniques, and the capability to gather and analyze data in real time from numerous electronic sources (e.g., the Internet and mobile devices) are facilitating novel methods to collect and analyze immense amounts of complex data in ways that were not possible in the past. As noted by [2], technology is not the sole driving force behind big data, but also the change in the mindset of how data can be used. This is the realization that data itself has economic value, and can be reused rather than destroyed after its

[1]Department of Psychiatry and Behavioral Sciences, University of Washington School of Medicine, Seattle, WA, USA
[2]Patterns and Predictions LLC, Boston, MA, USA

initial collection and use. Indeed, the rapid rise in capabilities and practical uses of big data has provided opportunities across diverse industries and sciences.

Big data also brings important capabilities to the field of public health, particularly in health surveillance, research, and intervention. We believe that it is essential for public health professionals to be aware of these capabilities as big data represents one of the most significant technological advancements for the field. By drawing from our experience with public health surveillance systems for suicide prevention and an analytic review of the literature, we present need-to-know information about big data methods in public health. While the general ethical issues associated with big data have been discussed in other recent articles and reports [3–6], we aim to further guide and advance the practical application of Big Data in public health by discussing these core issues and providing specific recommendations for professionals and organizations who desire to make use of big data.

3.2 Overview of big data analytics

With big data, hundreds of thousands of measurements may have been collected for each person thereby resulting in massive and complex data sets. "Big data analytics" entails the analysis of that data in order to determine patterns and predict future outcomes and trends [2,7]. Big data analytics consists of more than just the application of traditional statistical techniques, such as linear regression or Bayesian analysis to large data sets: it involves the use of novel enabling technologies to collect, aggregate, compile, and analyze data in much more sophisticated and powerful ways. Furthermore, big data analytics involves the capability to process *unstructured data*. In traditional relational databases with structured data, data resides in fields that are arranged in the familiar row-column format. *Unstructured data* typically refers to data that has not been quantified so that it can reside in a traditional row-column database, but may very well be "human readable" (e.g., text). Examples of unstructured data include e-mail messages, word-processing documents, audio files, video files, and digital images. There is also *semi-structured data* – information that doesn't reside in a traditional relational database, but has some organizational properties that make it easier to analyze (e.g., formats for www) [2].

3.3 Enabling technologies

The computational and data processing power that was once only possible with expensive super computers, can now be accomplished with desktop personal computers, and especially groups of personal computers. Improvements in specialized statistical software with the ability to process multiple large data sets assist analysts with applying advanced statistical models. Moreover, the use of cloud computing has enabled data to be stored and analyzed on network computers, rather than on local machines. Thus, data from multiple sources can be aggregated to the cloud, processed, and then made available for users to access.

AI techniques are used to assist with data-intensive tasks, such as the analysis of unstructured data that would otherwise be too difficult and time consuming for humans to accomplish [8]. Machine learning is a core branch of AI that involves giving machines the ability to learn without being explicitly programmed [9]. A typical machine learning model first learns the knowledge from the data it is exposed to (i.e., training) and then applies this knowledge to provide predictions about future data (i.e., inference) [8,10]. Data mining is a familiar example of the use of machine learning algorithms to identify patterns in data.

The Durkheim Project [11] is one example of the application of the aforementioned techniques in public health. The Durkheim Project began as a Defense Advanced Research Projects Agency (DARPA)-sponsored study for estimating suicide-risk among U.S. military veterans. The project entails the collection of data from several inputs, including smartphone and social media use, which is processed and then sent into a secure analytics network. The text and mobile device data collected from these sources is continuously updated and analyzed by machine learning processes that monitor the content and behavioral patterns that are statistically associated with suicidal behavior. Ultimately, the system allowed for identification of persons at heightened-risk and thus identify opportunity for immediate intervention.

Natural language processing (NLP) – the ability for computers to process human written or spoken language – is dependent on underlying machine learning techniques. Natural language processing can be used to analyze free text and audio recordings, which can be useful for quantifying and analyzing data in these formats (e.g., The Durkheim Project). Natural language processing can also be used in genomics research to phenotype patients [12] or to analyze free-text in electronic health records (EHRs), such as "chief complaints" data collected by Emergency Departments to detect, localize, and predict emerging outbreaks of disease [13,14]. Furthermore, specific machine perception techniques that make use of machine learning and artificial neural networks can be used to analyze visual images. For example, machine perception can be used to analyze large-scale medical image databases, such as population-based image analyses of MRI scans [15].

Data visualization (or business intelligence software) is another advancing technology that makes use of high tech data manipulation techniques to analyze, present, and disseminate knowledge data in ways that are more sophisticated. For example, visualization tools and news aggregators can be used to create disease-surveillance "mashups". Mashups are web application hybrids that take the functionality of two information sources, merge certain aspects of each, in order to create a novel third source [16]. These can be used to mine, categorize, filter, and visualize online intelligence about epidemics in real time [17]. HealthMap (www.healthmap.org), for example, is an openly available public health intelligence system that uses data from different sources to produce a global view of ongoing infectious disease threats. Other similar systems include Argus (http://biodefense.georgetown.edu), EpiSPIDER (www.epispider.org), BioCaster (http://biocaster.nii.ac.jp), MediSys (http://medusa.jrc.it), and the Wildlife Disease Information Node (http://wildlifedisease.nbii.gov).

3.4 Data sources and collection methods

3.4.1 Traditional databases

Big data is facilitated by the numerous data sources and methods for collection. Data used in public health can be sourced from existing enterprise databases such as health registries, mortality databases (e.g., the National Death Index), laboratory or epidemiological databases, public records, and other databases of collected data such as from surveys. Other sources of data include environmental sensor data (i.e., weather patterns, pollution levels, allergens, land use change, forest fires, airborne particulate matter, traffic patterns, pesticide applications, or water quality).

3.4.2 Electronic health records

EHRs are a core source of clinical data for big data analytics [12]. EHRs typically include current diagnostic information and history, number of medical visits, medications lists, history of procedures, standardized measures (such as behavioral health) and health outcomes. EHR data can be structured (e.g., BMI index), as well as unstructured (including free text fields and image data). Finally, there is also the potential for EHRs to be linked to other big data sources such as database systems that contain information about military service, income, education, diet, exercise, and social habits [12].

3.4.3 Internet and social media

The Internet and social media also provide a source of data for big data analytics in public health. Infodemiology (also called "infoveillance") is the science of distribution and determinants of information in an electronic medium, specifically the Internet, or in a population, with the ultimate aim to inform public health and public policy [18]. For example, data on Internet searches (such as the signs and symptoms of a disease or any health condition) and social media posts can provide information on the outbreak of disease [17].

One of the first high profile examples of big data in public health is when Google (Google Flu Trends) claimed to predict an influenza outbreak [19]. The analysis entailed examining how 50 million of the most common Internet search terms (between 2002 and 2008) were associated with a list of seasonal flu symptoms based on Centers for Disease Control and Prevention (CDC) data. Analysts claimed to determine where the flu had started and to do so while it was happening, rather than after the fact. However, a paper published in Science [20] disputes Google's success at predicting influenza outbreaks, including failure to successfully predict an outbreak in 2013. Nonetheless, big data analytics potentially provides for the analysis of previously unavailable data in real time, providing alerts to health agencies when a risk arises.

Data can also be collected from online purchases (such as for medications) and social media use, including emails and SMS texting, can provide information regarding the behavior of individuals and a population, such as the amount of social interaction. Semantic analysis can reveal information about emotional states and cognitive processes that can serve as social determinants of health risks [21]. For example, the real-time analysis of social media data can provide insights into the patterns of users, such as suicidal behavior (e.g., expressions of intent), as well as information about risk factors, such as cyberbullying [22].

3.4.4 Mobile and wearables devices

Mobile devices such as smart phones or wearable devices, such as biosensors, can collect survey instruments, physiological data, and other information, all in real time. These devices can also be used to determine social behavior, such as locations frequented (via GPS tracking), the amount of social interaction, and whom people are communicating with [23]. As noted by Luxton and colleagues [23], mobile technologies will serve as the underpinning of the big data movement given their ubiquitous use and integration with other technologies, such as cloud computing.

3.4.5 Genomics data

Advances in genomics are also providing useful information for big data analysis. For example, the Electronic Medical Records and Genomics Network uses big data methods by allowing for the integration of genetics data with other data, such as that in EHRs as well as social and behavioral data collected from surveys or mobile/wearable devices [12]. Fortunately, genetic information is becoming increasingly easy and inexpensive to collect. The capability to affordably link genetics data with other data has the potential to greatly expand the capabilities of medical and public health research.

3.5 Advantages of big data in public health

Barrett and colleagues [24] describe two primary ways in which big data can uniquely improve the discovery of new risk factors for disease. First, massive data sets allow not only population-level analyses, but also analysis of subpopulation (and individual-level analyses). An advantage of this is that such data enables the identification of personalized risk factors that take into account the various additional variables that might confer susceptibility or resistance to a given risk factor. Identifying personalized risk factors holds the promise of giving people more effective information about how to prevent disease, and doing so in a way that is more compelling for them to act upon because it is targeted to them specifically as opposed to the "average person". Second, new passive sensors (e.g., for physical activity or sleep) can allow collection of richer, more detailed data on potential risk factors over longer periods of follow-up than is currently possible using standard epidemiologic questionnaires. This will also strengthen the capacity to extract new insights from this big (and personal) data.

The self-collection of data is an important opportunity for big data public health applications. The "Quantified Self" movement entails individuals using wearable sensors and self-monitoring devices to measure and improve their own health and behavior [25]. Data is collected from various inputs (e.g., food consumed, quality of surrounding air), internal states (e.g., mood, arousal, blood oxygen levels), and performance (mental and physical). These technologies allow for the potential discovery of new, personalized disease risk factors related to lifestyle or the environment, and also help people to successfully modify their risk behaviors [24,26]. The Quantified Self-concept can be expanded and aggregated to a population level, leading to what Barrett and colleagues [24] call "quantified communities" that measure the health and activities of their population and institutions, thereby improving collective health with a data-driven approach. And, we are seeing functioning examples of this in the modality of mental health (e.g., Durkheim Project). In this case, a time series tracking of linguistic intent provides a "ticker" of psychometric state. This state can be used to ascertain appropriate action (i.e., intervention) by mental health professionals.

In summary, big data analytics can help identify meaningful patterns in data that were not observable previously and help us understand complex relationships, including risk factors for disease and other health conditions as well as exposure to risks. It is the capability to collect and analyze data in real time that provides the unique advantage over traditional methods of detection, surveillance, and intervention.

3.6 Ethics and Risks

3.6.1 Privacy and misuse of data

Privacy concerns are now one of the most discussed risks associated with big data [5]. We are living in a world in which data is constantly collected on individuals by commercial businesses and governments. The public has been made aware of widespread domestic surveillance, including monitoring of all cell phone and email traffic of everyday people that occurred behind the scenes and with presumed legal precedence [27]. Commercial businesses also collect information about individuals, including shopping preferences and habits, and other behavioral characteristics on a regular basis. There has even been recent advancements in technologies that directly sense human emotional states, and also headway in the design of human thought detection, directly through the skull using electromagnetic sensors [8]. Keep in mind too that physiological data, collected from ubiquitous consumer mobile or wearable devices, such as heart rate monitors, can also be used to identify an individual [28]. The concerns and implications regarding the loss of privacy have been dramatized for decades in science fiction novels and films, but alarmingly, are a reality in this modern age.

It is clear that sensitive data about behavioral health and diagnoses can be extremely damaging to individuals when it is misused by others. Data breaches and misuse of data can harm personal or corporate reputations as well as be detrimental to the field of public health by damaging public trust. In the United States, laws such as the Privacy Act, The Health Insurance Portability and Accountability Act of 1996 (HIPAA), and the The Health Information Technology for Economic and Clinical Health (HITECH) Act help assure a level of privacy to protect both consumers and public health and healthcare professionals [29]. Updated policies, such as the Consumer Privacy Bill of Rights Act [6], have been proposed. Unfortunately, risks to privacy and misuse of data exist regardless of laws and guidelines, as evidenced by high profile and high-volume breaches of health data [30].

Even when data is stripped of standard personal identifiers (e.g., name, social security number, address, etc.), the identities of anonymous persons can be determined, given that enough data is collected about them. This is sometimes called "re-identification". Moreover, with enough information over time, there is the opportunity to predict events in an individual's life, and if one observes how an individual reacts to such events, one can predict that individual's future behavior [4].

3.6.2 *Informed consent and transparency*

An enormous amount of data is collected from individuals every moment, every day. Data is collected fluidly, and not necessarily with awareness or consent of the consumer. Companies that collect data are both adept and not always transparent about what and how data is used. For example, corporate policies may be changed after a user has opted-in to a service and users may miss those changes or find that it is too difficult to opt-out of. Moreover, users can be manipulated into providing data that they may otherwise not have provided if they were more aware of how that data may be used (e.g., an offer to provide more features of a service, such as in a mobile app game, if personal information is provided).

Even if an individual has consented to some information to be collected on them, the data collected may be linked to data collected from another source, with or without the person's consent. When data is merged with other data, it can be used to generate new data, such as whether a person may or may not have a specific medical condition. Electronic data can also exist in perpetuity. Unless there is a policy for scheduled destruction, and if that destruction is carried through, electronic data will exist forever and can used (for good or for bad) at any time in the future.

3.6.3 *Risk associated with discrimination and inaccurate prediction*

Another risk of big data analytics is the labeling of a class of people based on characteristics that may portend risk for a certain condition, such as a particular disease or mental health condition. This could result in unintended stigmatization of individuals or members of groups with particular characteristics [6]. One example of this scenario in public health and healthcare is the classic ethical issues associated with genetic testing. A gene may be discovered that indicates an underlying medical condition or propensity to acquire a specific disease. With this information, an insurance company may adjust an individual's medical insurance costs or deny coverage all together. Furthermore, apparent or perceived genetic variation from the "normal" can result in real genetic discrimination that extends from an individual to the family or subset of the population [31].

The potential for discrimination based on the vast amounts of information from big data, whether it be behavioral data or latent indicators of disease, is a serious emerging ethical issue. If predictive models based on particular behaviors on social media (e.g., Facebook posts and interactions) may suggest particular chance for particular sexual identity or activity, it could cause unwanted stigmatization of person with those characteristics. As our own research suggests [4], we must also consider the psychological impact at the individual level. If data suggests back to a person a heightened risk for suicide, for example, will the person be *more likely* to engage in the behavior? This line of questioning raises additional ethical considerations when deciding whether to and at what time it is appropriate to inform individuals of potential risk that data may suggest at any given time. Meanwhile, targeting an intervention on "false positives" is a waste of resources and possible stigmatization. The hope is adequate testing and research will help prevent misplacement or redirection of resources and waste.

3.6.4 Other considerations

Who owns the data, and how providers of data are compensated or receive some benefit for the exploitation of their data is another issue. Consider that personal data may never be, or have been, within one's possession if data is acquired passively from external sources such as public cameras and sensors, or public disclosures by others via social media [6]. Meanwhile, if an individual provides information, what benefit does it have (or should be provided) to that individual? Will the collective benefit extend to additional or entire groups in the population? Some countries, regions, and populations do not have the technical infrastructure, smartphones, even electricity, therefore limiting data collection. Thus, people in areas without the appropriate infrastructure will not be able to contribute to data collection and thus benefit from it [32]. Furthermore, inferences and decisions based upon such data can also be biased by this problem.

Whether and how rights to data is transferred from one entity (i.e., a corporation or government agency) to another is also to be considered [33]. Concerns that have legal and ethical implications include whether the same privacy standards will be used with that data. For example, one organization may have different standards as to what constitutes personally identifiable information (PII) compared to another. Finally, is there also an increased risk for data security to be compromised the more times data is shared and merged with other data?

At the time of this chapter going to print, the authors do note the recent emergence of the General Data Protection Regulation (GDPR) in Europe (see https://www.eugdpr.org/). But while rectifying a few issues mentioned above, it remains to be seen if the regulations will have a lasting impact, especially with larger companies and if so, that there is also substantive improvement outside of the European Union (EU).

3.7 Recommendations

All public health professionals should become familiar with the ethical risks that are associated with the collection and use of private data, regardless of pending regulation. This includes awareness of the capabilities of big data analytics, as well as the ethics involved. As such, public health and healthcare training programs should include such topics in their curriculums. Moreover, organizations and individuals who are planning to make use of the capabilities of big data should consider the risks from the planning stage forward. Many government projects involving large data collection, such as the Precision Medicine Initiative (https://www.whitehouse.gov/precision-medicine), have included a committee to determine the ethical implications, such as privacy considerations, when collecting data. Guidance based on ethical principles and standards should be standard operating procedures; and we have mentioned the EU's GDPR.

Wyber and colleagues [32] (2015) note that an appropriate governance framework must be developed and enforced to protect individuals and assure healthcare delivery is tailored to the characteristics and values of the target communities. As noted by Larson [34], trusted partnerships must be established among institutions that collect healthcare data so they can share it in ways that best serve consumer (e.g., patients) needs. Public health surveillance and research are governed by national and international legislation and guidelines (e.g., HIPAA, HITECH Act); however, these laws and guidelines were developed in response to the conditions and technologies of the past. Health research that had made use of social media and other modern technologies have pushed the need to expand research guidelines and ethics [5]. What is needed is legislation and guidelines that begin to address the modern technologies and the ways data is collected and used in public health applications. We recommend that public health and professional groups and organizations review the current and emerging ethical issues as they modernize their ethical standards. The Council for Big Data, Ethics, and Society (http://bdes.datasociety.net/) is one example of an organization that brings together multidisciplinary researchers to study and disseminate knowledge associated with the ethical, legal, policy and social issues of the big data movement.

Appropriate and user-friendly "opt-in" procedures should also be the standard. Our Durkheim Project is an exemplar of the use of informed consent and an "opt-in" network [11]. Sophisticated "privacy profiles" have also been proposed to enable consumers to predefine and select what personal data they are willing to be collected and shared with any given service or purpose (i.e., context) [6]. Standard consent forms can be too long and many of large companies' terms of use have been criticized because they are in small print and may be changed without informing the users [4]. Pages upon pages of small print legal jargon are not feasible for thorough review, or probably not ethical. Lengthy clinical/research consent forms may also obfuscate risks. To be ethical, the consent process requires transparency, readability, and options for consumers to get more information should be provided. In regard to transparency, why, how, when, and for who data is collected should be disclosed. Finally, we also recommend legal review before any data collection.

3.8 Conclusion

Big data is a promising game-changer for improving public health. The efficacious use of big data has the potential to dramatically improve population health and reduce healthcare costs. However, public health professions must adapt a new mindset of how data can be collected and analyzed to help with disease detection and prevention. Public health professionals, and all healthcare professionals, need to be cognizant of the risks and must be advocates for the ethical use of these modern techniques. The personal privacy implications of the big data movement should be of paramount concern. Historically, the signatories of the U.S. Constitution considered the protection of privacy from state intrusion a fundamental principle of a free society, and this is reflected in the 4th Amendment of the Bill of Rights. The signatories understood that a free and enlightened society is one that respects the rights of individuals and promotes the health and welfare of the population. As such, the authors herein believe we can maximize the benefits of big data while also respecting rights to privacy. We, as a global society, can accomplish this by educating ourselves on how data is collected, influencing policy decision making, advocating for transparency, and by being responsible stewards of data that is collected and employed for significant outcomes.

References

[1] Manyika J, Chui M, Brown B, *et al.* (2011). Big Data: The Next Frontier for Innovation, Competition, and Productivity. McKinsey Global Institute.

[2] Mayer-Schönberger V. & Cukier K. (2013). Big Data: A Revolution that Will Transform how We Live, Work, and Think. Eamon Dolan/Houghton Mifflin Harcourt.

[3] Myers J, Frieden TR, Bherwani KM., & Henning K.J. (May 2008). Ethics in Public Health Research. Am J Public Health. 98(5), 793–801. doi: 10.2105/AJPH.2006.107706.

[4] Poulin C. (2014). Big Data Custodianship in a Global Society. SAIS Review of International Affairs, Volume 34, 1, Winter-Spring, pp. 109–116 Published by The Johns Hopkins University Press DOI: 10.1353/sais.2014.0002.

[5] Vayena E, Salathé M, Madoff LC, & Brownstein JS. (Feb. 9, 2015). Ethical Challenges of Big Data in Public Health. http://dx.doi.org/10.1371/journal.pcbi.1003904

[6] President's Council of Advisors on Science and Technology. (May 2014). Report to the President Big Data and Privacy: A Technological Perspective. Available at: https://www.whitehouse.gov/sites/default/files/microsites/ostp/PCAST/pcast_big_data_and_privacy_-_may_2014.pdf

[7] National Research Council. (2013). Frontiers in Massive Data Analysis, National Academies Press.

[8] Luxton, DD. (Ed.) (2015). Artificial Intelligence in Behavioral and Mental Health Care. San Diego: Elsevier/Academic Press.

[9] Samuel AL. (2000). Some studies in machine learning using the game of checkers. IBM J Res Dev. 44(1.2.), 206–226.

[10] Mitchell TM. (1997). Machine Learning. Burr Ridge, IL: McGraw Hill. p. 45.
[11] Poulin C, Thompson P, & Bryan C. (2016). Public health surveillance: predictive analytics and Big data. In: Luxton DD, ed. Artificial Intelligence in Behavioral and Mental Health Care. New York: Elsevier/Academic Press.
[12] Murdoch TB., & Detsky AS. (2013). The inevitable application of big data to health care. J Am Med Assoc. 309(13):1351–1352. doi:10.1001/jama.2013.393.
[13] Neill DB. (2012). New Directions in AI for Public Health Surveillance. Available at: http://lifesciences.ieee.org/articles/120-new-directions-in-ai-for-public-health-surveillance
[14] Liu Y. & Neill, D.B. (2011). Detecting previously unseen outbreaks with novel symptom patterns. Emerging Health Threats J. 4: 11074 - DOI: 10.3402/ehtj.v4i0.11074. Available at: http://www.cs.cmu.edu/~neill/papers/isds2011a.pdf
[15] Gonzalez FA., & Romero E. Biomedical Image Analysis and Machine Learning Technologies: Applications and Techniques. Medical Information Science Reference. Hershey, PA.
[16] Cho A. (2007). An introduction to mashups for health librarians. J Can Hel Lab Assoc / JABSC. 2007;28(1):19–21.
[17] Brownstein JS, Clark C. Freifeld CC., & Madoff LC. (2009) Digital disease detection — Harnessing the web for public health surveillance. N Engl J Med 360:2153–2157 May 21, 2009 DOI: 10.1056/NEJMp0900702.
[18] Eysenbach G. (2009). Infodemiology and infoveillance: framework for an emerging set of public health informatics methods to analyze search, communication and publication behavior on the Internet. J Med Internet Res. 11 (1):e11.
[19] Ginsberg J, Mohebbi MH, Patel RS, Brammer L, Smolinski MS, & Brilliant L. (2009). Detecting influenza epidemics using search engine query data. Nature. 457(7232):1012–4. doi:10.1038/nature07634.
[20] Lazer D, Kennedy R, King G, & Vespignani A. (2014). The parable of Google flu: Traps in big data analysis. Science. 343, 6176;1203–1205. DOI: 10.1126/science.1248506.
[21] Poulin C., Shiner B, Thompson P., *et al.* (2014). Predicting the risk of suicide by analyzing the text of clinical notes. PLoS ONE. 9(1), e85733.
[22] Luxton DD., June JD., & Fairall, JM. (2012). Social media and suicide: A public health perspective. Ame J Pub Health. 102(2), 195–200. doi:10.2105/AJPH.2011.300608.
[23] Luxton, DD., June, JD., Sano A., & Bickmore T. (2015). Mobile, wearable, and ambient intelligence in behavioral health care. In D. D. Luxton (Ed). Artificial Intelligence in Behavioral and Mental Health Care. San Diego: Elsevier Academic Press.
[24] Barrett MA, Humblet O., Hiatt, R.A., and Adler, NE. Big Data and Disease Prevention: From Quantified Self to Quantified Communities DOI: 10.1089/big.2013.0027.

[25] Lupton, D. The Quantified Self. Wiley.
[26] Swan. M. (June 2013). The quantified self: Fundamental disruption in big data science and biological discovery big data. Big Data.1(2): 85–99. doi:10.1089/big.2012.0002.
[27] Savage C. F.B.I. (Jan. 11, 2015). Is Broadening Surveillance Role, Report Shows. The New York Times.
[28] Luxton, D. D., Kayl, R. A., & Mishkind, M. C. (2012). mHealth data security: The need for HIPAA-compliant standardization. Telemed e-Health. 18, 284–288. doi: 10.1089/tmj.2011.0180.
[29] O'Connor J, & Matthews G. (2011). Informational privacy, public health, and state laws. Am J Public Health. 101(10), 1845–1850. http://ajph.aphapublications.org/doi/abs/10.2105/AJPH.2006.107706
[30] U.S. Department of Health and Human Services Office for Civil Rights Breach Portal: Notice to the Secretary of HHS Breach of Unsecured Protected Health Information US Department of Health and Human Services Office for Civil Rights. Available at https://ocrportal.hhs.gov/ocr/breach/breach_report.jsf
[31] Billings PR. Kohn MA. de Cuevas M. Beckwith J, Alper, JS, & Natowicz MR. (1992). Discrimination as a consequence of genetic testing. Am J Hum Genet. 50,476–482.
[32] Wyber R, Vaillancourt S, Perry W, Mannava P, Folaranmi T, CeliLA. (Mar. 1, 2015). Big data in global health: improving health in low- and middle-income countries. Bull World Health Organ. 93(3):203–8. doi: 10.2471/BLT.14.139022. Epub 2015 Jan 30.
[33] Davis K. Patterson D. (2012). Ethics of Big Data. O'Reilly Media, Inc., Sebastopol, CA.
[34] Larson EB. (2013). Building trust in the power of "big data" research to serve the public good. J Am Med Assoc. 309:2443–2444.

Chapter 4

Preferential hyperacuity perimetry: home monitoring to decrease vision loss due to age-related macular degeneration

David M. Kleinman, M.D., M.B.A.[1]*, Susan Orr, O.D.*[2]*, Jeff Heier, M.D.*[3]*, Gidi Benyamini, M.B.A.*[2]*, Jon Johnson*[2] *and Muki Rapp, Ph.D.*[2]

4.1 Introduction

Vision is one of the most valued of human sensory perceptions, and vision loss is associated with a significant decrease in quality of life as well as serious medical, psychological, social and financial consequences. Due to the high value people place on vision, ophthalmologists often find that patients are motivated to take an active role in reducing their risk for vision loss. Age-related macular degeneration (AMD) is the leading cause of irreversible vision loss in the western world. Despite major advances in treating this condition over the past two decades, additional efforts are needed to significantly alter current rates of visual decline due to AMD. This unmet need provides an opportunity to utilise home monitoring technology to enable self-aware AMD patients to preserve their vision.

Remote patient monitoring is growing in clinical applicability generally, and AMD is an excellent target for this valuable approach to patient care. The ForeseeHome® preferential hyperacuity perimeter is a telemedicine home-based monitoring system and has been proven to improve visual outcomes in patients suffering from AMD.

The development of ForeseeHome is the result of a global cooperative effort to change the lives of people with AMD by using a simple at-home test. As is true for other successes in biomedicine, this program was founded on excellent basic science, strong engineering, an experienced, dedicated team and well-designed clinical trials showing unquestionable efficacy.

[1]Flaum Eye Institute, University of Rochester School of Medicine, Rochester, NY, USA
[2]Notal Vision Ltd., Tel Aviv, Israel
[3]Ophthalmic Consultants of Boston, Boston, MA, USA

Notal Vision has its roots in the innovative culture of Tel Aviv, an internationally recognized center of hardware and software disruption. The pioneering research & development (R&D) team remains in Israel under the leadership of Gidi Benyamini and Muki Rapp, PhD. Mr. Benyamini, who has over 15 years of experience in ophthalmology, serves as the Chief Technology Officer and Director of Notal Vision Innovation Center and Dr. Rapp, who has over 16 years of experience in heading research in ophthalmology, serves as the Executive Vice President of R&D.

Today, Notal Vision headquarters is located in Manassas, Virginia, where the strength of the Tel Aviv R&D is combined with a veteran industry leadership team led by CEO Kester Nahen, who has a deep pedigree of ophthalmic diagnostic successes in companies. Dr. Susan Orr, OD, was the former Chief Medical Officer and Vice President of Medical Affairs. She has more than 19 years of ophthalmic strategy and operational experience. Jeffrey Heier, MD, is a key opinion leader in ophthalmology and was an early investigator who advanced the preferential hyperacuity perimetry technology in the clinics. Dr. Heier serves as Co-President and Medical Director, Director of the Vitreoretinal Service and Director of Retina Research at Ophthalmic Consultants of Boston.

Commentary is provided in this chapter by some of these key leaders in AMD to add real-world context to this discussion.

Mr. Benyamini: 'The commitment our team has shown over the years to this program is now saving people's sight, which is rewarding.'

Dr. Rapp: 'Our scientists, engineers, and clinicians all recognized the value inherent to the visual science of hyperacuity, and we kept our sights on the goal of bringing a technology based upon this to improve the early detection of eye disease. The clinical data has really validated these efforts.'

4.2 Background

4.2.1 The eye 58

The eye is a transparent biological optical system that focuses electromagnetic radiation in the visible spectrum (wavelength 390 to 700 nm) on the light-sensitive human retina. The retinal photoreceptors convert this light energy into electrochemical signals that are then processed and transmitted as neurological input via the optic nerve to the visual cortex of the brain where the perception of sight is generated. Problems with almost any part of the eye can lead to visual disturbances (see Figure 4.1).

Problems of the retina are of particular concern because this very thin, fragile tissue can be damaged in multiple ways – often with permanent consequences. On a per milligram basis, the retina is the highest oxygen-consuming tissue in the body [1]. In addition, unaltered microanatomical architecture and healthy function of photoreceptors are critical components of normal retinal function. The centre of the retina is called the macula, and the macula is responsible for providing the fine visual acuity integral to reading, recognising faces and performing detailed visual tasks. The macula is especially a high- oxygen-consuming watershed region relying

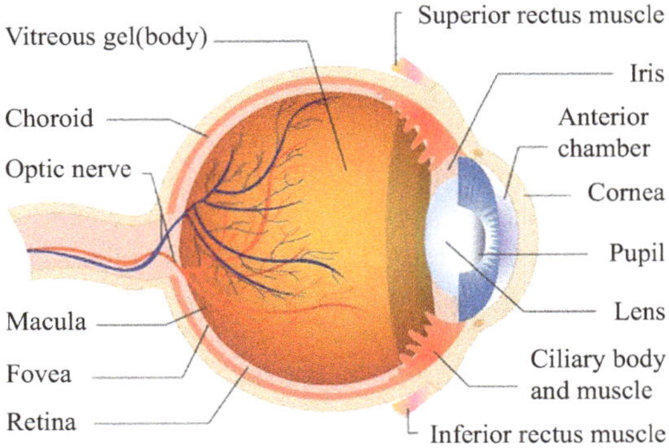

Figure 4.1 Basic human eye anatomy

in large part on diffusion from the choroidal circulation. There is minimal tolerance for pathological changes here without an effect on visual function, and macular disease accounts for very high rates of decreased vision globally.

4.3 Diagnostic testing

Multiple diagnostic technologies are widely available to assist ophthalmologists in the diagnosis and management of retinal disease. Both functional and imaging modalities play important roles. The majority are beyond the scope of this discussion, and only the most relevant approaches are described here. AMD decreases visual performance. Testing to elicit declines in function includes acuity measurements (minimum angle of resolution), assessments of central scotomas (areas where the vision is missing akin to the well-known natural blind spot due to the optic nerve head) and evaluations for metamorphopsia (areas of the visual field where the quality of vision shows waviness or distortion).

Visual acuity is commonly measured and referred to as Snellen acuity. The basic principle is that patients report the smallest letter they can read at distance with spectacle correction in a high-contrast setting. The chart has multiple lines of letters with a set of letters of all one size on a single line. The letters of each line subtend an angle of 5 min and parts of the letter subtend an angle of 1 min of arc at a given distance. The result is reported as a fraction where the numerator is the distance tested and the denominator is the number associated with the line with the smallest letters the patient can read correctly. A normal seeing eye can resolve letters between 30 seconds and 1 minute of arc. In the United States, for example, this result is tested at a distance of 20 feet and the eye would be recorded as seeing 20/20. Snellen acuity works well in a real-world clinical setting, but is less than ideal for clinical trials where visual acuity is the endpoint because of inconsistent numbers of letters on each line and a variable progression rate between letter sizes [2]. Visual acuity in clinical trials is measured using the early treatment of diabetic retinopathy study best-corrected visual acuity (ETDRS BCVA) methodology, which corrects for these weaknesses. Each line has five letters. Acuity scores using this system are reported as total number of letters read correctly, or in a log minimum angle of resolution (logMAR) format. In this system, every three lines (or 15 letters) represent a doubling of the minimum angle of resolution. A change of three or more lines, whether better or worse, is considered to be clinically meaningful. Many studies report their findings in ETDRS BCVA nomenclature, so it is important to have some facility with the concept of letters read and logMAR acuity.

Changes in central scotomas are most commonly assessed using the Amsler chart. The Amsler chart is a simple test that has been widely available since the 1960s. Basically, the patient views a square grid with each side 10 cm in length containing multiple horizontal and vertical crossing lines. There is a centre dot.

The grid is viewed at 30 cm with near correction and assesses the central 20 degrees of the patient's visual field. Patients are instructed to fixate on the central dot and perceive the gridlines. Areas of metamorphopsia and scotomas can be mapped out and even marked with ink on paper versions of the grid. The performance of Amsler charts is negatively affected by issues including cortical completion where the patient's visual system fills in missing areas of small sizes and crowding where multiple lines in the periphery decrease sensitivity. Also, fixation is not forced or verified and, thus, the Amsler test frequently doesn't faithfully map retinal distortions. Thus, the Amsler chart has limited ability to accurately detect new, small areas of visual change. In addition, the Amsler chart is noninteractive, so compliance may suffer [3,4]. Figure 4.2 shows Snellen, ETDRS, and Amsler charts.

Metamorphopsia, however, can be assessed at very minute levels through advanced testing algorithms.

Specifically, the ForeseeHome methodology is a functional test for analysing preferential hyperacuity perimetry (PHP), and it has demonstrated clinical effectiveness in a randomised, controlled trial. This topic will be addressed in greater detail later.

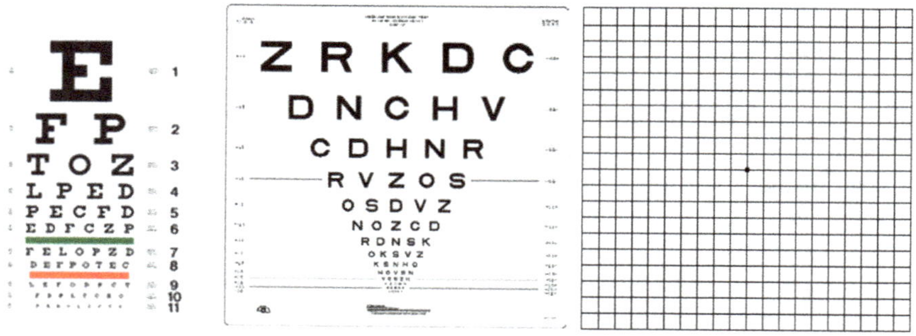

(a) (b) (c)

Figure 4.2 Assessing visual function: Snellen chart (left), ETDRS chart (centre) and Amsler grid (right)

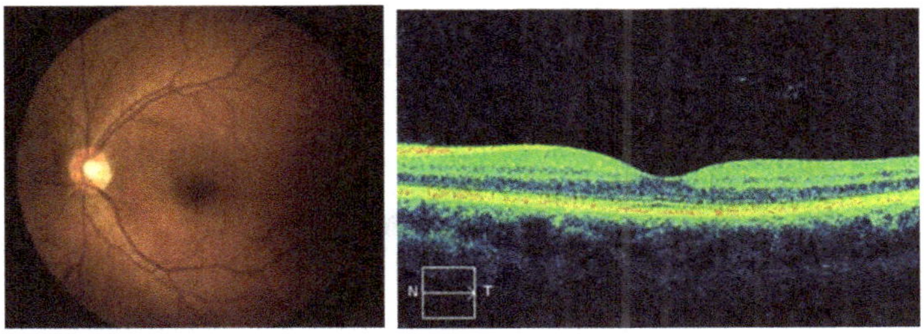

Figure 4.3 Fundus photograph of normal eye and normal OCT scan
[Reprinted, with permission, from Flaum Eye Institute, Rochester NY.]

Moving from functional testing to more objective assessments, fundus photography and optical coherence tomography (OCT) make up the mainstay of clinical retinal imaging approaches. These tests are only performed in in-office settings. Fundus photography provides a high-quality colour image of the macula. OCT is a more recent addition to the retinal imaging armamentarium, and is based on the principle of interferometry and combined with advanced software to generate detailed cross-sectional images of the retina. By analysing the fundus and assessing the macular OCT, a great deal can be learned about eye health. Intravenous fluorescein angiography (which is also a photographic technique) remains an important approach to assessing macular pathology, and, prior to OCT, it was used much more frequently in the clinical setting. As OCT has improved, the utilisation of fluorescein angiography has declined. A normal macula by fundus photography and OCT is shown in Figure 4.3.

Mr. Oswald: 'While imaging is extremely important in managing AMD, currently retinal imaging is an in-office assessment only. By bringing a sensitive and specific diagnostic test assessing macular function to patient's homes, visual outcomes can be improved to advance the quality of medical care in ophthalmology.'

4.4 Age-related macular degeneration

AMD is a multifactorial condition whereby macular function declines due to a combination of pathological processes including decreased choroidal perfusion, oxidative damage, inflammation, alterations in the metabolic support of photoreceptors, thickening of supporting membranes, development of excrescences (drusen), cell death (atrophy), and ischemia and neovascularisation. This condition typically first shows up as small hard drusen which then grow over time and can be associated with pigmentary changes.

A grading scale has been established for AMD. Initially, AMD is described as early when small hard drusen are present in the macula, and the presence of greater and greater amounts of drusen and their confluence lead to the determination of intermediate AMD (see Figure 4.4.). Intermediate AMD is usually associated with good or acceptable visual acuity (driving legal or better), although metamorphopsia

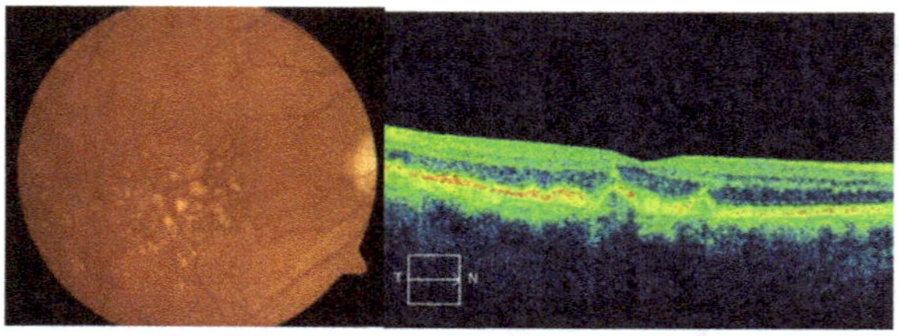

Figure 4.4 Fundus photograph of left eye with multiple soft drusen and intermediate AMD. The OCT shows subretinal drusen
[Reprinted, with permission, from Flaum Eye Institute, Rochester NY.]

can develop at this stage. Intermediate AMD is also termed nonexudative or dry AMD.

Once AMD progresses beyond the intermediate stage into the advanced stages, visual acuity drops off significantly and can eventually lead to legal blindness. Advanced AMD is associated with either central retinal atrophy (geographic atrophy) or exudative (wet) AMD. AMD with geographic atrophy is the preferred term for the advanced stage of dry AMD. Although a nutraceutical formulation can decrease expected rates of progression to advanced AMD in patients with intermediate AMD, there are currently no effective pharmaceutical therapies to treat or prevent the development of geographic atrophy.

Geographic atrophy develops slowly over time from the earlier stages of AMD, and accounts for a minority of the cases of blindness due to AMD. Exudative AMD, on the other hand, accounts for the majority of severe vision loss due to AMD – 70 percent by some accounts [5].

Exudative AMD is diagnosed by identifying a subretinal or choroidal neovascular membrane in an eye with underlying dry AMD. These neovascular membranes alter the retinal tissue structure by leaking fluid into or under the retina, and they can also bleed. Untreated, these lesions rapidly have adverse effects on visual function and can eventually lead to scarring. A fundus photograph and OCT revealing intra- and subretinal fluid is shown in Figure 4.5. The schematic in Figure 4.6. shows the morphological changes associated with progression of AMD. For the sake of clarity, wet AMD, exudative AMD, neovascular AMD and choroidal neovascularisation in AMD all describe the same condition that by definition is one component of advanced AMD. When patients develop fluid under or within the retina and when the macula is otherwise disturbed by exudative lesions or small amounts of haemorrhage, vision is adversely affected. Visual acuity can decrease, small bind spots can develop and, often, some degree of metamorphopsia is present.

Dr. Orr: 'Although it may take a generation to develop new medications to prevent AMD and affect changes in diet and lifestyle to reduce the current high rates of this condition, executives in biotechnology are working hard to address practical approaches to help preserve sight in cases where primary prevention of AMD is not possible.'

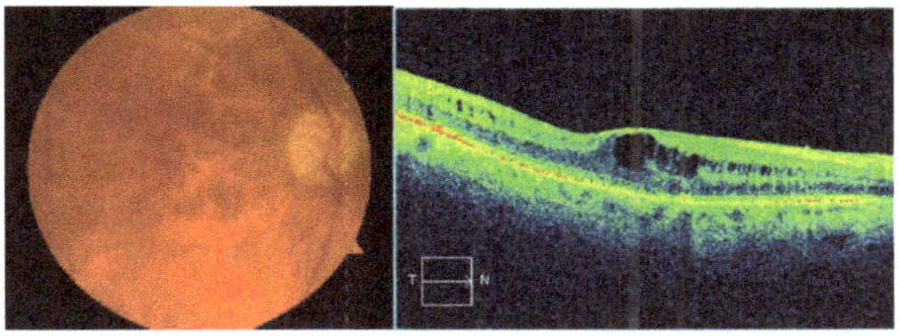

Figure 4.5 Exudative AMD with drusen, pigment and choroidal neovascularisation visible by photography and intraretinal oedema seen by OCT
[Reprinted, with permission, from Flaum Eye Institute, Rochester, NY.]

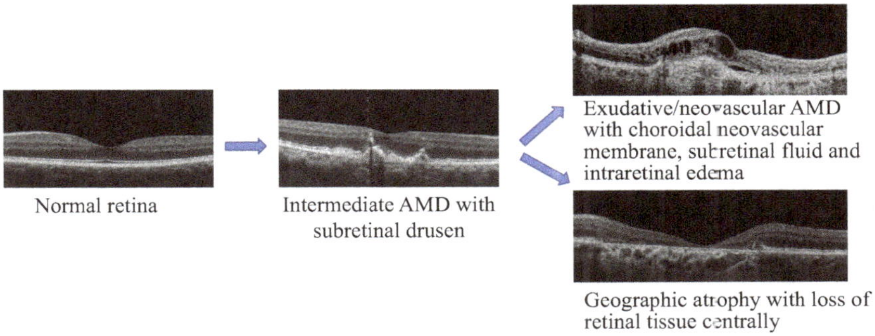

Figure 4.6 Morphological changes associated with progression of AMD as demonstrated through OCT images
[Reprinted, with permission, from of the Flaum Eye Institute, Rochester, NY.]

Dr. Heier: 'In my clinical practice in Boston, the volume of patients with wet AMD is astounding—and it continues to grow almost daily.'

4.5 Treatment for exudative age-related macular degeneration

Retinal inflammation and ischemia lead to the production of vascular endothelial growth factor (VEGF) in the retina, and VEGF is the driving factor related to the progression of exudative AMD from an incipient neovascular process to a large, leaking, vision-threatening lesion. VEGF is a highly potent hyperpermeability agent that also stimulates the growth of new blood vessels (angiogenesis).

Fortunately, retinal VEGF can be antagonised pharmaceutically via an intravitreal injection of VEGF binding agents, and this form of anti-VEGF therapy (which became available just over 10 years ago) has revolutionised the treatment of patients with exudative AMD, and many untoward effects have been reduced.

Currently, the three main therapeutic options are bevacizumab, ranibizumab and aflibercept. These agents are safe and effective. The first two are based on monoclonal antibody technology, while the latter is a fusion protein. Multiple large-scale, high-quality clinical trials of these agents demonstrate that they have similar efficacy in treating exudative AMD. Generally speaking, at the time of diagnosis of exudative AMD, anti-VEGF therapy is initiated. Patients have about a 33 percent chance of showing a clinically significant improvement in vision (15 or more ETDRS letters gained), and a 95 percent chance of maintaining their vision over 2 years (less than 15 ETDRS letters gained or lost) [6–9]. Longer-term outcomes based on formal follow-up data is not as favourable. For example, by 5 and 7 years many patients suffer a clinically significant worsening of visual acuity in the affected eye [10–12]. Anti-VEGF usage in clinical trials was more regimented (more frequent injections and more total injections over the study duration) than standard of care clinical utilisation, thus real-world outcomes tend to be somewhat less favourable. Clinical experience, however, supports an overall conclusion that these agents provide great benefit to patients, and recent research on AMD blindness shows that the rates of blindness due to AMD are decreasing [13].

Dr. Heier: 'Anti-VEGF agents represent one of the most important developments in the history of ophthalmology. Nevertheless, there is still an opportunity to better utilise this therapeutic intervention to reduce the loss of good vision.'

Dr. Orr: 'Clearly these agents have made a huge difference in the lives of people with AMD. From the diagnostic standpoint, however, opportunities exist to improve individual patient results.'

4.6 The importance of early detection of exudative age-related macular degeneration to improve visual outcomes

One consistent theme in the treatment of patients with choroidal neovascularisation due to AMD is that, untreated, these lesions have an increasingly adverse effect on vision [14]. Furthermore, modest vision gain is only experienced in one third of cases. Early detection, when the patient's vision is better, is a critical factor in generating favourable short and long-term results [15]. This point is best represented graphically. As can be seen in Figure 4.7., those patients from the large comparison of age-related macular degeneration treatment trials (CATT) study categorised as having the best visual acuity at baseline had the best vision at 1 year. These findings were recapitulated on a much longer timeline in a large observational study that evaluated 1,212 eyes and 24,547 intravitreal injections [11]. Patients who were treated initially with better vision showed a much higher likelihood of not having visual impairment – which is commonly defined as seeing 20/60 (~63 letters) or worse – at 5 years [11].

Choroidal neovascular membranes can be seen clinically in a very wide distribution of sizes – from a pinpoint lesion to a membrane occupying a significant portion of the entire macula. Larger lesions are associated with poorer vision. Once

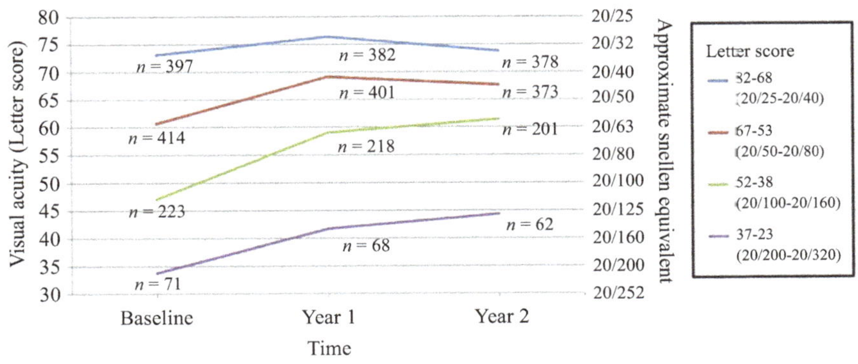

Figure 4.7 Mean visual acuity at 1 and 2 years in the comparison of age-related macular degeneration treatment trials (CATT) study [15]

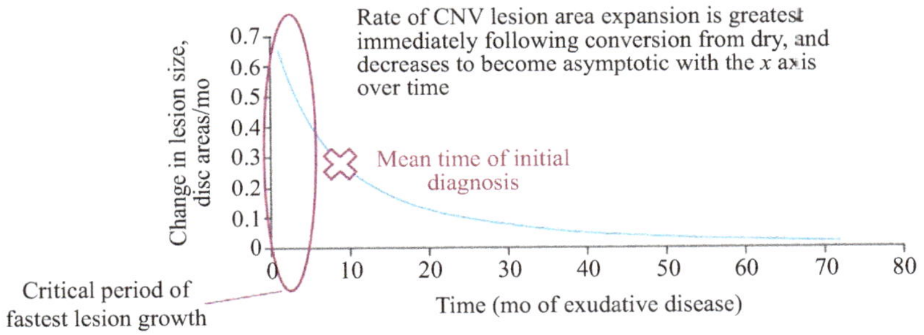

Figure 4.8 Lesion progression, and associated vision loss, is most rapid at disease onset [14]

a choroidal neovascular membrane begins to leak (when it is early and small), it initially grows most rapidly, as seen in Figure 4.8. In the CATT study, patients with smaller lesions at baseline had better outcomes following 1 year of anti-VEGF treatment, supporting the idea that treating earlier in the disease process yields better results [16].

Clearly, early identification of exudative lesions and initiation of anti-VEGF therapy is a key component of optimising outcomes in AMD. Many more patients have nonexudative than exudative AMD, and progression rates to neovascularisation on an annualised rate are not high. For example, even for subjects considered at high risk for progression to advanced AMD (either geographic atrophy or exudative AMD) by a scale known as the AREDS 5-step scale, 45 percent will progress to advanced AMD over 5 years, which translates to a 9 percent risk of progression per year. Individuals with lower scores on the 5-step scale have even lower rates of progression to advanced disease. When patients are seen in a retina clinic, comprehensive testing with functional assessments and imaging modalities can accurately identify the presence of an early exudative lesion. Unless patients already have exudative AMD in one eye, however, it is not practical to perform routine ophthalmic evaluations more frequently than every 6 months. Early detection using conventional methods is inadequate though. Patients are just not able to detect subtle visual changes without advanced diagnostics. Simply relying on symptoms, including home use of the Amsler grid, is a suboptimal method for early detection. For example, in reviewing six major trials evaluating anti-VEGF therapy in clinical trials of treatment-naïve choroidal neovascularisation in AMD (initial conversion from intermediate to exudative AMD), it was consistently found that subjects presented with a mean visual acuity of 20/63 or worse [6–9,17]. As has been demonstrated, a significant change in disease status can occur over just a few months. Nevertheless, the ophthalmic community currently must rely on patients' symptoms as a primary driver for detection of new onset exudative AMD. Optimally, patients would be evaluated frequently with a sensitive and specific assessment that is convenient (e.g. at home), and in-office visits would be scheduled when some sensitivity threshold is crossed.

Such a monitoring approach would be beneficial for patients. Early treatment in better seeing eyes leads to better outcomes. In a study designed to evaluate the relative effectiveness of treating eyes with good (6/12 or better – which is the metric method for reporting a US Snellen acuity of 20/40) visual acuity, compared to eyes that started therapy with vision between 6/12 (20/40) and 6/24 (20/80), 12,951 eyes and 92,976 injections were evaluated. The results were compelling. All eyes in the better-seeing group maintained a better mean visual acuity at all-time points over 2 years [18]. At this time, there is no standardised and widespread utilisation of technology to improve the early detection of exudative AMD in at-risk subjects.

4.7 The unmet needs for better early detection of exudative AMD

Early detection of exudative AMD remains a significant unmet need in AMD and demands a solution.

There exists great opportunity to improve visual outcomes by improving the detection of visual function compromise at home as an indicator for the development of exudative AMD. If AMD patients could be notified just before or at the point they are showing subtle declines in visual performance and were then instructed to see an ophthalmologist, for those that developed neovascularisation, treatment could be initiated and the long-term visual performance could be maximised. With an estimated global prevalence of AMD of 196 million people in 2020 increasing to 288 million in 2040, there is a vast opportunity to substantially improve overall outcomes through an earlier detection of choroidal neovascularisation and thereby preserve functional vision for millions of people with this condition. In order to inform an individual patient of a subclinical change in vision and motivate them to seek an ophthalmic examination, some type of reliable assessment tool is required. Fortunately, there is a technology amenable to widespread home deployment that has shown efficacy in detecting exudation and leading to earlier intervention. That technology utilises PHP.

Dr. Heier: 'We have made great strides in streamlining the in-office evaluation of patients at risk for transition to exudative AMD, and if indicated, treatment can be seamlessly integrated into the same visit. At this time, however, the vast majority of routine follow-up evaluations in patients with dry AMD show no evidence of such a change or, on the other hand, have evidence that a neovascular process has been present for some time. Unfortunately, and for a variety of reasons, patients often do not seek care immediately when symptoms develop, or they are unaware of their onset due to a normal functioning fellow eye. If we could better determine when a patient should be seen, we can improve visual outcomes, decrease costs, enhance patient convenience, increase the efficiency of a busy practice, and provide overall better health care.'

Dr. Orr: 'At Notal Vision, we are incredibly aware of this significant unmet need and are dedicated to helping retina specialists meet these very achievable goals. The ForeseeHome telemedicine platform can detect early macular dysfunction and serve as the vital link between AMD patients, their physicians, and practice administrators (to enable easy scheduling). The technology is now refined and available for commercial use. We are working hard to improve patient and physician access to this sight-saving system.'

4.8 Preferential hyperacuity perimetry (PHP)

PHP is a proprietary diagnostic technology for use in quantifying, in a repeatable manner, the amount and depth of central visual field defects resulting in metamorphopsia (distortions in vision) or scotomas (missing sections of the visual field). The visual disturbances detected can be attributable to new-onset exudation in AMD patients or to other morphological changes in the retina. Similar to other human sensations, such as changes in taste or smell, pain or vertigo, it is a significant challenge to quantify subtle alterations in central vision, and examiners typically rely on subjective self-reporting which can be biased by factors such as personality, scales and the depth of questioning. One of the key goals driving the development of a preferential hyperacuity perimeter was to detect earlier new onset choroidal neovascularisation, also known as conversion to exudative AMD.

The device is sensitive and specific in this regard. The ForeseeHome platform, cleared by the Food and Drug Administration (FDA), is unique because of its ergonomic design, ease of use, machine-learning algorithms utilised to detect an asymptomatic change in visual performance and its telemedicine capabilities.

The foundational principle behind hyperacuity testing is that the eye has a much greater ability to resolve very small misalignments between objects, such as changes in the integrity of a straight dotted line than separating out and discriminating objects, for example, in perceiving a letter (see Figure 4.9.).

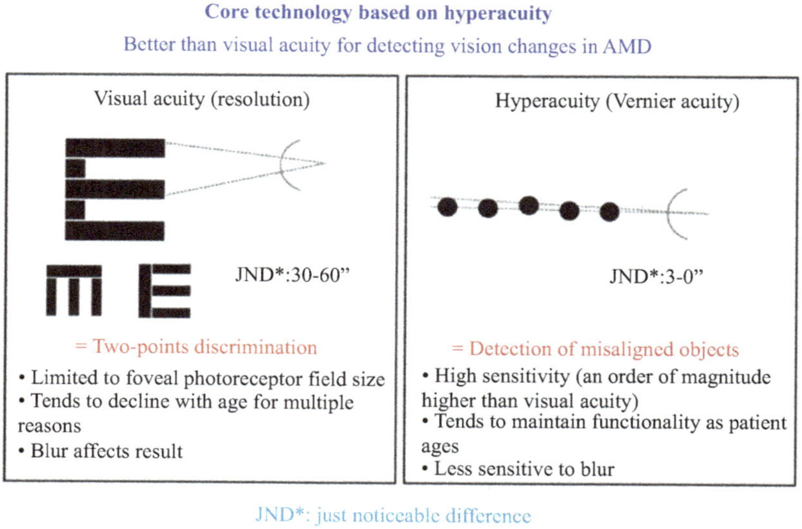

Figure 4.9 Visual acuity compared to hyperacuity

Visual physiology involves the stimulation of receptive fields in the retina and their interpretation by the visual cortex. A straight line appears straight because when a collinear set of receptive fields are stimulated, the brain can recognise their relationship and interpret seeing a straight line. If the macular photoreceptors are displaced because of the accumulation of fluid in the retina, a neovascular membrane, and/or subretinal blood, noncollinear sets of photoreceptors are stimulated and the brain perceives a line as distorted, and metamorphopsia is present. The preferential hyperacuity perimeter relies on this process to detect early evidence of neovascularisation.

The term hyperacuity is used because the relative ability to identify misalignment between the borders of objects is extremely sensitive and greater than other acuity measures. Another term for this type of visual acuity is Vernier acuity, and has been described as the smallest perceptible offset between presented stimuli. This acuity is far more refined than Snellen acuity by a factor of up to ten. While the best visual acuity in identifying letters is roughly 30 s of arc, Vernier acuity can perceive differences at levels of three to 6 s of arc. This characteristic makes this approach very valuable in identifying early-stage macular pathology [3].

Unlike resolution (e.g. identifying letters) which is based on visual acuity, hyperacuity relies on the object's alignment and thus, tolerant of impaired visual acuity or obscured media opacity, typical to AMD patients. The PHP technology also relies on 'attention competition' as a method to quantify the degree of distortion. In other words, instead of simply displaying straight lines across the central 14 degrees of the macula and relying on a patient to notice the onset of distortion

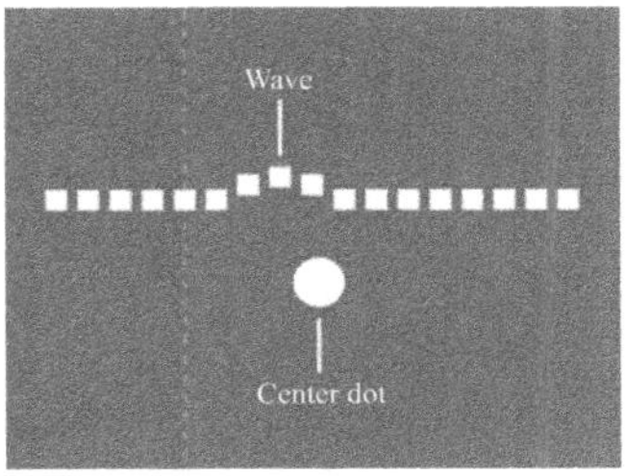

Figure 4.10 An artificial distortion in a dotted line is briefly projected onto the patient's central 14 degrees of vision. This artificial distortion 'competes' with any pathological metamorphopsia that may be present and the subject marks the largest wave noticeable. Then, the process repeats

rarely and reliably, the device briefly (a 160-ms duration) displays dotted lines with an artificial distortion which the patient must then identify while fixating on a central dot. The magnitude of the artificial distortions is varied thereby allowing for the generation of a map of the patient's central Vernier acuity (hence, the term perimetry). Once a patient develops metamorphopsia, due to cognitive competition, also known as preferential looking, the subject tends to notice (e.g. 'prefers') the largest distortion while ignoring other stimuli, hence the process has been named 'Preferential Hyperacuity Perimetry.' Once a location different than the artificial distortion is marked by the subject, the device can map out metamorphopsia.

The map reveals not only the visual field defect's location but also its severity. Figure 4.10. shows an example of the type of stimulus presented to a patient with PHP. This approach has been developed into a user-friendly, clinically tested and commercially available medical device called ForeseeHome.

4.9 ForeseeHome

The ForeseeHome device has been designed specifically to be self-operated at home by elderly patients. It is easily accessible and can be used on a table top (Figure 4.11). The eye piece is adjustable so that it is comfortable for the people of different heights and preferred positions for use. Subjects can perform the test using their own distance glasses. The test requires only about 3 min per eye.

Results are transmitted automatically to Notal Vision's propriety cloud-based servers. The device can transmit the data using cellular, Wi-Fi or landline communication.

The results of the patient's responses are analysed utilising a machine-learning algorithmic approach.

The location of the responses by the patient in relation to the presented signal (or lack thereof), and the relation to the amplitude of the presented distortion are all considered in the calculation of a test score.

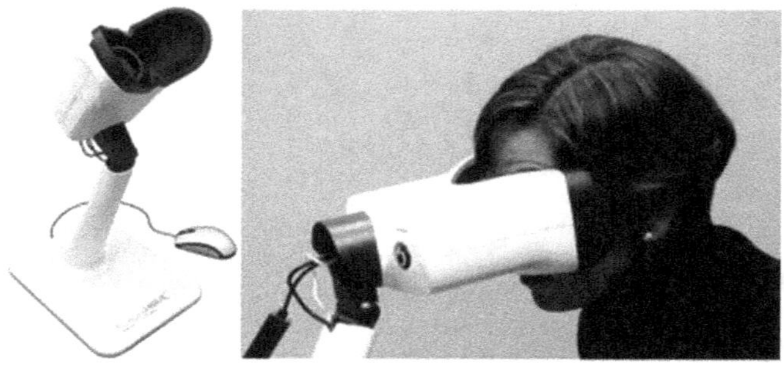

Figure 4.11 Left: ForeseeHome device. The mouse is used by the subject to point to the distortion. Right: A patient using the ForeseeHome device

The test score is compared with a normative database of test scores of non-exudative AMD and exudative AMD eyes, and is classified as 'negative' or 'positive' with a p-value. Each eye will go through an initial period to establish a baseline that informs the system about the eye's average scores and variability surrounding that average. Once a baseline is established, an additional algorithmic layer monitors for statistically significant change in the test score compared to the baseline. The application also generates a visual field defects map, representing areas of metamorphopsia and scotomas. An example of the analysis and results output is provided in Figure 4.12.

If it appears a new choroidal neovascular lesion is likely, the patient's physician is notified immediately so an appointment can be scheduled, usually within days. In addition, the patient's physician is provided with monthly reports on each patient to monitor performance and compliance. The system automatically monitors usage and calls the patient to remind them to take the test if no communication of new results is made within an adjustable time frame based on patient and physician preferences. The ForeseeHome program is described in detail online at www.foreseehome.com.

4.10 Clinical trial results

The story of clinical evaluations of PHP is actually quite long and predates the development of the ForeseeHome device. PHP has been well studied in the clinic for over 15 years, and the most recent clinical data is the most powerful. When evaluating the importance, applicability and validity of clinical trials results, the type of trial is critical.

Level 1 evidence is the highest-quality clinical data. It is derived out of well-designed, adequately powered, large, randomised, controlled trials with clear-cut results [19]. The ForeseeHome device safety and efficacy is well supported by Level 1 data.

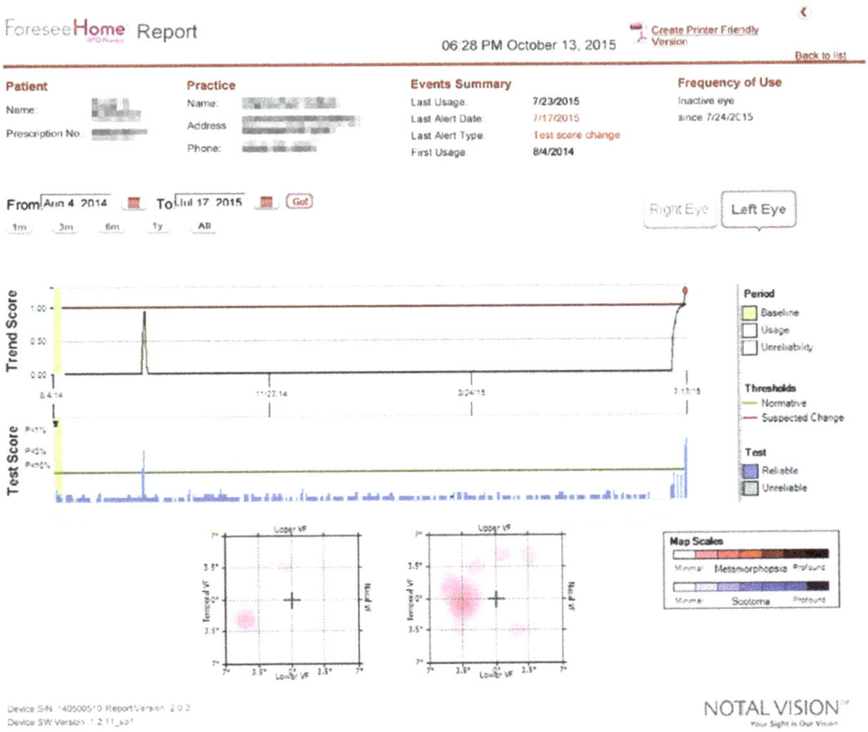

Figure 4.12 ForeseeHome results and analysis for left eye for which an alert was triggered on 30 April 2012. This example shows an established baseline and 86 tests over 4.5 months prior to the alert. The baseline visual acuity was 20/20, and the alert visual acuity was 20/25

Clinical trials evaluating PHP technology were initiated in 2001 on a desktop system designed for in-office use. At that time, OCT technology was less advanced and the resolution didn't provide as much information regarding the presence of an early neovascular membrane. In this first study [20] of 32 patients with choroidal neovascularization (CNV) due to AMD, hyperacuity testing identified 30 (94 percent) while the Amsler grid testing identified 11 (34 percent). In a 2005 multicentre study of 150 subjects with varying AMD status (33 healthy, 98 with nonexudative AMD and 19 with exudative AMD), PHP showed favourable sensitivity (100 percent) for identifying exudative AMD compared to Amsler testing (53 percent) which was the comparator and, importantly, administered in the office by a trained technician [21]. Amsler grid testing in the hands of a patient in a home environment typically shows even lower rates of sensitivity [4,21,22].

Another 2005 study designed specifically to evaluate the value of PHP in discriminating between intermediate AMD and new onset exudative AMD evaluated PHP results in 122 subjects – 65 with exudative AMD and 57 with intermediate AMD. Fluorescein angiography was used as the gold standard for classifying AMD as either neovascular or not. PHP showed a sensitivity and specificity* of 82 percent and 88 percent, respectively, suggesting the value of PHP in this setting as it identified the vast majority of exudative cases with few false positives [23]. And, similarly, a study which enrolled 200 subjects with non-exudative AMD, who were all part of the multicentre, randomised, controlled clinical trial 'Carotenoids and Co-antioxidants in Patients with Age-Related Maculopathy,' showed similar favourable outcomes associated with PHP. Groups that used the device had better vision by a mean of 9.7 letters and smaller choroidal neovascular membranes as measured by fundus photography. Both outcomes were statistically significant. Furthermore, 66 percent of the subjects in the device arm were asymptomatic at conversion to exudative AMD, while only 20 percent in the control arm were asymptomatic [24].

During the mid-2000s, the resolution of and ease of testing with office-based OCT improved significantly, and OCT technology has become the preferred method for differentiating between exudative and nonexudative cases during in-office clinical evaluation. This development presented commercial challenges for the office-based PHP device. However, patients still need to be seen by a physician to make determinations regarding AMD utilising OCT, and as mentioned, patients do not present to ophthalmologists at the optimal time for initiating anti-VEGF therapy under this paradigm.

The results for the clinical trials clearly indicated that PHP had the potential for improving early detection of new onset exudation. It was clear that the real advantage of this technology – early detection – would be maximised and would enable a close monitoring by transferring the PHP technology from the clinic to patient's homes. Notal Vision developed the low-cost, self-installed and self-operated tele-connected ForeseeHome version of PHP to drastically increase early detection rates of exudative AMD.

In 2010, a pilot evaluation of the ForeseeHome device in the home monitoring environment effectively identified two subjects who had converted to exudative AMD. It was the first time the technology was used for ongoing monitoring at home of eyes with intermediate nonexudative AMD for a significant change indicative of conversion to exudative AMD (in contrast to single encounter testing in the office). At the time of detection by ForeseeHome, about 2 years after starting the monitoring, one subject was asymptomatic (did not perceive any visual changes). The other subject caught by the ForeseeHome for exudative AMD reported the symptoms retrospectively but did not act upon them. At the time of diagnosis, the visual acuity in the affected eye of one subject was 20/20 and in the other, it was 20/32 – which is considered an early detection. In both cases, anti-VEGF therapy

*Sensitivity is the number of true positives detected by the test over a denominator of all true positives in the sample. Specificity is the number of true negatives identified by the test over a denominator of all true negatives in the sample. The results are typically reported as percentages.

was initiated earlier than would have occurred without ForeseeHome, and both subjects maintained their presenting acuity when the report was written [25].

In parallel, a large, pivotal, randomised and controlled trial was initiated to definitively assess the value of the ForeseeHome telemedicine platform in identifying new choroidal neovascularisation in AMD. This trial was named home monitoring of the eye (HOME) and compared the outcome of the ForeseeHome system plus standard of care (the device arm) and standard of care alone (the control arm), in detecting exudative AMD in at-risk eyes. The HOME study was a sub-study of the age-related eye disease trial study 2 (AREDS2), an National Institutes of Health (NIH)-sponsored clinical trial of more than 4,000 people between the ages of 50 and 85 at risk for advanced AMD at 82 clinical sites across the United States. AREDS2 was designed to evaluate the effectiveness of a nutraceutical formulation at reducing progression rates of AMD [26]. The HOME study enrolled 1,520 subjects from 44 clinical sites. All patients had intermediate AMD in one or both eyes. Patients were randomised 1:1 to the device arm (home monitoring with ForeseeHome together with standard care) and the control arm – (standard of care only). Subjects were encouraged to use the device on a daily basis. When a clinically meaningful change was detected, the subject's study site was alerted, and a visit was scheduled within 72 h to evaluate the clinical condition of that eye.

Subjects randomised to either ForeseeHome or standard of care received instructions from their investigator to contact the clinical site if they detected a change in their vision and an appointment was scheduled. Amsler charts were permitted but not mandated [27,28].

Visual acuity and fundus photography were standardised and obtained at baseline. At follow-up visits, triggered by either an alert from the ForeseeHome device, a new symptom development, or at scheduled visits for which the examining physician suspected a conversion to exudation, fluorescein angiography and OCT testing were obtained to determine if choroidal neovascularisation was present.

The study's primary outcome was to determine whether ForeseeHome led to earlier detection of exudative AMD than standard of care as reflected by the visual acuity at the time of new onset exudative AMD diagnosis. The investigator utilised the testing results at the applicable visit to determine if choroidal neovascularisation was present in the affected eye, and obtained confirmation from masked evaluators at a reading centre. Interim analyses were set at points when 50 percent and then 75 percent of the number of planned exudative AMD events occurred. It was predetermined that the study would be stopped early for either efficacy or futility [29].

Seven hundred and sixty-three patients were enrolled in the device arm, and 757 were enrolled in the control arm. The average age was 72 years in each group. Ethnicity was 96 percent white and the ratio of females to males was roughly 60:40 in each group. Likewise, baseline AMD category and mean visual acuity were similar in the two groups. The second interim analysis was conducted 2 years and 9 months after study initiation, and at that point the mean follow-up was 1.4 years.

Six hundred nine of the 763 subjects randomised to the device arm used the device regularly for a mean of 4.4 times per week. Fifty-seven of these subjects used the device less frequently than twice weekly.

Five days was the median interval between a ForeseeHome alert to an examination at the clinic in the device arm; in the control arm, subjects were seen at the clinic a median of 7.5 days after they reported new symptoms.

At the second interim analysis, 82 subjects in the study had progressed to exudative AMD in at least one eye. Fifty-one cases were in the device arm, while 31 were in the control arm. Subjects in the device arm showed a statistically significant smaller decrease in visual acuity than the control arm (Figure 4.13). Data analysis showed that the perception of higher conversion rates to exudative AMD in the device arm was due to earlier detection. In the device arm, a median of four letters were lost at the time of choroidal neovascular membrane detection in the study eye compared to baseline. In the control arm, a median of nine letters were lost at diagnosis of exudation compared to baseline. The difference between the groups was statistically significant. A key secondary visual function endpoint was the proportion of patients maintaining 20/40 or better vision at presentation, and the rates were 94 percent in the device arm and 62 percent in the standard-of-care arm, which was also statistically significant.

In real-world settings, the visual acuity is less likely to be 20/40 or better at presentation of exudative AMD. Data from a large US registry of 150,000 real-world cases AMD patients revealed that only 31 percent meet this criterion [29], as seen in Figure 4.14. Moreover, the choroidal neovascular membrane lesion median area in the HOME study [30] was significantly and statistically smaller in the device arm compared to the control arm. Based on the favourable primary outcome for subjects randomised to device in the HOME study, the independent safety monitoring committee recommended early termination of the trial [28].

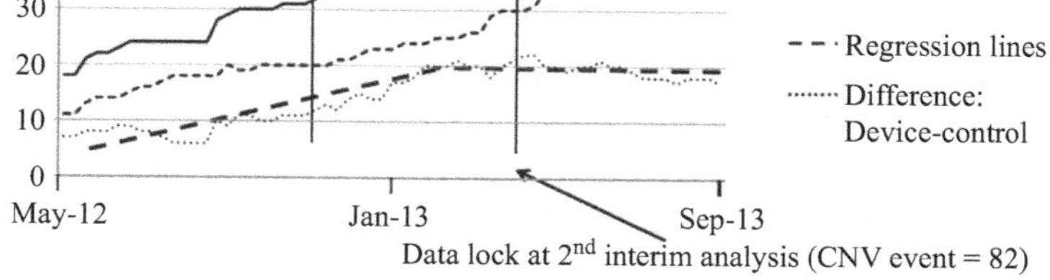

Figure 4.13 Differences in accumulation of exudative AMD cases by treatment arm in the HOME study. Initially, it appears that the rates of choroidal neovascularisation are higher in the device group, but that is an artefact of early detection. Before the second interim analysis, the incidence between the two groups became the same [28]

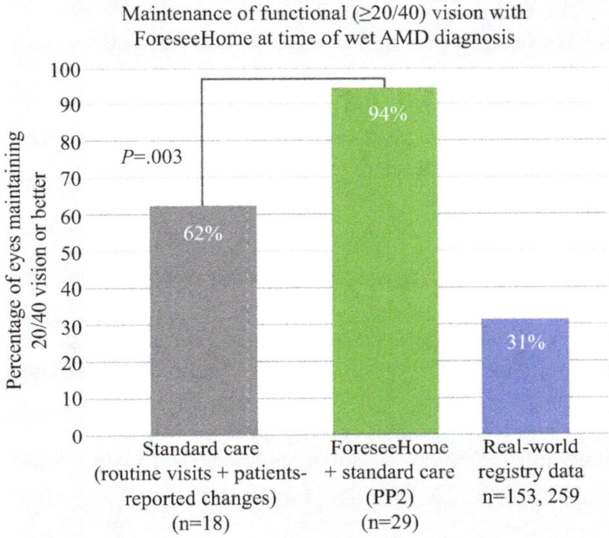

Figure 4.14 Proportion of subjects with 20/40 Snellen acuity in the HOME study compared to real-world data from the American Academy of Ophthalmogy's IRIS Registry database [28,29]

These results are clear and compelling: the home use of ForeseeHome in eyes at risk for exudative AMD is a valuable diagnostic intervention. It is rare that clinical trials are stopped for efficacy, yet HOME was stopped by an independent committee for this reason. ForeseeHome is FDA cleared for use in AMD to monitor patients at the risk of vision loss from exudative AMD.

Moreover, the HOME study was the first time telemonitoring was evaluated within a randomised controlled trial, comparing self-monitoring with a telemedicine instrument and standard care. This result is favourable for the potential for telemedicine in ophthalmology.

4.11 Impact, reimbursement and cost effectiveness of ForeseeHome monitoring

ForeseeHome has the potential to make a major impact on the quality of life of patients at risk for exudative AMD, and its benefits are recognised by payers. In an analysis based on the HOME study, monitoring was shown to reduce expected life-years lived with blindness by 10.8 percent [31,32].

Medicare, the largest insurer of adults over 65 years in the United States, reimburses ForeseeHome use in AMD. The costs to individuals are manageable, and depending on a patient's supplemental insurance, the per month charge ranges from no charge to ~$15 per month for a patient. It has also been shown that the use of the ForeseeHome technology in at-risk patients is cost effective.

Furthermore, the use of ForeseeHome for AMD patients at risk for exudative disease led to an increase in quality-adjusted life years for users [32]. Data from a recent survey showed that most patients expressed interest in using home monitoring if their central vision was at risk [33]. All these economic and logistical components to ForeseeHome telemedicine monitoring suggest great value is placed on the technology.

4.12 Additional applications for ForeseeHome

Patients with non-AMD macular diseases that typically involve symptoms of visual distortion may benefit from PHP assessments as well. There is a potential applicability of monitoring patients at risk for hydroxychloroquine toxicity, assessing patients with epiretinal membranes in the pre- and postoperative setting, and evaluating patients at risk for diabetic macular oedema [34,35]. Patients with central serous chorioretinopathy or macular telangiectasia may also benefit from PHP diagnostic testing. There is ample opportunity for further study and increasing the indications for the ForeseeHome platform.

4.13 Conclusions and future of home monitoring in ophthalmology

ForeseeHome has shown a great potential to help patients at risk for conversion to exudative AMD.

With the increasing implementation of this telemedicine system, patients and society at large should benefit.

Although there are other products with capability of providing home monitoring of vision (e.g. Paxos Mobile App from Digisight and myVisionTrack from Vital Art and Science), none of these approaches is supported by Level 1 evidence, none are covered by Medicare, and only ForeseeHome is indicated for home monitoring of patients with intermediate AMD at risk for developing exudative AMD.

Telemedicine in the form of in-home monitoring with ForeseeHome will become an important aspect of AMD patient management.

Beyond functional visual testing at home, however, there is a potential for at-home retinal imaging.

Home-based OCT systems are under development, but it has yet to be seen whether these devices can reach a price point acceptable for home use. Effectiveness of such an approach in macular disease management will need to be borne out in clinical trials. Until that time, functional vision testing via ForeseeHome will be a key diagnostic approach to reducing vision loss in AMD.

Without a doubt, the era for home monitoring telemedicine in ophthalmology is critically at hand. This important development will improve the quality of life and vision in AMD populations. ForeseeHome is economical, designed for easy use by the elderly, clinically proven, covered by insurers, and will improve patient management and practice-flow processes for retina specialists. ForeseeHome represents an advanced technological, home-based approach to helping people maintain their vision.

References

[1] Schmidt M., Gissel A., Laufs T., Hankeln T., Wolfrum U., and Burmester T. 'How does the eye breathe? Evidence for neuroglobin-mediated oxygen supply in the mammalian retina.' *Journal of Biological Chemistry*. 2003;278 (3):1932–1935.

[2] Kaiser P.K. 'Prospective evaluation of visual acuity assessment: a comparison of Snellen versus ETDRS charts in clinical practice (An AOS Thesis).' *Transactions of the American Ophthalmological Society*. 2009;107:311.

[3] Keane P.A., de Salvo G., Sim D.A., Goverdhan S., Agrawal R., and Tufail A. 'Strategies for improving early detection and diagnosis of neovascular age-related macular degeneration.' *Clinical Ophthalmology* (Auckland, NZ). 2015;9:353.

[4] Crossland M., and Rubin G. 'The Amsler chart: absence of evidence is not evidence of absence.' *British Journal of Ophthalmology*. 2007;91(3): 391–393.

[5] Friedman D.S., O'Colmain B.J., Muñoz B., *et al.* 'Prevalence of age-related macular degeneration in the United States.' *Archives of Ophthalmology*. 2004;122(4):564–572.

[6] CATT Research Group. 'Ranibizumab and bevacizumab for neovascular age-related macular degeneration.' *New England Journal of Medicine*. 2011; (364):1897–1908.

[7] Rosenfeld P.J., Brown D.M., Heier J.S., *et al.* 'Ranibizumab for neovascular age-related macular degeneration.' *New England Journal of Medicine*. 2006;355(14):1419–1431.

[8] Brown D.M., Michels M., Kaiser P.K., Heier J.S., Sy J.P., and Ianchulev T. 'Ranibizumab versus verteporfin photodynamic therapy for neovascular age-related macular degeneration: two-year results of the ANCHOR study.' *Ophthalmology*. 2009;116(1):57–65.

[9] Heier J.S., Brown D.M., Chong V., *et al.* 'Intravitreal aflibercept (VEGF trap-eye) in wet age-related macular degeneration.' *Ophthalmology*. 2012;119(12):2537–2548.

[10] Rofagha S., Bhisitkul R.B., Boyer D.S., Sadda S.R., Zhang K; and SEVEN-UP Study Group. 'Seven-year outcomes in ranibizumab-treated patients in ANCHOR, MARINA, and HORIZON: a multicenter cohort study (SEVEN-UP).' *Ophthalmology*. 2013;120(11):2292–2299.

[11] Gillies M.C., Campain A., Barthelmes D., *et al.* 'Long-term outcomes of treatment of neovascular age-related macular degeneration: data from an observational study.' *Ophthalmology*. 2015;122(9):1837–1845.

[12] CATT Research Group, Maguire M.G., *et al.* 'Five-year outcomes with anti–vascular endothelial growth factor treatment of neovascular age-related macular degeneration: the comparison of age-related macular degeneration treatments trials.' *Ophthalmology.* 2016;123(8):1751–1761.

[13] Schmidt-Erfurth U., Chong V., Loewenstein A., *et al.* 'Guidelines for the management of neovascular age-related macular degeneration by the European Society of Retina Specialists (EURETINA).' *British Journal of Ophthalmology.* 2014;98(9):1144–1167.

[14] Liu T.A., Ankoor R.S., and Del Priore L.V. 'Progression of lesion size in untreated eyes with exudative age-related macular degeneration: a meta-analysis using Lineweaver-Burk plots.' *JAMA Ophthalmology.* 2013;131 (3):335–340.

[15] Ho A.C., Albini T.A., Brown D.M., Boyer D.S., Regillo C.D., and Heier J.S. 'The potential importance of detection of neovascular age-related macular degeneration when visual acuity is relatively good.' *JAMA Ophthalmology.* 2017;135(3):268–273.

[16] Ying G.S., Huang J., Maguire M.G., *et al.* 'Baseline predictors for one-year visual outcomes with ranibizumab or bevacizumab for neovascular age-related macular degeneration.' *Ophthalmology.* 2013;120(1):122–129.

[17] IVAN Study Investigators, Chakravarthy U., Harding S.P., *et al.* 'Ranibizumab versus bevacizumab to treat neovascular age-related macular degeneration: one-year findings from the IVAN randomized trial.' *Ophthalmology.* 2012;119(7):1399–1411.

[18] Lee A.Y., Lee C.S, Butt T., *et al.* 'UK AMD EMR USERS GROUP REPORT V: benefits of initiating ranibizumab therapy for neovascular AMD in eyes with vision better than 6/12.' *British Journal of Ophthalmology.* 2015;99(8):1045–1050.

[19] Burns P.B., Rohrich R.J., and Chung K.C. 'The levels of evidence and their role in evidence-based medicine.' *Plastic and Reconstructive Surgery.* 2011;128(1):305–310.

[20] Loewenstein A., Malach R., Goldstein M., *et al.* 'Replacing the Amsler grid: a new method for monitoring patients with age-related macular degeneration.' *Ophthalmology.* 2003;110:966 –970.

[21] Goldstein M., Loewenstein A., Barak A., *et al.* 'Results of a multicenter clinical trial to evaluate the preferential hyperacuity perimeter for detection of age-related macular degeneration.' *Retina.* 2005;25(3):296–303.

[22] Crossland M., and Rubin G. 'The Amsler chart: absence of evidence is not evidence of absence.' *British Journal of Ophthalmology.* 2007;91(3):391–393.

[23] Preferential Hyperacuity Perimetry Research Group. 'Preferential Hyperacuity Perimeter (PreView PHP) for detecting choroidal neovascularization study.' *Ophthalmology.* 2005;112(10):1758–1765.

[24] Lai Y., Grattan J., Shi Y., Young G., Muldrew A., and Chakravarthy U. 'Functional and morphologic benefits in early detection of neovascular age-related macular degeneration using the preferential hyperacuity perimeter.' *Retina.* 2011;31(8):1620–1626.

[25] Chaikitmongkol V., Bressler N.M., and Bressler S.B. 'Early detection of choroidal neovascularization facilitated with a home monitoring program in age-related macular degeneration.' *Retinal Cases and Brief Reports*. 2015;9(1):33–37.

[26] https://www.nih.gov/news-events/news-releases/nih-study-provides-clarity-supplements-protection-against-blinding-eye-disease

[27] Chew E.Y., Clemons T.E., Bressler S.B., *et al.* 'Randomized trial of the ForeseeHome™ monitoring device for early detection of neovascular age-related macular degeneration. The HOme Monitoring of the Eye (HOME) study design—HOME Study report number 1.' *Contemporary Clinical Trials*. 2014;37(2):294–300.

[28] Chew E.Y., Clemons T.E., Bressler S.B., *et al.* 'Randomized trial of a home monitoring system for early detection of choroidal neovascularization home monitoring of the Eye (HOME) study.' *Ophthalmology*. 2014;121(2):535–544.

[29] Ho A.C., 'Retrospective Analysis of Real-World Disease Detection and Visual Acuity Outcomes in Patients with Dry AMD Converting to Wet AMD Using the AAO IRIS Registry Database.' Presented at the Annual Meeting of the American Society of Cataract and Refractive Surgeons; Washington, DC, 2018

[30] Kim, J. 'The HOME Study: Lesion Characteristics of Early Choroidal Neovascularization.' Presented at the Annual Meeting of the American Society of Retinal Specialists; San Diego, CA, 2014

[31] Chew, E.Y., Clemons T.E., Harrington M., *et al.* 'Effectiveness of different monitoring modalities in the detection of neovascular age-related macular degeneration: the home study, report number 3.' *Retina*. 2016;36(8):1542–1547.

[32] Wittenborn J.S., Clemons T., Regillo C., Rayess N., Liffman Kruger D., and Rein D. 'Economic evaluation of a home-based age-related macular degeneration monitoring system.' *JAMA Ophthalmology*. 2017;135(5):452–459.

[33] Wong R.W., Franklin M., Day S., *et al.* 'Patient utilization of web-based health data management technology in an outpatient ophthalmology practice setting.' *Investigative Ophthalmology & Visual Science*. 2016;57: 5536.

[34] Anderson C., Pahk P., Blaha G.R., *et al.* 'Preferential hyperacuity perimetry to detect hydroxychloroquine retinal toxicity.' *Retina*. 2009;29(8):1188–1192.

[35] Bae S.H., Kim D., Park T.H., Han J.R., Kim H., and Nam W. 'Preferential hyperacuity perimeter and prognostic factors for metamorphopsia after idiopathic epiretinal membrane surgery.' *American Journal of Ophthalmology*. 2013;155(1):109–117.

Chapter 5

Incorporating mobile resources to enhance the impact of behavioral health services for suicidal persons

Courtney L. Crooks, Ph.D.[1], *Sallie Mack*[2], *Julie Nguyen*[3] *and Nadine J. Kaslow, Ph.D.*[3]

In keeping with the technology explosion, there has been a multitude of strides in the provision of healthcare and supplemental assistance pertinent to treatment through smartphone technology. Mobile health (mHealth) has gained popularity in recent years and has only recently been gaining empirical support. Mobile phone applications (apps) are a particularly valuable form of mHealth, as they have many advantages not true for websites and text messaging. Apps have been used in numerous ways to assist in behavioral health assessment and intervention. One domain in which they have been shown to be particularly promising is with individuals who are suicidal. This chapter reviews the current behavioral health technology landscape and focuses specifically on one form of technology, mHealth apps, for one serious public health concern, suicidal behavior. Based on the existing state-of-the-field, we conclude with future recommendations for researchers and behavioral health practitioners.

The primary focus of this chapter is on the value of mHealth technology for behavioral healthcare, with a specific focus on suicide prevention. To set the stage, we overview the current landscape, with attention to the growing role of technology in healthcare and to the state-of-the-field of technology and behavioral healthcare. This is followed by a more detailed exploration of the nature of and evidence of the various forms of mHealth in improving people's behavioral health, including

[1]Georgia Tech Research Institute, Advanced Concepts Laboratory, Atlanta, GA, USA
[2]Department of Psychology, College of Education and Human Services, Utah State University, Logan, UT, USA
[3]Department of Psychiatry and Behavioral Sciences, Emory University School of Medicine, Atlanta, GA, USA

mobile phone applications (apps), text messaging, social media usage, ecological momentary assessments and interventions (EMA, EMI), and sensory technology. We particularly highlight apps because of their growing popularity and many advantages. Subsequently, we turn our attention to the current literature and evidence-base for suicide-prevention apps as one exemplar. We conclude with future recommendations.

5.1 Technology landscape

Technology has altered our everyday lives. The smartphone, one of the most distinguishable devices that has contributed to the technological revolution, has given us the capability to do almost everything. No longer a simple means of communication, smartphones assist us in our everyday lives to accomplish ordinary tasks. Access to mobile phones has increased drastically over the past two decades, and approximately 77% of Americans currently own smartphones [1]. One form of technology rapidly gaining in popularity is apps. People spend an average of 5 hours per day on their mobile devices, and 92% of that time is spent using apps (http://flurrymobile.tumblr.com/post/157921590345/us-consumers-time-spent-on-mobile-crosses-5), which are discrete and independent software that can be used on a mobile device [2]. There are over 2.8 million apps available for smartphones, a number that is growing continuously (https://www.statista.com/statistics/276623/number-of-apps-available-in-leading-app-stores/).

5.1.1 Technology and healthcare

One reflection of this technology explosion is the dramatic increase in the use of different internet technologies (e.g., digital gaming, virtual reality, robotics) for health promotion and intervention services, collectively referred to as "ehealth" [3]. Concomitant with this, there has been a growing use of mobile devices (e.g., smartphones, tablets, personal digital assistants, wearable devices) within the healthcare context that can support the promotion, maintenance, and intervention of health-related concerns (i.e., "mHealth") [3–6]. mHealth includes apps, text messaging, social media usage, EMA and EMI, and sensory technology [3].

Apps are the most common form of mHealth and a plethora of apps have been developed related to physical and behavioral health, healthcare management, fitness, and wellness [7]. These apps, which are rated positively by users, offer a realistic and appropriate platform for accessing health information [7]. There is recent evidence that people indicate a strong preference for accessing such information in this manner [8,9]. mHealth apps also provide valuable health interventions [7]. For example, apps have been created to target health behavior change goals, such as diet and exercise (e.g., MyFitnessPal) and sleep (e.g., Sleep Cycle). Often visually engaging and user-friend, apps can be personalized, facilitate symptom evaluation, offer psychoeducation, provide interventions in real time, and track progress [5,6,10,11]. In addition, apps are an effective technological approach for providing health services to minority populations, who frequently experience disparities with regard to accessing quality healthcare [12].

5.2 Technology and behavioral healthcare

The prevalence of smartphone usage paired with the surge in apps offers a promising new approach to healthcare intervention that has the potential to make behavioral health treatment more accessible, convenient, and effective [4,6,13,14]. This development is very timely and important given that one in six individuals are diagnosed with a mental illness [15] and the global burden of mental illness is significant in terms of years lived with a disability [16]. Unfortunately, however, only half of these individuals actually access behavioral health services (https://www.nimh.nih.gov/health/statistics/index.shtml) due to barriers such as low-perceived need; a desire to resolve symptoms on one's own; attitudinal barriers such as privacy and stigma-related concerns; negative beliefs about the effectiveness of treatment and negative experiences with treatment providers; and logistics including difficulties with access due to cost, transportation, lack of therapists, lack of insurance, and long waitlists [17,18].

mHealth technologies can help overcome these and other barriers [5,19,20]. These technologies are convenient and portable and as a result, behavioral health interventions can be delivered any time or place. Because these technologies can be accessed by a greater number of individuals than can access formal healthcare services, they have the potential to bypass stigmatizing attitudes toward the seeking of behavioral health resources and are associated with a lessened financial burden. In addition, they may offer an approach that helps reduce the disparities related to access to quality services commonly found in minority populations [20,21]. mHealth tools for behavioral health are similar to those for health more generally [3].

5.2.1 Apps

In recent years, considerable progress has been made in the creation of a broad array of mHealth apps (https://www.nimh.nih.gov/health/topics/technology-and-the-future-of-mental-health-treatment/index.shtml). These apps can be used for psychoeducational purposes, to provide patients and the general public with information on various disorders. mHealth apps may promote early identification of individuals who could benefit from behavioral health services [6] and can be used for shared decision-making between patients and their providers [22]. Self-management apps enable the user to input information into the app and receive reminders, information about pertinent coping strategies, and to track progress in various domains. For example, T2 Mood Tracker, an app developed for military personnel returning from deployment, tracks symptoms associated with deployment-related behavioral health issues (e.g., stress, depression, anxiety, post-traumatic stress disorder (PTSD), general well-being, head injury) [23]. As another example, a review of self-management apps for bipolar disorder suggested that the apps with the best evidence based are those that focus on ongoing monitoring, maintaining hope, providing education, and planning for and taking action [24]. Apps for improving thinking skills assist the user in bolstering their cognitive abilities. Skill-training apps assist the user in developing new or more effective coping strategies or approaches to thinking and these apps have been shown to have advantages. For example, apps that provide instructions on deep breathing (e.g., Breathe2Relax (B2R)) are more cost effective than in-person treatment for stress management [25], although their clinical effectiveness has yet to be determined. In addition, a series of apps (e.g., Headspace, VGZ Mindfulness Coach, Calm) have been developed to support meditation and mindfulness practice and there is support for these apps [26,27]. Illness-management apps allow the user to interact with others, such as peers or trained behavioral health specialists, and receive support and guidance. They specifically increase patient engagement with peer support and directly connect people with resources, especially in times of extreme distress or crisis [28]. Passive symptom–tracking apps in which sensors record throughout the day patterns of movement, social interactions, vocal tone and speed, etc., have the potential to detect changes in behavior that may be associated with a significant behavioral health problem (e.g., depressive, manic, or psychotic episode) before it actually occurs. As a result, passive-tracking apps may be able to alert the individual, the caregiver(s), and the behavioral health professionals that the person needs additional attention and evaluation. Research suggests that creative use of smartphone sensing apps can provide effective and efficient monitoring of an array of behavioral health problems [29].

Mobile apps offer therapeutic interventions that can be a primary intervention tool, accompany existing interventions including evidence-based approaches by equipping individuals with strategies and tools to make everyday living easier (e.g., mindfulness techniques, behavioral activation, acceptance, and commitment therapy), or serve a valuable function after a formal in-person intervention occurs (e.g., post discharge) [5,6,30–33]. A multitude of mobile apps have been created to target a broad array of behavioral health disorders including but not limited to: mood, anxiety, post-traumatic stress, obsessive-compulsive, eating, schizophrenia spectrum, and alcohol and substance use [24,34–38]. In addition, there are apps to bolster the implementation, fidelity, and adherence to various evidence-based interventions, such as prolonged exposure [39,40]. Recently, efforts have been made to evaluate the efficacy of these apps. For example, a mobile app version of PRIME-D has been found to be associated with sustained improvements in depressed individuals and enhanced interactions with coach [41]. PTSD Coach, produced by the Department of Defense (DoD) and the Veterans Administration (VA), is an app that is associated to some extent with greater improvements in PTSD treatment than a wait-list control [42]. There is some initial evidence to suggest that this app yields greater benefits if utilized in conjunction with clinician support [43]. Despite preliminary evidence that mobile apps are acceptable to patients and effective in treating behavioral health symptoms, the limited research investigating their efficacy means that it is premature to conclude that they are effective for behavioral health treatment [35,36].

5.2.2 Text messaging

The short messaging service (SMS) provided by mobile phones allows for direct communication between patient and provider, which allows for the potential increase of patient engagement in outpatient services and following inpatient discharge [35]. SMS technology has been used to remind people of upcoming appointments, support illness management, provide coping techniques and skills practice, offer motivational messages, and detail emergency contacts [35,44]. It also has been used as an adjunctive intervention, such as to enhance cognitive behavioral therapy (CBT) for the treatment of depression [45]. Its inclusion has been associated with better treatment outcomes. For example, in one study, individuals diagnosed with bulimia nervosa receiving outpatient treatments were less likely to be readmitted to inpatient services in the SMS intervention group that featured individualized feedback than in the treatment as usual eating disorders group without the SMS component [46]. Further, there are some promising data to suggest the effectiveness of an intervention that combines SMS and web-based messaging. As an example, one recent study found that a combined web- and text-messaging-based intervention was more effective than assessment only in reducing risky singly occasion drinking [47]. However, no between-group differences were found on other relevant outcome variables [47]. Finally, there is growing evidence that SMS interventions are found to be acceptable and satisfactory to users [35].

5.2.3 Social media usage

Evidence is also growing that suggests social media may be a valuable tool for individuals with behavioral health concerns. In particular, some data indicate that individuals with serious and persistent mental illnesses increasingly are utilizing various forms of social media (e.g., Facebook, YouTube, Twitter) to share their experiences and/or hear from others with similar challenges [48]. People are forming peer-to-peer support networks in online communities in which they receive information and support and doing so makes them feel less alone and stigmatized [48]. However, to date, these efforts require further systematic evaluation.

5.2.4 Ecological momentary assessment/intervention: EMA and EMI

EMA allows for the collection of large amounts of data in real-life, in-the-moment situations. Through EMA, individuals are prompted in-the-moment through use of their mobile devices to evaluate current thoughts, behaviors, and symptom characteristics [49]. For example, EMA has been used to gather information on substance use and adherence to recording such information appear to be adequate to good [50]. EMA with youth with borderline personality disorder show that they have limited self-awareness with regard to their motives or environmental triggers for nonsuicidal self-injurious behavior [51]. Further, specific information that can gleaned from EMA is either not able to be measured by other methodologies or is more effectively assessed via EMA [50]. For example, one study found that EMA outperformed traditional paper-and-pencil measures in terms of sensitivity to change in some (e.g., depression) but not all (e.g., anxiety) symptoms, as well as mindfulness, in response to a mindfulness-based intervention for older adults [52].

EMI, also called "just in time adaptive interventions" (JITAI), refers to an approach to intervention that can be used to enhance self-management. A recent meta-analysis of EMI for three behavioral health problems (anxiety, depression, perceived stress) and positive psychological outcomes (e.g., acceptance) revealed a small to medium impact of EMIs on all variables [53]. This benefit was bolstered by the addition of a behavioral health professional [53]. There is the potential for EMIs in the future to be developed so that they are more engaging and more responsive to the user and the contexts in which that individual is embedded [54].

There is evidence that experience sampling methods, such as EMA and EMI, can bolster people's resilience by augmenting their ability to access natural rewards [55]. Receiving information about one's own illness and recovery trajectory can enable patients to gain insight and become more able and willing to engage in decision-making with their providers. Thus, these technologies can be empowering and associated with improved outcomes and satisfaction with care.

5.2.5 Sensor technology

Sensor technology encompasses the use of mobile devices or wearable technology (e.g., FitBits, Google watches) to monitor physical symptoms, bodily movements, sleep quality and characteristics, and physical locations. Recently, it has been integrated with app usage to increase symptom monitoring and intervention efficacy. Specifically, sensor technology has been used to monitor behavioral markers and "multimodal behavioral sensing" (e.g., physical movement through the use of Global Positioning System (GPS); bodily movements through "multi-axial accelerometers," sleep quality, and speech characteristics) to better assist in psychiatric assessments [29]. This technology has been found to be acceptable and helpful to individuals with serious mental illness in terms of targeting their weight loss efforts [56]. It has also been employed for symptom management with the goal of predicting psychotic relapse in individuals discharged from clinical services [57]. Conversation and voice data, including via phone call recordings and analysis of audio features (e.g., pitch, tone), have been utilized for monitoring individuals recovering from mood disorders [58]. Sensor technology provides the opportunity to move psychiatric assessment to natural environments outside of clinics, which may increase accuracy of diagnoses and ecological validity [29]. While sensor technology is relatively new in its usage for psychiatric purposes, it provides a promising new approach for symptom monitoring and potential intervention or prevention of relapse. However, additional research is needed in testing the accuracy of information collected by sensor technology.

5.3 Evidence for behavioral health apps for suicide prevention

5.3.1 Suicide-prevention apps

One behavioral health problem for which there has been considerable focus vis-à-vis behavioral mHealth technology is suicide prevention, with the most progress related to app development and evaluation. This reflects in large part mounting recognition of suicide as a major public health problem and, thus, suicide prevention as a high priority. Indeed, there have been clarion calls for scalable and sustainable suicide-prevention efforts [59]. In response, there has been a recent proliferation of suicide-prevention apps, many of which are in the app stores free of charge [60]. At the present time, there are close to 150 of such apps available and the number keeps going up [61,62]. Some of the most popular suicide-prevention apps include: A Friend Asks, My3, Guard Your, Ask & Prevent Suicide, Suicide Crisis Support, HELP Prevent Suicide, Stay ALIVE, and Operation Reach Out (https://www.tomsguide.com/us/suicide-prevention-apps,review-2397.html) [60].

Most of these apps include components that target identifying warning signs, securing crisis support, engaging in safety planning, using coping strategies, and accessing social support and professional help [62]. There is the strongest empirical evidence for apps or app components that facilitate accessing crisis support [62]. The majority of the existing apps incorporate a focus on a single suicide-prevention strategy and, typically, the strategy is in keeping with the pertinent evidence-base or best practice guidelines [62]. Unfortunately, some of these apps also include content that is potentially deleterious to the user, such as listing lethal access to means or encouraging risky behavior [62].

Despite the wealth of available apps, there has been little empirical study of the efficacy of this mHealth tool for suicide prevention. Not surprisingly, therefore, there have been recent efforts to create guidelines for the development, implementation, and evaluation of new suicide-prevention apps [61]. In addition, the case has been built for using other forms of technology, in addition to apps, for suicide prevention, such as video (e.g., YouTube) and podcasts [63].

5.3.2 Examples of specific suicide-prevention apps that have feasibility or efficacy data

The following offers a brief review of popular suicide-prevention apps that have been subjected to feasibility and/or efficacy evaluations.

MyPlan. Safety planning is an evidence-based tool for suicide prevention. It involves identifying warning signs for a suicidal crisis, delineating coping strategies that may be helpful, and listing available resource personal. The advantage of having a safety app available via smartphone ensures its accessibility whenever the smartphone itself is available. MyPlan is a mobile app on which people can create an individualized safety plan that includes strategies, actions, and direct links to key support people [64]. This is a frequently downloaded suicide-prevention app for which there is considerable positive feedback. Thus, while there is no formal evaluation of this app, systematic feedback about its value and utility has been gathered.

Virtual Hope Box. A common element of cognitive therapy (CT) and dialectical behavior therapy (DBT) is the Hope Box, a therapeutic tool that houses items that serve as a reminder of reasons for living that a patient can refer to when feeling hopeless. Each box varies from patient to patient, but may contain items such as important pictures, memorable letters, and future goals. The box has shown to be useful but has its limitation such as being physically difficult to carry, inaccessible or no private access in times of crisis. As result, the Virtual Hope Box (VHB) smartphone app was created by the National Center for Telehealth & Technology and is currently being tested with military and veterans. It is designed to help identify and affirm personalized reasons for living [65,66]. The VHB app currently includes six primary sections that are designed to provide support, comfort, distraction, or relaxation. The app includes audio, video, pictures, games, mindfulness exercises, messages, inspirational quotes, and coping statements. Patients have found the VHB to be convenient and easy to set up, beneficial, and helpful in reducing their suicidal thoughts, as well as increasing their capacity for emotion regulation, distress tolerance, and resilience. In 2014, the VHB project was awarded the Department of Defense (DoD) Innovation Award (U.S. Department of Veterans Affairs, 2018). Although users noted some drawbacks (e.g., missing the sensory experience of the traditional Hope Box), they indicated a high likelihood that they would use it again and would recommend it to their peers [65].

Therapeutic Evaluative Conditioning (TEC). This game-like app was designed to address self-injurious thoughts and behaviors (SITBs) by increasing aversion to these thoughts and behaviors and decreasing aversion to the self [67]. Use of this app as compared to no app is associated with moderate reductions on all SITBs, most notably self-cutting, suicidal plans, and suicidal behaviors, but not in suicidal ideation. Although the findings were promising, the positive impact of TEC was not evident at follow-up [6].

ReliefLink™. Another mobile app showing promise is Emory University's ReliefLink™, which is available as a free download for iPhone. ReliefLink™ addresses the issue of staying connected to mental health resources, and can be used in conjunction with standard care models including post discharge from acute/emergency care. It was developed by our clinical team as a free, user-centered mHealth tool, through a competitive grant from the 2013 Suicide Prevention: Continuity of Care and Follow-up App Challenge (SAMHSA) and was awarded $50,000 at a White House Conference (http://news.emory.edu/stories/2013/09/kaslow_relieflink_app/campus.html). ReliefLink™ provides information links to follow-up care, and includes an emergency 911 alert, appointment reminders, mood rating, locations of nearby services, tweet alerts, and coping activities.

A recently completed usability study of patient and non-patient experiences with ReliefLink™ was funded through the Emory-GaTech ACTSI Healthcare Innovations Program [79]. This study assessed the feasibility of ReliefLink™ for use in conjunction with standard care to promote psychological health and prevent suicidal behavior. The primary purpose was to inform the continued development of ReliefLink™, and explore how well-designed mobile apps can contribute to connectedness to care and resources that lead to clinically and socially relevant outcomes. To determine the usability of ReliefLink™, a brief semi-structured interview gathered users' adherence to assigned feature related tasks and qualitative, experiential commentary through a ReliefLink™ paper diary table, and quantitative ratings pertaining to user experience the System Usability Scale (SUS) indicators [68]. Strengths-based behavioral outcome measures also were obtained [69]. Over a 2-week timeframe, we collected our preliminary data from eight non-patient participants, to ensure software met stated design requirements. We then repeated the 2-week procedure with five patients already enrolled in standard care through our affiliated clinic following a suicide attempt/ideation. To ensure access to the ReliefLink™ app, which at this time is only available from the iOS platform, we assessed iOS and internet access during patient recruitment. Any patients without smartphones were assigned to a loaned study phone, and limited data plan if necessary. When the study was complete, participants returned borrowed study phones. Personal device access with an active phone/data plan was a stated requirement for non-patient to participate. In each sample, the ten outcome measures were used to measure psychological strengths and perceived access to resources, at baseline and then again at a 2-week follow-up. The SUS was also completed, and user experience paper diary was reviewed, during the final measurement period at the 2-week follow-up for both non-patients and patients.

All participants were assigned ReliefLink™ daily mood tracking and completion of a minimum of one stress-management activity per day, and trained on app function. Relaxation exercises to choose from on the current version of ReliefLink™ were audio files, and consisted of: Guided Meditation, Energizing Breath, Guided Visualization for Relaxation, Progressive Relaxation, Mindfulness Meditation Body Scan, and Mindfulness of Breathing. Usage data was tracked with a weekly diary sent home with users to record their app experience. Frequency of feature use and nature of comments were examined during the follow-up assessment.

No significant changes in outcome measurements were expected or assessed in either sample, over the 2-week study period, given the short length of the time period between measurements and small number of participants. Both non-patient and patient participants successfully completed the outcome and usability measurement battery in 2 hours or fewer. Re-usable spreadsheet-based templates for data analysis were successfully created and manipulated to upload data from the paper-and-pencil measurement battery. This suggested that the composition, quality, and length of the instruments contained in the measurement packet were appropriate, and no impediment to data analysis or interpretation was caused by these instruments. This also indicated that the measurement battery is viable for future studies with similar aim. A qualitative analysis revealed that the overall user acceptability was high, but the patient sample expressed more impediments to user acceptance. The greatest number of comments within each of the two samples were made for relaxation exercises: 23 (positive) and 9 (negative) – non-patients; 17 (positive) and 26 (negative) - patients. Qualitative comments yielded several areas for potential functional improvement of ReliefLink™ related to ensuring that the app is accessible to a broader array of users, is kept current, and that all features function well. The intent of the clinical research team is to implement ReliefLink™ into standard behavioral healthcare for patients at high risk of self-harm. We hope to integrate viable and effective, value-added features of ReliefLink™ with other mobile tools, toward a comprehensive toolkit for enhancing mental healthcare services. We would like to extend ReliefLink™ capabilities through integration with successfully fielded support programs, such as the Caring Contacts program [70]. The Caring Letters Project involves sending brief communications (e.g., letters, emails, or for an app could be text messages) that convey caring concern to suicidal persons, such as those recently discharged from the hospital, and it has been found to be feasible [71] and possibly associated with a statistically significant reduction in suicidal behavior [72]. We also intend to enhance it with a secure text-messaging feature that is compliant with current regulations, including the Health Insurance Portability and Accountability Act (HIPAA) and standards for telehealth [73]. Ultimately, the aim of future ReliefLink™ development projects is to develop and demonstrate a fully functional, cross-platform ReliefLink™ web-based product, including enhanced functionality in specific areas reflecting feedback provided directly from the intended user community.

5.4 Discussion

mHealth apps in general and for suicide prevention more specifically offer considerable promise in terms of expanding the accessibility and affordability of behavioral health services, overcoming common barriers to service utilization, and empowering people to take control of their own behavioral health. Indeed, there is a proliferation of behavioral health-related apps that offer assessment, symptom tracking, and/or interventions for a broad array of behavioral health problems, including suicidal behavior [38]. However, despite the increasing dependence on technology, behavioral health professionals have not capitalized on the potential of mHealth apps with regard to the provision of personalized assessments and interventions that ultimately can improve outcomes [74]. Doing so will require behavioral health professionals to ascertain what mHealth app best meets the suicidal person's needs, the patient's preference with regards to technology, the extent to which various apps meet appropriate regulatory and data security standards, the data in support of the app's efficacy [60]. They will also need to have a plan or protocol for the incorporation of the mHealth app into their care of the suicidal patient [60].

In addition, although there are many advantages of mHealth apps and preliminary results are promising, it is important to bear in mind that there is a dearth of data supporting their efficacy and their use in a psychotherapy context requires further research [5]. We need a stronger commitment to researching the effectiveness of mHealth apps, not just their feasibility. Such evaluations must consider the voices of patients, clinicians, researchers, and policymakers [75].

More research is necessary to test the efficacy of mHealth apps generally, as well as specifically related to suicide prevention and intervention, to ensure this form of assistive technology is providing additive benefits to mental health treatments. With the possibility of using mHealth applications in support of typical, current behavioral health treatments, or possibly in lieu of them, additional research will help determine which forms of assistive technology have the greatest efficacy. Agreed-upon standards need to be developed so that consumers can be informed about the extent to which a particular mHealth app has been shown to be effective for a given behavioral health concern. In addition, while we appreciate and share the excitement about the value of technology for advancing behavioral health care, we do not believe that technology can or should replace the key elements of quality behavioral health services, such as the therapeutic relationship including its motivational elements, collaborative decision-making, and personalized adjustments to care [76].

Despite the growing number of advantages of mHealth apps related to behavioral healthcare, there are still challenges on implementation using this new medium that need to be addressed going forward. These are related to ensuring the security of patient data, the transferability of data when mobile software is updated or phones or switched, and the operation of apps on different interfaces (Apple versus Android) [39,77]. More attention needs to be paid to guaranteeing privacy for mHealth app users and creating apps that can be utilized in the provision of behavioral health services in accord with federal privacy guidelines. For a suicidal person is particular, it is important to ensure that they do not become overly dependent on an app for assistance in a crisis and risk, feeling hopeless when the app fails [78].

Future efforts related to the development and efficacy evaluation of apps and other forms of mHealth could be optimized if there was greater collaboration among app developers, software engineers, clinical-researchers, and the patient population for whom the apps are designed to serve. Finally, in keeping with the technology evolution, the field is moving beyond apps to the use of avatars as vehicles for empowering people to take control of their own behavioral health concerns (https://www.washingtonpost.com/news/to-your-health/wp/2018/07/02/from-apps-to-avatars-new-tools-for-taking-control-of-your-mental-health/?noredirect=on&utm_term=.0b62b782e93f&wpisrc=nl_tech&wpmm=1). For example, there is now a humanoid robot (Pepper), who purportedly can "read" people's emotions and who has conducted mindfulness and meditation classes. In addition, there is some promising support for avatars that embody people's auditory hallucinations with regard to assisting individuals diagnosed with schizophrenia. This is a new frontier that will receive increasing clinical and research attention for individuals who both want assistance coping with everyday life stresses and those who are experiencing significant psychological distress and symptoms including suicidal behavior and attempts.

Conflict of interest

The authors have no conflict of interest to report.

Acknowledgements

The research presented in reference to ReliefLink™, was supported in part by the National Center for Advancing Translational Sciences of the National Institutes of Health under Award Number UL1TR000454. The content is solely the responsibility of the authors and does not necessarily represent the official views of the National Institutes of Health.

References

[1] Pew Research Center. (2018). Mobile fact sheet. Retrieved March 20, 2018 from http://www.pewinternet.org/fact-sheet/mobile/

[2] Sherwin-Smith, J., & Pritchard-Jones, R. (2012). Medical applications: The future of regulation. *Annals of the Royal College of Surgeons of England*, 94, 12–16. doi: 10.1308/147363512X13189526438512

[3] Borrelli, B., & Ritterband, L. M. (2015). Special issue on eHealth and mHealth: Challenges and future directions for assessments, treatment, and dissemination. *Health Psychology*, 34, 1205–1208. doi: 10.1037/hea0000323

[4] Donker, T., Petrie, K., Proudfoot, J., Clarke, J., Birch, M.-R., & Christensen, H. (2013). Smartphones for smarter delivery of mental health programs: A systematic review. *Journal of Medical Internet Research*, 15, e247. doi: 10.2196/jmir.2791

[5] Lui, J. H. L., Marcus, D. K., & Barry, C. T. (2017). Evidence-based apps? A review of mental health mobile applications in a psychotherapy context. *Professional Psychology: Research and Practice*, 48, 199–210. doi: 10.1037/pro0000122

[6] Luxton, D. D., McCann, R. A., Bush, N. E., Mishkind, M. C., & Reger, G. M. (2011). mHealth for mental health: Integrating smartphone technology in behavioral healthcare. *Professional Psychology: Research and Practice*, 42, 505–512. doi: 10.1037/a0024485

[7] Payne, H. E., Lister, C., & Bernhardt, J. M. (2015). Behavioral functionality of mobile apps in health interventions: A systematic review of the literature. *JMIR Mhealth Uhealth*, 3, e20. doi: 10.2196/mhealth.3335

[8] Casey, L. M., Joy, A., & Clough, B. A. (2013). The impact of information on attitudes toward e-mental health services. *Cyberpsychology, Behavior, and Social Networking*, 16, 593–598. doi: 10.1089/cyber.2012.0515

[9] Klein, B., & Cook, S. (2010). Preferences for e-mental health services amongst an online Australian sample. *E-Journal of Applied Psychology*, 6, 28–39. doi: 10.7790/ejap.v6i1.184

[10] Bircker, J. B., Mull, K. E., Kientz, J. A., *et al.* (2014). Randomized, controlled pilot trial of a smartphone app for smoking cessation using acceptance and commitment therapy. *Drug and Alcohol Dependence*, 143, 87–94. doi: 10.1016/j.drugalcdep.2014.07.006

[11] Gustafson, D. H., McTavish, F. M., Chih, M. Y., *et al.* (2014). A smartphone application to support recovery from alcoholism: A randomized clinical trial. *JAMA Psychiatry*, 71(566–572). doi: 10.1001/jamapsychiatry.2013.4642

[12] López, S. R., Barrio, C. A., Kopelowicz, A., & Vega, W. A. (2012). From documenting to eliminating disparities in mental health care for Latinos. *American Psychologist*, 67, 511–523. doi: 10.1037/a0029737

[13] Free, C., Phillips, G., Watson, L. B., *et al.* (2013). The effectiveness of mobile-health technologies to improve health care service delivery processes: A systematic review and meta-analysis. *PLOS Medicine*, 10, e1001363. doi: 10.1371/journal.pmed.1001363

[14] Mohr, D. C., Burns, M. N., Schueller, S. M., Clarke, G. N., & Klinkman, M. (2013). Behavioral intervention technologies: Evidence review and recommendations for future research in mental health. *General Hospital Psychiatry*, 35, 332–338. doi: 10.1016/j.genhosppsych.2013.03.008

[15] Substance Abuse and Mental Health Services Administration. (2017). Key substance use and mental health indicators in the United States: Results from the 2016 National Survey on Druge Use and Health). (HHS Publication No. SMA 17-5044, NSDUH Series H-52). Rockville, MD: Center for Behavioral Health Statistics and Quality, Substance Abuse and Mental Health Services Administration. Retrieved from https://www.samhsa.gov/data/.

[16] Vigo, D., Thornicroft, G., & Atun, R. (2016). Estimating the true global burden of mental illness. *The Lancet Psychiatry*, 3, 171–178. doi: 10.1016/S2215-0366(15)00505-2

[17] Andrade, L. H., Alonso, J., Mneimneh, Z., *et al.* (2014). Barriers to mental health treatment: Results from the WHO World Mental Health surveys. *Psychological Medicine*, 44, 1313–1317. doi: 10.1017/S0033291713001943

[18] Clement, S., Schauman, O., Graham, T., *et al.* (2015). What is the impact of mental health-related stigma on help-seeking? A systematic review of quantitative and qualitative studies. *Psychological Medicine*, 45, 11–27. doi: 10.1017/S0033291714000129

[19] Kazdin, A. E., & Rabbitt, S. M. (2013). Novel models for delivering mental health services and reducing the burdens of mental illness. *Clinical Psychological Science*, 1, 170–191. doi: 10.1177/2167702612463566

[20] Miner, A., Kuhn, E., Hoffman, J. E., Owen, J. E., Ruzek, J. I., & Taylor, C. B. (2016). Feasibility, acceptability, and potential efficacy of the PTSD Coach app: A pilot randomized controlled trial with community trauma survivors. *Psychological Trauma: Theory, Research, Practice, and Policy*, 8, 384–392. doi: 10.1037/tra0000092

[21] Shalev, A. Y., Ankri, Y., Israeli-Shalev, Y., Peleg, T., Adessky, R., & Freedman, S. (2012). Prevention of posttraumatic stress disorder by early treatment: Results from the Jerusalem Trauma Outreach And Prevention

study. *Archives of General Psychiatry*, 69, 166–176. doi: 10.1001/archgenpsychiatry.2011.127

[22] Korsbek, L., & Tonder, E. S. (2016). Momentum: A smartphone application to support shared decision making for people using mental health services. *Psychiatric Rehabilitation Journal*, 39, 167–172. doi: 10.1037/prj0000173

[23] Bush, N. E., Ouellette, G., & Kinn, J. (2014). Utility of the T2 mood tracker mobile application among army warrior transition unit service members. *Military Medicine*, 179, 1453–1457. doi: 10.7205/MILMED-D-14-00271

[24] Gliddon, E., Barnes, S. J., Murray, G., & Michalak, E. E. (2017). Online and mobile technologies for self-management in bipolar disorder: A systematic review. *Psychiatric Rehabilitation Journal*, 40, 309–319. doi: 10.1037/prj0000270

[25] Luxton, D. D., Hansen, R. N., & Stanfill, K. (2014). Mobile app self-care versus in-office care for stress reduction: A cost minimization analysis. *Journal of Telemedicine and Telecare*, 20, 431–435. doi: 10.1177/1357633X14555616

[26] Bennike, I. H., Wieghorst, A., & Kirk, U. (2017). Online-based mindfulness training reduces behavioral markers of mind wandering. *Journal of Cognitive Enhancement*, 1, 172–181. doi: 10.1007/s41465-017-0020-9

[27] van Emmerik, A. A. P., Berings, F., & Lancee, J. (2018). Efficacy of a mindfulness-based mobile application: A randomized waiting-list controlled trial. *Mindfulness*, 9, 187–198. doi: 10.1007/s12671-017-0761-7

[28] McColl, L. D., Rideout, P. E., Parmar, T. N., & Abba-Aji, A. (2014). Peer support intervention through mobile application: An integrative literature review and future directions. *Canadian Psychology/Psychologie Canadienne*, 55, 250–257. doi: 10.1037/a0038095

[29] Ben-Zeev, D., Scherer, E. A., Wang, R., Xie, H., & Campbell, A. T. (2015). Next-generation psychiatric assessment: Using smartphone sensors to monitor behavior and mental health. *Psychiatric Rehabilitation Journal*, 38, 218–226. doi: 10.1037/prj0000130

[30] Ly, K. H., Asplund, K., & Andersson, G. (2014). Stress management for middle managers via an acceptance and commitment-based smartphone application: A randomized controlled trial. *Internet Interventions*, 1, 95–101. doi: 10.1016/j.invent.2014.06.003

[31] Ly, K. H., Carlbring, P., & Andersson, G. (2012). Behavioral activation-based guided self-help treatment administered through a smartphone application: Study protocol for a randomized controlled trial. *Trials*, 13, 62. doi: 10.1186/1745-6215-13-62

[32] Ly, K. H., Truschel, A., Jarl, L., *et al.* (2014). Behavioural activation versus mindfulness-based guided self-help treatment administered through smartphone application: A randomised controlled trial. *BMJ Open*, 4, e003440. doi: 10.1136/bmjopen-2013-003440

[33] Mani, M., Kavanagh, D. J., Hides, L., & Stoyanov, S. R. (2015). Review and evaluation of mindfulness-based iPhone apps. *JMIR Mhealth and Uhealth*, 3, e82. doi: http://dx.doi.org/10.2196/mhealth.4328

[34] Ben-Zeev, D., Kaiser, S. M., Brenner, C. J., Begale, M., Duffecy, J., & Mohr, D. C. (2014). Development and usability testing of FOCUS: A smartphone system for self-management of schizophrenia. *Psychiatric Rehabilitation Journal*, 36, 289–296. doi: 10.1037/prj0000019

[35] Clough, B. A., & Casey, L. M. (2015). The smart therapist: A look to the future of smartphones and mHealth technologies in psychotherapy. *Professional Psychology: Research and Practice*, 46, 147–153. doi: 10.1037/pro0000011

[36] Sucala, M., Cuijpers, P., Muench, F., *et al.* (2017). Anxiety: There is an app for that. A systematic review of anxiety apps. *Depression and Anxiety*, 34, 518–525. doi: 10.1002/da.22654

[37] Torous, J., & Powell, A. C. (2015). Current research and trends in the use of smartphone applications for mood disorders. *Internet Interventions*, 2, 169–173. doi: 10.1016/j.invent.2015.03.002

[38] Van Ameringen, M., Turna, J., Khalesi, Z., Pullia, K., & Patterson, B. (2017). There is an app for that! The current state of mobile applications (apps) for DSM-5 obsessive-compulsive disorder, posttraumatic stress disorder, anxiety and mood disorders. *Depression and Anxiety*, 34, 526–539. doi: 10.1002/da.22657

[39] Reger, G. M., Browne, K. C., Campellone, T. R., *et al.* (2017). Barriers and facilitators to mobile application use during PTSD treatment: Clinician adoption of PE coach. *Professional Psychology: Research and Practice*, 48, 510–517. doi: 10.1037/pro0000153

[40] Reger, G. M., Hoffman, J., Riggs, D., *et al.* (2013). The "PE Coach" smartphone application: An innovative approach to improving implementation, fidelity, and homework adherence during prolonged exposure. *Psychological Services*, 10, 342–349. doi: 10.1037/a0032774

[41] Scholosser, D. A., Campellone, T. R., Truong, B., *et al.* (2017). The feasibility, acceptability, and outcomes of PRIME-D: A novel mobile intervention treatment for depression. *Depression and Anxiety*, 34, 546–554. doi: 10.1002/da.22624RESEARCH

[42] Kuhn, E., Kanuri, N., Hoffman, J. E., Garvert, D. W., Ruzek, J. I., & Taylor, C. B. (2017). A randomized controlled trial of a smartphone app for posttraumatic stress disorder symptoms. *Journal of Consulting and Clinical Psychology*, 85, 267–273. doi: 10.1037/ccp0000163

[43] Possemato, K., Kuhn, E., Johnson, E., *et al.* (2017). Using PTSD Coach in primary care with and without clinician support: A pilot randomized controlled trial. *General Hospital Psychiatry*, 38, 94–98. doi: 10.1016/j.genhosppsych.2015.09.005

[44] Aschbrenner, K. A., Naslund, J. A., Gill, L. E., Bartels, S. J., & Ben-Zeev, D. (2016). A qualitative study of client-clinician text exchanges in a mobile health intervention for individuals with psychotic disorders and substance abuse. *Journal of Dual Diagnosis*, 12, 63–71. doi: 10.1080/15504263.2016.1145312

[45] Aguilera, A., & Munoz, R. F. (2011). Text messaging as an adjunct to CBT in low-income populations: A usability and feasibility pilot study. *Professional Psychology: Research and Practice*, 42, 427–478. doi: 10.1037/a0025499

[46] Bauer, S., Okon, E., Meermann, R., & Kordy, H. (2012). Technology-enhanced maintenance of treatment gains in eating disorders: Efficacy of an intervention delivered via text messaging. *Journal of Consulting and Clinical Psychology*, 80, 700–706. doi: 10.1037/a0028030

[47] Haug, S., Castro, R. P., Kowatsch, T., Filler, A., Dey, M., & Schaub, M. P. (2017). Efficacy of a web- and test messaging-based intervention to reduce problem drinking in adolescents: Results of a cluster-randomized controlled trial. *Journal of Consulting and Clinical Psychology*, 85, 147–159. doi: 10.1037/ccp0000138

[48] Naslund, J. A., Aschbrenner, K. A., Marsch, L. A., & Bartels, S. J. (2016). The future of mental health care: Peer-to-peer support and social media. *Epidemiology and Psychiatric Sciences*, 25, 113–122. doi: 10.1017/S2045796015001067

[49] Shiffman, S., Stone, A. A., & Hufford, M. R. (2008). Ecological momentary assessment. *Annual Review of Clinical Psychology*, 4, 1–32. doi: 10.1146/annurev.clinpsy.3.022806.091415

[50] Shiffman, S. (2009). Ecological momentary assessment (EMA) in studies of substance use. *Psychological Assessment*, 21, 486–497. doi: 10.1037/a0017074

[51] Andrewes, H. E., Hulbert, C., Cotton, S. M., Betts, J., & Chanen, A. M. (2017). Ecological momentary assessment of nonsuicidal self-injury in youth with borderline personality disorder. *Personal Disord.* 8(357–365). doi: 10.1037/per0000205

[52] Moore, R. C., Depp, C. A., Wetherell, J. L., & Lenze, E. J. (2016). Ecological momentary assessment versus standard assessment instruments for measuring mindfulness, depressed mood, anx anxiety among older adults. *Journal of Psychiatric Research*, 75, 116–123. doi: 10.1016/j.jpsychires.2016.01.011

[53] Verslius, A., Verkuil, B., Spinhoven, P., van der Ploeg, M. M., & Brosschot, J. F. (2016). Changing mental health and positive psychological well-being using ecological momentary interventions: A systematic review and meta-analysis. *Journal of Medical Internet Research*, 18, e152. doi: 10.2196/jmir.5642

[54] Schueller, S. M., Aguilera, A., & Mohr, D. C. (2017). Ecological momentary interventions for depression and anxiety. *Depression and Anxiety*, 34, 540–545. doi: 10.1002/da.22649

[55] van Os, J., Verhagen, S., Marsman, A., *et al.* (2017). The experience sampling methods as an mHealth tool to support self-monitoring, self-insight, and personalized health care in clinical practice. *Depression and Anxiety*, 34, 481–493. doi: 10.1002/da.22647

[56] Naslund, J. A., Aschbrenner, K. A., Barre, L. K., & Bartels, S. J. (2015). Feasibility of popular m-Health technologies for activity tracking among individuals with serious mental illness. *Telemedicine and e-Health*, 21, 213–216. doi: 10.1089/tmj.2014.0105

[57] Ben-Zeev, D., Brian, R., Wang, R., *et al.* (2017). CrossCheck: Integrating self-report, behavioral sensing, and smartphone use to identify digital indicators of psychotic relapse. *Psychiatry Rehabilitation Journal*, 40, 266–275. doi: 10.1037/prj0000243

[58] Or, F., Torous, J., & Onnela, J.-P. (2017). High potential but limited evidence: Using voice data from smartphones to monitor and diagnose mood disorders. *Psychiatric Rehabilitation Journal*, 40, 320–324. doi: 10.1037/prj0000279

[59] Kreuze, E., Jenkins, C., Gregoski, M., *et al.* (2017). Technology-enhanced suicide prevention interventions: A systematic review. *Journal of Telemedicine and Telecare*, 23, 605–617. doi: 10.1177/1357633X16657928

[60] Luxton, D. D., June, J. D., & Chalker, S. A. (2015). Mobile health technologies for suicide prevention: Feature review and recommendations for use in clinical care. *Current Treatment Options in Psychiatry*, 2, 349–362. doi: 10.1007/s40501-015-0057-2

[61] Aguirre, R. T. P., McCoy, M. K., & Roan, M. (2013). Development guidelines from a study of suicide prevention mobile applications (apps). *Journal of Technology in Human Services*, 31, 269–293. doi: 10.1080/15228835.2013.814750

[62] Larsen, M. E., Nicholas, J., & Christensen, H. (2016). A systematic assessment of smartphone tools for suicide prevention. *PLOS ONE*, 11, e0152285. doi: 10.1371/journal.pone.0152285

[63] Luxton, D. D., June, J. D., & Kinn, J. T. (2011). Technology-based suicide prevention: Current applications and future directions. *Telemedicine and e-Health*, 17, 50–54. doi: 10.1089/tmj.2010.0091

[64] Larsen, J. L., Frandsen, J., & Erlangsen, A. (2016). MYPLAN – A mobile phone application for supporting people at risk for suicide. *Crisis*, 37, 1–5. doi: 10.1027/0227-5910/a000371

[65] Bush, N. E., Dobscha, S. K., Crumpton, R., *et al.* (2015). A virtual hope box smartphone app as an accessary to therapy: Proof-of-concept in a clinical sample of veterans. *Suicide and Life-Threatening Behavior*, 45, 1–9. doi: 10.1111/sltb.12103

[66] Bush, N. E., Smolenski, D. J., Denneson, L. M., Williams, H. B., Thomas, E. K., & Dobscha, S. K. (2017). A virtual hope box: Randomized controlled trial of a smartphone app of emotional regulation and coping with distress. *Psychiatric Services*, 68, 330–336. doi: 10.1176/appi.ps.201600283

[67] Franklin, J. C., Fox, K. R., Franklin, C. R., *et al.* (2016). A brief mobile app reduces nonsuicidal and suicidal self-injury: Evidence from three randomized controlled trials. *Journal of Consulting and Clinical Psychology*, 84, 544–557. doi: 10.1037/ccp0000093

[68] Brooke, J. (1986). *System usability scale: A quick-and-dirty method of system evaluation user information*. Reading, UK: Digital Equipment Co Ltd.

[69] Wagstaff, C. R. D., & Leach, J. (2015). The value of strengths-based approaches in SERE and sport psychology. *Military Psychology*, 27, 65–84. doi: 10.1037/mil0000066

[70] Luxton, D. D., Thomas, E. K., Chipps, J., *et al.* (2014). Caring letters for suicide prevention: Implementation of a multi-site randomized clinical trial in the U.S. military and Veteran Affairs Health Systems. *Contemporary Clinical Trials*, 37, 252–260. doi: 10.1016/j.cct.2014.01.007

[71] Luxton, D. D., Kinn, J. T., June, J. D., Pierre, L. W., Reger, M. A., & Gahm, G. A. (2012). Caring Letters Project: A military suicide-prevention pilot program. *Crisis*, 33, 5–12. doi: 10.1027/0227-5910/a000093

[72] Luxton, D. D., June, J. D., & Comtois, K. A. (2013). Can post discharge follow-up contacts prevent suicide and suicidal behavior? A review of the evidence *Crisis*, 34, 32–41. doi: 10.1027/0227-5910/a000158

[73] Luxton, D. D., Kayl, R. A., & Mishkind, M. C. (2012). mHealth data security: The need for HIPAA-compliant standardization. *Telemedicine and e-Health*, 18, 284–288. doi: 10.1089/tmj.2011.0180

[74] Aung, M. H., Matthews, M., & Choudhury, T. (2017). Sensing behavioral symptoms of mental health and delivering personalized interventions using mobile technologies. *Depression and Anxiety*, 34, 603–609. doi: 10.1002/da.22646

[75] Torous, J., & Roberts, L. W. (2017). Needed innovation in digital health and smartphone applications for mental health: Transparency and trust. *JAMA Psychiatry*, 74, 437–438. doi: 10.1001/jamapsychiatry.2017.0262

[76] Arean, P., & Cuijpers, P. (2017). Technology and mental health. *Depression and Anxiety*, 34, 479–480. doi: 10.1002/da.22636

[77] Maged, N., Boulous, K., Brewer, A. C., Karimikhani, C., Buller, D. B., & Dellavalle, R. P. (2014). Mobile medical and health apps: State of the art, concerns, regulatory control and certification. *Online Journal of Public Health Informatics*, 53, e229. doi: 10.5210/ojphi.v5i3.4814

[78] Ozdalga, E., Ozdalga, A., & Ahuja, N. (2012). The smartphone in medicine: A review of current and potential use among physicians and students. *Journal of Medical Internet Research*, 14, e128. doi: 10.2196/jmir.1994

[79] Crooks, C., Kaslow, N., & Luxton, D. (2016). *ReliefLink: A preventative mobile toolkit for follow-up care of behavioral health patients*. Poster presented at the 2016 Stanford MedX Conference, September 2016, Palo Alto, CA.

Chapter 6

The gamification of mental health prevention and promotion

Robert Anthony, M.B.A.[1] *and Nadja Reilly, Ph.D.*[2]

The World Health Organization defines mental health as the foundation for physical health and well-being and effective functioning. Mental health encompasses the self and others within an environment that promotes emotional, social, and cognitive well-being. Further, improvement of mental health is not an elusive ideal to be reached, but a priority to be intentionally addressed and maintained. Traditional mental health models are not reaching the amount of children and adolescents in need of services. Technology, however, may offer a unique platform for the creation of innovative solutions to reach a broader number of children globally given the number of children connected to various forms of digital platforms. Therefore, programming that integrates the fields of child development, psychology, learning, and gaming offer a significant potential to address the promotion of mental health and wellness.

6.1 Introduction

Play is so critical to child development that the United Nations Convention on the Rights of the Child, an international treaty that sets out universally accepted rights for children, identified play as a fundamental right of all children [1]. Play takes on many forms and definitions; however, as Yogman (2018) states, "there is a growing consensus that it is an activity that is intrinsically motivated, entails active engagement, and results in joyful discovery. Play is voluntary and often has no extrinsic goals; it is fun and often spontaneous" [2]. Play has many benefits for children, including socialization, learning of social norms, and regulation of emotions. It also has tremendous positive impacts on cognitive functioning. As Yogman (2018) describes, executive functioning, "which is described as the process of how we learn over the content of what we learn, is a core benefit of play and can be characterized by three dimensions: cognitive flexibility, inhibitory control, and working memory. Collectively, these dimensions allow for sustained attention, the

[1]Adolescent Wellness, Inc., Naples, FL, USA
[2]Freedman Center for Child and Family Development, William James College, Newton, MA, USA

filtering of distracting details, improved self-regulation and self-control, better problem solving, and mental flexibility" [3]. Interestingly, these dimensions are also critical for children's healthy emotional regulation and management, as well as for the development of active coping skills [4]. Furthermore, it is these skills that are the focus of mental health–promotion activities.

Why is it so critical to address fundamental activities of children, such as play, and focus on mental health promotion? Presently, the typical development of 1:5 children under the age of 18 is interrupted by some form of developmental, emotional, or behavioural problem. In fact, 10–20% of children and adolescents worldwide experience mental disorders [5]. Additionally, there is a large discrepancy between the proportion of children who need services and those who are actually diagnosed and subsequently receive services [6,7]. The mental health needs of many young people remain undetected and unaddressed on a global level [8]. When left unaddressed, mental health disorders can have long-lasting negative consequences, including higher risk of developing physical and mental disorders, substance use, lower educational attainment, and poorer overall quality of life [9,10]. Knowing these adverse long-term effects, we must transition from the common focus of individual treatment to an intentional focus on mental health prevention and promotion [11].

According to the Institute of Medicine's 2009 publication, "Preventing Mental, Emotional, and Behavioral Disorders Among Young People," the terms prevention and promotion are often used interchangeably, but important differences exist. Prevention refers to programs and activities designed to reduce incidence of harmful circumstance that target a population. Promotion refers to programs that promote attitudes, behaviours, and lifestyles that enable people to achieve and maintain physical, mental, social well-being [12]. Mental health–promotion strategies are typically used with a whole population, so they are particularly well suited for platforms that allow access to large groups of people. Furthermore, mental health–promotion strategies benefit everyone, regardless of presence or symptoms of mental illness, making them particularly beneficial when implemented on a large scale.

According to Beals (2011), the internet can be both a tool and a setting for improving mental health and well-being as children are immersed in media that shape the way they live and learn [13]. Access to the internet is increasing globally, largely through smartphones. In Ghana, over a third of children (36%) age 12 and older are able to access the internet; in Brazil it is 85% of children age 9–17 years (Global Kids Online) [14]. In the United States, 88% of teens ages 13–17 say they have access to a computer at home; 95% have access to a smartphone [15]. For comparison, a global survey completed in the Spring of 2018 summarized the median percentage of adults who report owning a smartphone at 45% in emerging economies and 76% in advanced economies [16].

Sixty-two percent of smartphone owners have used their phone in the past year to look up information about a health condition [17]. The rapid growth in the use of online technologies among youth provides a unique opportunity to increase access to mental health resources through apps and games. Multiple apps aimed at promoting health and wellness are available. Examples range from the US commercial products on mindfulness called iBreathe [18] and Headspace [19] to High Res [20] from the Australian government that adapts evidence-based cognitive behaviour therapy tools for daily stress management and resilience training. Combining lessons learned from the successful aspects of wellness focused apps and with developmentally appropriate mental health–promotion strategies presents a particularly interesting and helpful approach to promoting emotional health among youth.

6.2 Making it playful

Given the inherent importance of play for children, the benefits of play upon critical components of emotional health, and the increased access to information and play through online platforms, it is essential to find opportunities to create accessible and responsible digital programming to promote children's mental health and wellness. Such an opportunity arose in 2011, when conversations with James Bowers, Ph.D., and Jennifer Sun, Ph.D. from Numedeon, Inc., and the two authors of this book chapter sparked an idea for providing mental health and wellness resources directly to children through an educational game platform called Whyville [21]. Whyville is a cooperative learning site designed for users ages 7 and older across the world. Whyville was launched in 1999 to provide a socially interactive space for children to engage in science, technology, engineering, and mathematics (e.g., "STEM")-related activities hosted by several organizations including NASA, Toyota, and the Getty foundation [22]. It includes both science-based and recreational games as well as chat and intra-Whyville email. Over the lifetime of the website, the cumulative user population of Whyville is over 8 million "citizens" or unique registered users. The current count for active users is 142,000 [23]. The population of Whyville is comprised of 27% boys and 73% girls with an average of 6,500 visitors per month [23]. The virtual world of Whyville is set up as individual locations within a larger map, and each location focuses on a specific activity. Virtual worlds offer a unique setting for learning given their interactive gaming component, and are a great setting for teaching skills, as they include engaging activities, encourage cooperative play, and challenge players to use creativity to solve problems [24,25] (Figure 6.1).

The idea was to use Whyville as the virtual location where users could access activities specifically created to promote mental health and wellness and the development of active coping skills. To test the idea, Adolescent Wellness, Inc. (AWI), funded a pilot project with the platform owner, Numedeon, and William James College to learn whether children would a) recognize a stressed avatar and b) care to help it get better.

Winning the stressed avatar game occurs by selecting enough helpful questions and suggestions to reduce the avatar's stress level (from highest "three" to lowest "zero" level of stress) before time expires. In the pilot version, the avatar's stress related to difficulties with peers and school. Unhelpful questions and suggestions are rejected by the avatar with a comment as to why they are unhelpful. Winning a game successfully reduces the stress level to zero and generates rewards (a "clam

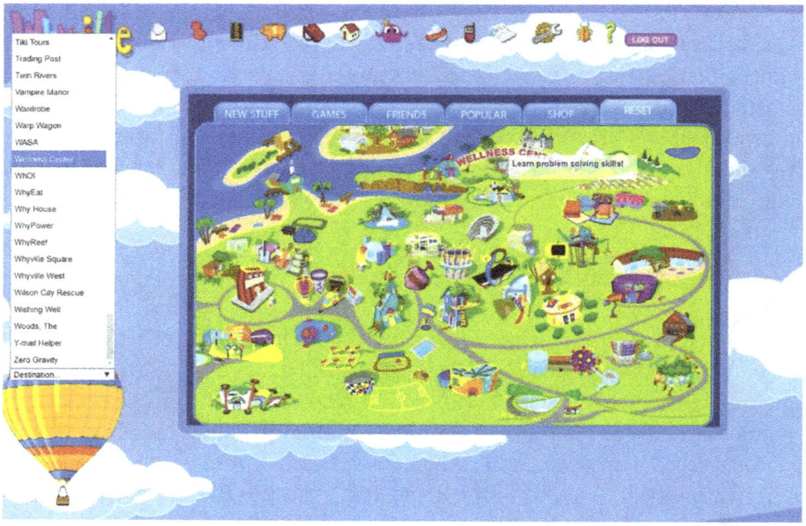

Figure 6.1 Overview of the Whyville map of activity locations

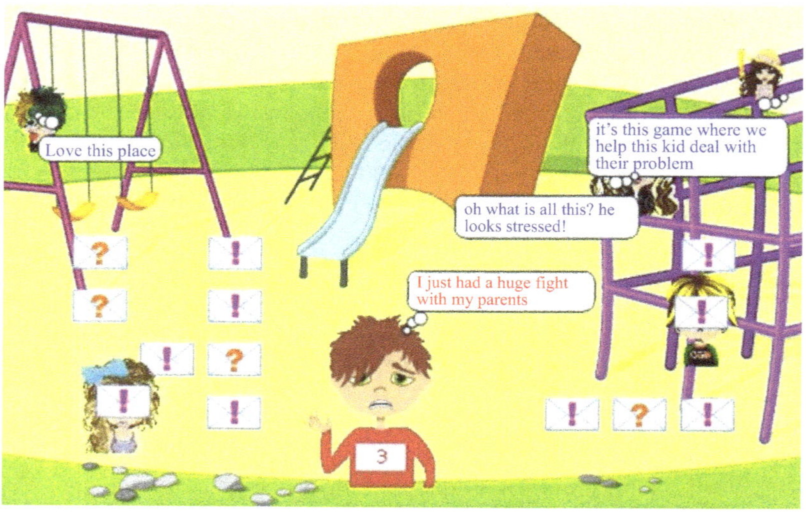
Love this place
it's this game where we help this kid deal with their problem
oh what is all this? he looks stressed!
I just had a huge fight with my parents
3

Figure 6.2 Stressed avatar

storm" – clams are the virtual currency of Whyville) for all game participants and observers. This feature of the game is important, as it not only maintains interest for the observers, but also offers an opportunity to learn through the observation of what others do even before trying the activity (Figure 6.2).

Responses to the stressed avatar were overwhelmingly positive, and from that initial idea and activity, a larger project was created. A new destination within the virtual Whyville world, the Wellness Center, was developed and launched in June 2013. The aim of the Wellness Center was to create a safe space with interactive opportunities for children to develop social and self-awareness, effective ways to manage their emotions and achieve their goals, positive communication and relationships, and effective problem-solving skills.

The inviting design of the Wellness Center, as well as the topics addressed within it, were based on direct feedback from adolescents ages nine to sixteen. All activities within the Wellness Center focus on mental health promotion and are available to all Whyville users. An important component of the development of the Wellness Center was the partnership among experts in different fields to create accessible, translatable activities. Within the Wellness Center, all mental health–related content was created by mental health providers with expertise in child development, disorders of childhood and adolescence, and promotion and prevention strategies. The gaming experts at Whyville then translated these concepts into engaging, accessible activities (Figure 6.3).

When the Wellness Center was created, the stressed avatar game was enhanced to specifically address additional themes that Whyville users, through a focus group, identified as topics of particular interest. These topics are: bullying, depression, eating disorders, empathy, grief and loss, making friends, social anxiety, and stress. Entirely new interactive games and activities were also created for the Wellness Center, including a journaling activity, the PIP (Problems, Ideas, Plans), and various relaxation activities. Activities were created with learning and

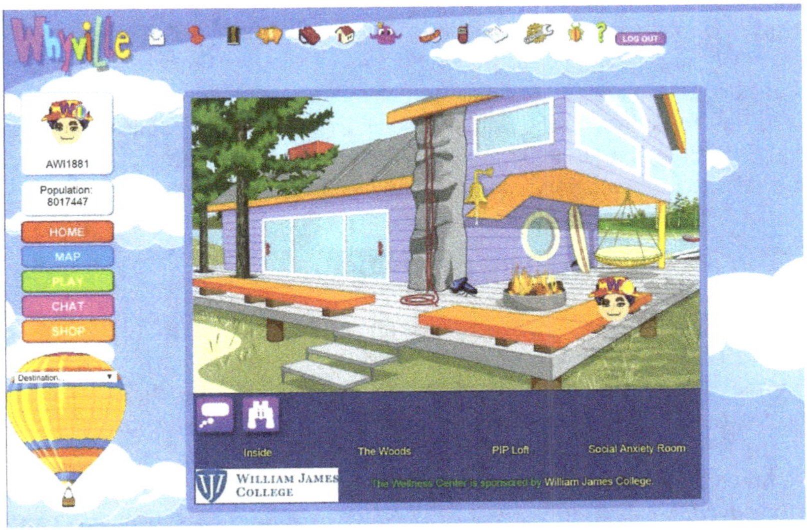

Figure 6.3 Outside the Wellness Center

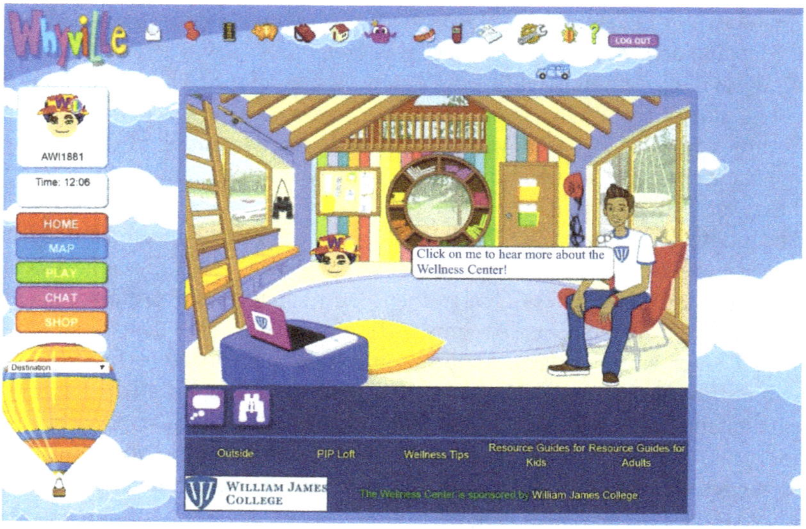

Figure 6.4 Inside the Wellness Center, first floor

development in mind, offering multiple formats to account for different learning styles and preferences. In addition to the activities, the Wellness Center houses supplemental resources on emotions and coping through downloadable tip sheets and links to existing resources (Figure 6.4).

An important component of mental health promotion is the intentional awareness of mood on a daily basis. Using past information for learning is also important. Therefore, the Wellness Center includes a format to identify and journal mood on a daily basis (through the Mood Ring activity), as well as a repository of information that keeps track of each player's participation in the games, ideas for problem solving, and access to tip sheets through the user's personal log, called the Wellness Book. These additional features give users access to their progress, daily learning, and, therefore, create a vehicle for practicing regular mental health and wellness strategies.

6.3 Use of Wellness Center activities

Over 20,000 youth have exercised at least one of the games in the Wellness Center since 2012 (Figure 6.5). Several hundred children participated in a survey, confirming the Wellness Center to be useful for coping with life challenges. As one youth reported, "*When my friends were fighting, I stopped them and said a thing that a distressed avatar said.*"

Another explained, "*I've used the PIP, tip sheets and resource sheets. I've recently moved to a new city on my own, both my parents have passed away, so I've been struggling with depression a lot. Using the information really helped me understand my feelings and cope. I had a counselor back in my previous city but*

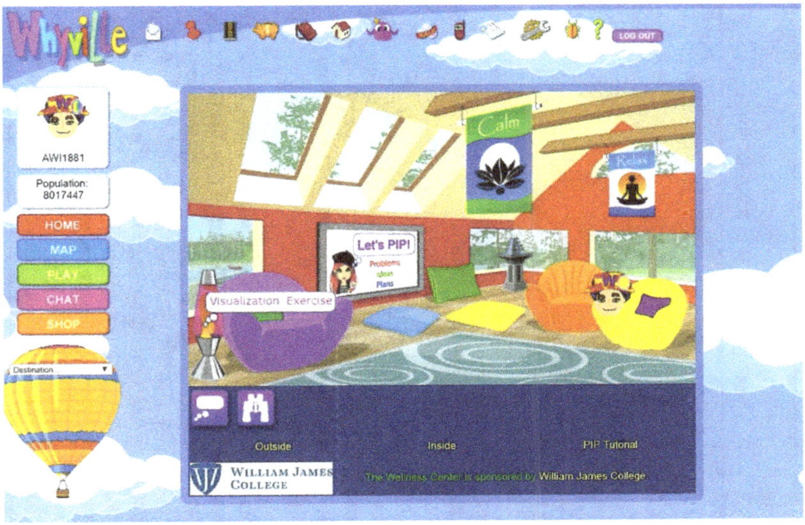

Figure 6.5 Inside the Wellness Center, PIP loft

haven't had the chance to find one here so the information available on Whyville was an amazing find. I particularly like the (PIP Problems-Ideas-Plans) *sheets you fill out to determine a process to act upon. I'd like to thank Whyville for bringing the wellness center here, it's a gem.*" Selected responses to a poll of users following completion of the PIP tutorial for creative problem solving are shown in Tables 6.1 and 6.2.

6.3.1 Generalizing online use to real-world scenarios

An important consideration of promoting mental health and wellness among children and adolescents is how to create a community that will support this learning in various settings and will help children generalize the skills they learned to new situations.

To examine the feasibility of using Whyville in different contexts, Adolescent Wellness and William James engaged different partners to use Whyville with the children with whom they interacted. One critical setting where mental health and wellness is promoted is the school setting. Schools are increasingly focusing on students' social and emotional competence as a critical component of academic success and have identified the science behind the connection of emotions to cognitive and academic functioning [26]. In 2016, the "Whyville Teacher's Tutorial: Adolescent Wellness Program"; was added to the Wellness Center to help teachers access lessons that teach social emotional learning skills to their students; 407 teacher accounts are now associated with the Adolescent Wellness program [27].

A middle school in Massachusetts piloted activities from the Wellness Center with its 6th, 7th, and 8th grade students. While there was definite interest from the

Table 6.1 PIP Problems-Ideas-Plans tutorial poll questions and responses

What did you think about the PIP?	What was it like to come up with a problem and define it?	What was helpful? Difficult?	Why does it make sense to break down large problems into smaller portions?
It helps me calm down without stressing out by taking it step by step	Made me felt more in control	It was difficult, but relieving	To identify what the real problem is and the best way to solve it.
I liked it, it helped me decide on a situation	Felt good to solve things out on my own	Helpful very, solved my own real life problem	It was calming to break it down like that, instead of bottling it up.
Easy way to break stuff down and help u concentrate	At first i was confused but then i thought "wow this is actually helping!"	The feeling of fixing it was awesome! it really was helpful!! picking ideas i wrote felt real good.	It helps lighten the load of what you are actually experiencing.
Really cool and helpful, and a good way to break down complex issues that seem hard to solve.	It would like dissecting my problem and pairing all the little problems with solutions.	It was helpful. I usually am not social and I do not like describing my problems but this was kind of like a diary!	Sometimes people can be so negative and not see that there is a way to come up with a solution to their problem
I think it helped me with finding a place to start with all my questions and how I can solve them on my own.	It's like, I feel smart. Like if I can figure out what my problem is, I can deal with it or solve it.	It was rather tough thinking of a problem's definition, usually I just avoid thinking about a problem altogether.	It gives you a better chance of slowing down and breathing so that you can solve the problem by easier means rather than stressing about the whole thing at once.
I think it was very helpful! It really helps you think about how to take control of problems	It was weird because I don't really think my problems out like this.	It was difficult at first thinking about the problem which for me is sad, but in the end it helped me cope.	Problems are circumstances that blocks our way and prevent us from stepping forward, PIP make sense because it gets rid of the blockage around our way.
I think the PIP is an amazing way to help people on the internet! It definitely helped me with my friend problems!	Its was like letting all the stuff building up in you and than pip lets it all out	PIP is actually helpful because I don't have anyone to talk to in real life so this is a good escape.	Instead of having this giant mass of a problem weighing down on you, you can pick it apart and set things aside to deal with later, which allows you to focus on how to solve the problem better.

Table 6.2 Cumulative unique (registered individual) users – March 2019

Activity or resource	Unique users	Boy / Girl %	Volume
Stressed Avatar	19,946	26.8 / 73.2	68,206 games successfully won (72.1% of games started)
Tip Sheets	4,262	21.9 / 78.1	11,776 views
PIP Problems-Ideas-Plans tutorial for creative problem solving	1,144	15.9 / 84.1	1,515 completed tutorial sessions
Deep breathing	1,096	15.2 / 84.8	2,027 exercised
Visualization	941	15.7 / 84.3	1,880 exercised
Emotions and Coping (chat) Forums	907	24.0 / 76.0	25,690 forum posts
Muscle relaxation	860	16.2 / 83.8	1,882 exercised
Journaling	660	15.4 / 84.6	1,436 exercised
Mood colour	n/a	18.8 / 81.2	24,127 changes

middle school students, both of these opportunities yielded important information about how to effectively use Whyville within a group setting. First, dedicated time must be allotted to learn how to navigate the Whyville virtual world. Whyville has a number of requirements for participation and chatting. While these requirements are important in maintaining the safety of its users, they do require time, and if children are under 13, permission from parents. Therefore, some time to establish user privileges is critical before scheduling time to actually engage with the activities. Second, there must be alignment with either a lesson or dedicated curriculum time so that students are able to contextualize the activities, discuss them, and follow a unified sequence.

As part of the authors' ongoing commitment to mental health and wellness globally, they partnered with individuals in Nigeria and India to introduce Whyville to students. In Nigeria, for example, the Whyville game activities are included during ongoing computer labs at Our Lady of Apostles Secondary Grammar Public School in Ibadan. The format of a computer lab provides the dedicated, ongoing time needed to fully engage with the activities. This intentional use of the Wellness Center is new to the school (as of April, 2019) and the hope is that the students benefit from the exercises, go on to introduce the resource to their peers outside of school, and the teachers find the repository of lessons helpful as supplements to the work they do in promoting social and emotional health in their students.

The first comments received from the teacher in Nigeria, Fr. Felix Kingsley Obialo, spoke to the safety elements built into Whyville (which are addressed in more detail in Section 6.5 of this chapter, "Mitigating Liabilities to Protect the End User"). Felix emailed,

> One thing I found intriguing on the day I introduced Whyville was when a student was asked her phone number. ... when I took a closer look, only then I realised that she had gone into the game proper and was being taught a huge lesson in not disclosing phone or house contacts to strangers. Then I remembered my own experience at Wellesley, when I was going through the game myself. I used the opportunity to call the attention of the group to the lesson inherent in that particular activity. i.e. to play safe by not disclosing personal details to strangers. This discovery was particularly important because there had been cases recently in Nigeria where people, who disclosed their personal details, had been deceived and killed by strangers they met on the internet. It was an A-ha moment for the student, who hitherto did not see anything wrong with giving out personal details to strangers, especially through the internet. Another lesson gained was 'disclosure of personal information' might not be a smart way to feel accepted by their peers. ... Conclusively, with the rate at which teens are gaining access to the internet and learning a lot of bad things, I believe Whyville will offer an alternative learning resource for our teens, who seem to learn so much evil on the internet these days.

Beyond schools, community settings such as youth groups and community centers (e.g., Boys and Girls Clubs) also offer opportunities for guided use of this

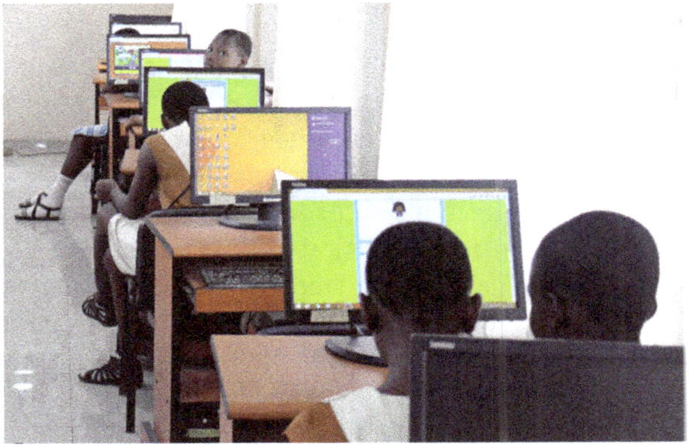

Figure 6.6 *Whyville in Nigeria – photograph by Iruobe Anakhu Photography*

resource (Figure 6.6). Whether it is as part of a group activity, or as part of one of the multiple resources youth have available to practice coping and self-regulation in a moment when they need it, the Wellness Center offers activities that are versatile to varied needs.

Finally, the therapy setting offers another unique opportunity to use Whyville with children and adolescents accessing mental health services. A pilot with a child psychologist using Whyville as a supplement to therapy with a client indicated that Whyville offered a helpful platform to practice skills in a way that did not feel like traditional homework. Therapeutic work with children often includes homework in the form of filling out forms, worksheets, and keeping track of using one's coping skills. The Wellness Center not only offered fun games to practice these skills, but also a way to keep track of progress. Additionally, the Wellness Center offers activities that can help with self-regulation (e.g., relaxation exercises) that children can access independently outside the therapy hour, therefore generalizing skills and increasing practice. For example, the PIP game is one of the activities found in the Wellness Center. The PIP focuses on creative problem solving through an interactive tutorial and game. Problem solving is an important strategy used in the treatment of mental illness and as a coping skill to promote wellness. Youth struggling with anxiety and depression often have a hard time with problem solving, given the strong tendency for avoidance, as well as due to feelings of low self-efficacy and helplessness. Problem solving assists in promoting more active coping, increasing self-efficacy, and control. Problem solving is also an important skill for children who do not struggle with mental illness to learn; in fact, it promotes the following for all youth:

- Withholding judgment and criticism in evaluating one's and other's ideas
- Importance of developing and examining multiple perspectives
- Promoting cognitive flexibility – generating many ideas and ways of thinking
- Promoting collaboration
- Use of creativity as it is defined by the individual

6.3.2 Emerging evidence

The joint endeavours of different fields, such as psychology, education, gaming, and public health, towards the creation of games that foster mental health and wellness will be essential in creating engaging and sustainable programs. These joint endeavours are also critical in creating opportunities for research that will examine the feasibility and effectiveness of such programs, as well as the creation of a work force with particular expertise to advance the field of mental health promotion. Two William James College students focused on the Wellness Center for completion of their doctoral projects. The first study examined the virtual delivery of mental health promotion programming to children and adolescents. Overall, results indicated the activities within the Wellness Center offer a feasible, acceptable, and adaptable way to deliver mental health–promotion programming to youth. Results also supported the creation of games to facilitate emotional awareness, problem solving, and coping skills among users. The second study sought to investigate the feasibility and effectiveness of using the stressed avatar activity to promote understanding of social anxiety and offer coping skills. Important findings indicated users completed the activity more than once and that there was a high completion success rate (83%). As a second method of activity evaluation, expert reviewers offered feedback about their experience with the activity and thoughts about its clinical utility. Overall, reviewers found the activity to be age appropriate, fun, engaging and interactive, and a helpful supplement to therapy.

6.4 Platform

Whyville runs on the Numedeon Interactive Community Engine (NICE), a proprietary software platform for developing virtual communities and environments. Numedeon, Inc., created and owns the (NICE) development platform and is the assignee of a related patent [28]. In addition to Whyville, Numedeon has created virtual worlds for NASA, Humana, and the University of Texas [29]. The NICE platform employs Java Flash to provide the development features requisite for immersive interaction and also simplifies the eventual end user access both by running through standard browsers without a need to load client software and also by operating over low-bandwidth networks. Using the NICE platform, Numedeon has also created virtual worlds and environments for NASA, Humana, and the University of Texas.

6.5 Mitigating liabilities to protect the end user

The Whyville site summarizes safety as follows: “We take safety seriously in Whyville and have been setting industry standards since 1999. We strive not only to keep children safe, but, most importantly, we also teach children how to be safe on the internet.

- Chat License: Before citizens can chat in Whyville, they have to earn their Chat License by taking a tutorial that teaches them the rules of chat safety and etiquette. In addition, citizens under 13 must send in a signed Parental Permission Slip before they are allowed to chat.
- Chat Filter: Whyville's proprietary chat filter blocks and tags inappropriate language, personal information, web links and more. If a citizen tries to communicate in ways that are against Whyville's rules, our city managers will be alerted, and the citizen may risk losing chat privileges or even banishment from Whyville.
- Safety Tools: In Whyville, citizens take an active role in assuring our city stays a safe place by using safety tools to report trouble. The 911 report tool allows citizens to alert city workers to situations that need investigation. We encourage responsible reporting by providing feedback on each and every report." [30].

Further details are posted in the Whyville document titled, "Whyville Safety – White Paper Our Philosophy and Processes" [31].

When it comes to children's mental health and wellness, it is imperative that we find ways to move away from models that focus on treatment only once a crisis has occurred or a diagnosis has been made. Instead, we need to focus on approaches that promote early health and wellbeing. The vast outreach of technology allows us the opportunity to find innovative ways to bring together thought leaders from various fields to create programming that is easily accessible, engaging, developmentally appropriate, ethical, and promotes skill building both in the short and long term. The pilot with Whyville allowed for a tremendous amount of learning and the development of the following recommendations:

- Children as young as 7 years old can be effectively engaged with games that promote mental health and wellness. While critical to keep in mind child safety and protection, the platform needs to be easy to find and readily accessible.
- Self-regulation and coping skills encompass a number of different aspects, including cognition, language (verbal and non-verbal) and practice of interactions. Therefore, the platform needs to be sophisticated enough to allow children to practice skills that involve non-verbal language (e.g., an avatar practicing appropriate eye contact or body movements), as well as interactions with others.
- Monitoring of the content, use, and update of the material is critical. Therefore, development plans should include ongoing monitoring and revision from all content and design experts.
- Ways to engage schools and parents are critical aspects of developing and maintaining successful mental health promotion games for youth. As mentioned earlier in the chapter, offering ways for children to generalize the information they learn to other settings and with other populations is important. By engaging the adults in their lives and offering ways to reinforce learning, we maximize youth's potential for sustained learning.

References

[1] 'Childs Right to Play', http://ipaworld.org/childs-right-to-play/uncrc-article-31/un-convention-on-the-rights-of-the-child-1/, accessed 29 April 2019.

[2] Yogman, M., Garner, A., Hutchinson, J., *et al.*: 'The power of play: A pediatric role in enhancing development in young children', Am Aca Ped, 2018, (142)3. doi:10.1542/peds.2018–2058

[3] Yogman, M., Garner, A., Hutchinson, J., *et al.*: 'The power of play: A pediatric role in enhancing development in young children', Am Aca Ped, 2018, (142)6.

[4] Reilly, N.: 'Anxiety and depression in the classroom: A teacher's guide to fostering self-regulation in young students' (WW Norton & Co., 2015, 1st edn.).

[5] Hosman, C., Jané-Llopis, E. & Saxena, S.: 'Prevention of Mental Disorders: Effective Interventions and Policy Options Summary Report', p 15. Available at https://www.who.int/mental_health/evidence/en/prevention_of_mental_disorders_sr.pdf accessed 29 April 2019.

[6] Merikangas, K., He, J., Burstein M., *et al.*: 'Service utilization for lifetime mental disorders in U.S. adolescents: Results of the National Comorbidity Survey-Adolescent Supplement (NCS-A)', J Am Acad Child Adolesc Psychiatry, 2011, 50(1), pp. 32–45. doi:10.1016/j.jaac.2010.10.006

[7] Mufson L., Rynn M., Yanes-Lukin P., *et al.*: 'Stepped care interpersonal psychotherapy treatment for depressed adolescents: A pilot study in pediatric clinics', Adm Policy Ment Health, 2018, 45(3), pp. 417–431. doi:10.1007/s10488-017-0836-8

[8] 'Mental Health Action Plan 2013–2020', p 8, http://www.who.int/mental_health/publications/action_plan/en, accessed 29 April 2019.

[9] Felitti, V., Anda, R., Nordenberg, D., *et al.*: 'Relationship of childhood abuse and household dysfunction to many of the leading causes of death in adults: The Adverse Childhood Experiences (ACE) study', Am J Preventive Med, 1998, 14(4), pp. 245–258. doi:10.1016/S0749-3797(98)00017-8

[10] Leitch, L.: 'Action steps using ACEs and trauma-informed care: A resilience model', Health Justice, 2017, 5(1). doi:10.1186/s40352-017-0050-5

[11] Merikangas K., He J., Burstein M., *et al.*: 'Lifetime prevalence of mental disorders in U.S. adolescents: Results from the National Comorbidity Survey Replication–Adolescent Supplement (NCS-A)', J Am Acad Child Adolesc Psychiatry, 2010, 49(10), pp. 980–989. doi:10.1016/j.jaac.2010.05.017

[12] O'Connell, M., Boat, T. & Warner, K.: 'Preventing mental, emotional, and behavioral disorders among young people: Progress and possibilities' (National Academies Press, 2009, 1st edn.).

[13] 'Beals 2011: A Framework for the Design and Evaluation of Virtual World Programs for Preadolescent Youth', http://ase.tufts.edu/DevTech/resources/Theses/LBeals_2011.pdf, accessed 29 April 2019.

[14] 'Global Kids Online', http://globalkidsonline.net/results/, accessed 29 April 2019.
[15] Pew Research Center, 'Teens, Social Media & Technology 2018' May 2018, p 7. Available at https://www.pewinternet.org/wp-content/uploads/sites/9/2018/05/PI_2018.05.31_TeensTech_FINAL.pdf, accessed 29 April 2019.
[16] Pew Research Center, 'Smartphone Ownership Is Growing Rapidly Around the World, but Not Always Equally', February 2019, p.4. Available at https://www.pewglobal.org/wp-content/uploads/sites/2/2019/02/Pew-Research-Center_Global-Technology-Use-2018_2019-02-05.pdf, accessed 29 April 2019.
[17] Pew Research Center, 'The Smartphone Difference', April, 2015. Available at http://www.pewinternet.org/2015/04/01/us-smartphone-use-in-2015, accessed 29 April 2019.
[18] 'Jade Lizard Software, LLC: iBreathe', https://www.jadelizardsoftware.com/ibreathe, accessed 29 April 2019.
[19] 'Headspace, Inc: Headspace', https://www.headspace.com, accessed 29 April 2019.
[20] 'Australian Government: High Res', https://highres.dva.gov.au/highres/#!/home, accessed 29 April 2019.
[21] 'Numedeon Inc: Whyville', http://www.whyville.net, accessed 29 April 2019.
[22] J. Sun, personal communication, 1 April, 2014.
[23] J. Sun, personal communication, 30 April, 2019.
[24] Anderson, C., Shibuya, A., Ihori, N., *et al.*: 'Violent video game effects on aggression, empathy, and prosocial behavior in Eastern and Western countries: A meta-analytic review', Psychol Bul, 2010, 136(2), pp. 151–173. doi:10.1037/a0018251
[25] Miller M, and Jensen R.: 'Avatars in nursing: An integrative review', Nurse Educ., 2014, 39(1), pp. 38–41. doi:10.1097/01.NNE.0000437367.03842.63
[26] Aspen Institute, 'A Practice Agenda in Support of How Learning Happens', 2018. Available at http://nationathope.org/wp-content/uploads/aspen_practice_final_web_optimized.pdf, accessed 29 April 2019.
[27] 'Whyville Teacher's Tutorial: Adolescent Wellness Program', https://www.adolescentwellness.org/wp-content/uploads/2011/06/Wellness-Center-Teacher-Tutorial.pdf, accessed 29 April 2019.
[28] Dinan, M., Sun, J., Pickard, A., Bowers, J.: 'Graphical interactive interface for immersive online communities'. United States Patent #7,925,703, April 2011.
[29] 'Numedeon, Inc.', http://www.numedeon.com, accessed 29 April 2019.
[30] 'Whyville safety', http://b.whyville.net/smmk/persPage/index#safety, accessed 29 April 2019.
[31] Numedeon, Inc.: *'Whyville Safety - White Paper Our Philosophy and Processes'* is available here: http://whyville.s3.amazonaws.com/frontpage/WhyvilleSafetyWhitePaper.pdf, accessed 29 April 2019.

Chapter 7

Minimally disruptive medicine: how mHealth strategies can reduce the work of diabetes care

Julie A. Perry, Ph.D.[1] *and*
Karen M. Cross, M.D., Ph.D., FRCSC[1,2,3]

7.1 Introduction

7.1.1 The coming tsunami: global rates of diabetes are reaching epidemic proportions

Diabetes is a chronic metabolic disease in which the body has trouble regulating blood sugar due to a lack of insulin production by the pancreas (Type I diabetes) or by a resistance to the insulin that is produced (Type II diabetes). Over time, elevated levels of blood sugar (glucose) can cause serious damage to the heart, blood vessels, eyes, kidneys and nerves. The global prevalence of diabetes is currently 8.5% (up from 4.8% in 1980) or 422 million adults worldwide and is expected to continue increasing as the world's population ages [1]. In the United States, the prevalence is slightly higher: 30.3 million people (or 9.4% of the general population) had diabetes in 2015 [2], but this is a problem that gets worse with age: an estimated 25.2% of adults over 65 in the United States are diabetic. European rates of Type II diabetes range from 2.4% in Moldova to 14.9% in Turkey, with an estimated rate of undiagnosed diabetes in high-income European countries (Denmark, Finland, and the United Kingdom) of a staggering 36.6% [3]. Although the rate of new diagnoses remains steady in higher income countries, diabetes prevalence continues to rise in low- and middle-income countries [1]. Unfortunately, the WHO reports that 1.5 million deaths were directly attributable to diabetes in 2012, and a further 2.2 million deaths were caused by higher than optimal blood glucose, which caused death by cardiovascular and other related diseases. As a result, diabetes is one of four priority noncommunicable diseases targeted for action by world leaders [1].

[1]Keenan Research Centre for Biomedical Science, Unity Health Toronto - St. Michael's Hospital, Toronto, Canada
[2]Department of Surgery, University of Toronto, Toronto, Canada
[3]Division of Plastic Surgery, Unity Health Toronto - St. Michael's Hospital, Toronto, Canada

7.1.2 High blood sugar leads to vascular damage

Diabetes carries with it a heightened risk of serious complications requiring hospitalization, including heart attack, stroke, kidney failure, vision loss, nerve damage and leg amputation. In 2014, 14.2 million emergency department visits in the United States were due to diabetes, and a further 1.5 million patients were admitted to hospital due to diabetes-related cardiovascular events [4]. These pathologies are all due to the effects of elevated blood glucose on the body's vascular system, which can be further classified into either macrovascular complications (coronary artery disease, peripheral arterial disease (PAD) and stroke) and microvascular complications (diabetic nephropathy, neuropathy and retinopathy) [5]. Our research focuses on the complications of diabetes that result from microvascular problems in the lower extremity (feet and legs). In particular, we treat the wounds that occur on the feet of diabetics (diabetic foot ulcers, or DFUs) that often lead to amputation.

Two vascular pathologies are relevant to our discussions because they contribute directly to the development of DFUs and subsequent amputations. Diabetic neuropathy is a lack of sensation in the feet, caused by injury to the peripheral nerves by sustained hyperglycemia (high blood sugar) and microvascular damage. Because the patient cannot feel their toes and feet, injuries occur more easily and may go unnoticed for a period of time. These injuries can result from something as innocuous as the rubbing of an ill-fitting sock or shoe over time, which can lead to a nonhealing wound and end in amputation. Once a DFU forms, the wound is more vulnerable to infection and less able to heal if the patient has compromised vascular supply to the leg, due to one of the macrovascular complications of diabetes, known as PAD. PAD is also developed due to uncontrolled glucose: in a prospective study done in the United Kingdom, each 1% increase in HbA_{1c} level was associated with a 28% increase in risk of PAD [6]. PAD results from narrowing of arterial walls due to chronic inflammation and injury to the arterial wall. In response to injury, oxidized lipids and immune cells accumulate on the walls of arteries forming an atherosclerotic lesion. Rupture of this lesion leads to infarction [5] and effectively cuts off blood supply in that vascular tree. As a result, a DFU that forms in a patient with PAD lacks the nutrients needed to heal and can remain open for months or even years. When caught early, DFUs are highly treatable. However, most ulcers are not treated until they become more advanced, such that one-third of ulcers never heal and require lower extremity amputation (LEA) [7,8]. The 3-year overall mortality rate following LEA due to DFU is as high as 70% [9], higher than cancers of the breast and colon. These devastating outcomes are preventable, but consistent monitoring of foot health and early reporting of problems are critical.

7.1.3 Overmanagement and underdiagnosis: two opposites of the spectrum in the global management of diabetes

Evidence supports the notion that early diagnosis and consistent, regular management leads to better outcomes in diabetes. Blood glucose control through diet and exercise (and medication if necessary), blood pressure control to reduce cardiovascular complications and regular evaluation of the eyes, kidneys and feet for damage are all necessary to improve outcomes. Much of this monitoring falls to the patient themselves, and conscious and consistent self-management is believed to play an important role in preventing the microvascular and macrovascular complications of diabetes [10]. Diabetes self-management education aims to improve a patient's capacity to make informed decisions, problem solve and make self-directed changes to behavior based on increasing levels of health literacy [11]. Unfortunately, the age of diabetic patients and the many complications and sequelae of this chronic disease mean that patients may be managing several conditions at once—a condition termed multi-morbidity. In an example cited by Tran *et al.* [4], a patient with diabetes, hypertension, osteoporosis and osteoarthritis and chronic obstructive pulmonary disease could be prescribed up to 12 medications: as a result, patients experience not only the burden of illness, but a large "burden of treatment" associated with managing their illnesses in the developed world. In fact, 60% of patients in a recent study of 1,053 participants from 34 higher income countries examining the burden of treatment on multi-morbid patients reported that the frequency of treatment exacerbated its burden, and many patients reported that treatment was "too much" [4]. The consequence of a high burden of treatment is that treatment compliance rates drop, the disease become poorly managed and outcomes decline. Patients may prioritize checking their blood sugar over checking their feet or give them a cursory superficial check once a week. As we discuss later in this chapter, only 14% of patients reported checking their feet everyday in a recent Canadian study [12], and there is no data to tell us how (or how carefully) those patients are checking. The "work" of health-related care can become a burden, and health-care practitioners are beginning to take this patient "work" load into account in order to improve outcomes.

The converse situation exists in low- and middle-income countries: according to the WHO, only one in three (low- and middle-income countries) reports having the technology to diagnose and manage diabetes in their primary health-care facilities. A recently introduced peer-education campaign for diabetes self-management in Mali yielded substantial improvements in glycemic control and anthropomorphic measures like mean waist circumference [13]. This program consisted of three courses of culturally tailored patient education, emphasizing proper eating habits, regular physical activity, adherence to medical treatment and regular monitoring of their condition. Giving patients the tools to manage their condition themselves may lead to better outcomes, but the success of this program is not universal: a study using text messages to reach diabetic patients in the Democratic Republic of Congo, Cambodia and the Philippines was not successful in improving blood sugar control in diabetics [14]. The authors found that it was difficult to address individualized and specific behavior beliefs via text message, suggesting that a more personalized approach may be needed.

The solution to the global management of diabetes therefore requires a simple, personalized and low-tech approach that can integrate care of multiple conditions in the developed world while retaining its usefulness in mid- and lower income countries.

7.1.4 Minimally disruptive medicine and mobile healthcare

A growing area of research with application to delivery of care in both developed and developing countries is the delivery of healthcare remotely via "apps" on mobile devices (called mobile healthcare/mHealth). Mobile phones are now ubiquitous in society, and several software platforms have been developed for the self-management of diabetes, mainly in higher income countries. Using a well-thought out mobile "app" to manage multi-morbidity may help one to simplify and streamline the management of disease and in so doing increase compliance to therapy and improve outcomes. In a recent survey, 58% of smartphone users reported downloading a health-related app, and more than half had downloaded an app to track physical activity and eating [15]. Much of mHealth's applications to diabetes have been focused on apps that track patients' blood glucose levels at home and have been shown to result in an increase in the frequency of monitoring, fewer hyperglycemic events and lower average glucose levels than nonmobile platform-using controls [16]. There is currently no mobile health tool for the diabetic lower extremity, although there is evidence that monitoring via telemedicine is as effective as standard outpatient monitoring in regards to healing and amputation rates [17]. Ideally, a foot-monitoring app could be integrated into the glucose-monitoring apps currently used by this patient population to further reduce treatment burden.

7.2 The diabetic lower extremity

7.2.1 The case for remote monitoring

Our diabetic foot practice is set in a large tertiary care hospital in the downtown core of the largest city in Canada. It includes a specialized multidisciplinary team of wound care nurses, internists, surgeons and podiatrists who see a patient with a DFU regularly as an inpatient or outpatient until their ulcer heals. Once in our care, patients are also seen by a travelling homecare nurse for dressing changes every few days and are called back to the hospital if their ulcer begins to deteriorate. Our limb salvage pipeline also includes vascular surgeons to address the underlying causes of failure-to-heal, including increasing efforts to promote revascularization of limbs with PAD.

This care system is state of the art and effective, but it is (1) reactionary (instead of preventative), (2) expensive (the cost of treating a DFU is approximately $52,360 CAD) and (3) inaccessible for Canadian diabetics living outside of the urban downtown core. The following sections present arguments for how these three issues can be addressed using an mHealth-based intervention.

7.2.1.1 An ounce of prevention is worth a pound of cure

There is a golden window of opportunity to treat a DFU when it first forms, but patients often miss this window because they are not able/do not know how to check their feet regularly enough. In clinical medicine, DFUs are classified using the validated University of Texas grading scale [18], where the size, depth and involvement of bone are taken into account. Texas Grade 1 ulcers are superficial and easy to heal, and Grades 2 and 3 are deeper, larger and more involved ulcers that can take months to treat. A recent retrospective cohort study of 105 patients showed what clinicians have long articulated: early detection and treatment of ulcers are crucial for optimal ulcer healing. Patients who had an untreated ulcer for >52 days had a 58% decreased healing rate compared to those treated earlier, and patients with more severe ulcers (Texas grade 2/3, stage C/D) also had a more difficult time healing [8]. These conclusions are supported by a larger retrospective study in the United States, which examined data from 5,239 ulcers with the goal of developing a comprehensive "healing index" [19]. The authors of this study found that wound duration in days, size and several other parameters indicating severity of diabetes in general were predictive of healing (or nonhealing as the case may be). This evidence suggests that we should be treating as many ulcers as possible when they are Texas Grade 1, but how do we catch them at that stage?

The current standard of care in Canada for diabetic foot is self-monitoring by patients themselves, with support as requested from family physicians. However, in a large cohort study recently completed in the Canadian province of Alberta, only 14% of respondents reported checking their feet 6 days a week or more, and only 41% and 34% had their feet checked regularly by a clinician for ulcers or sensory loss, respectively [12]. In a recent survey of our own patients [20], 77.4% reported checking their feet regularly, although the majority (51.3%) reported spending less than a minute checking, and only 13.9% use a mirror to check the bottoms of their feet. Moreover, 72.2% of respondents reported wearing corrective lenses that may affect their ability to see their feet clearly. As a result, ulcers often go undetected until they are larger and harder to treat; in the same study, clinicians reported that approximately one in three patients is only being seen once they have already developed a problem.

7.2.1.2 mHealth can be cost-effective in the diabetic lower extremity

Even if a patient is checking their feet regularly, it may be difficult for an untrained eye to make clinical decisions regarding when to seek treatment. An objective tool or decision aid could help one to reduce unnecessary doctors' visits while still catching ulcers early enough to facilitate treatment and healing. Ideally, all diabetics would have their feet checked regularly by a trained foot specialist, but the cost of hospital-based screening for all diabetics is not trivial. We recently examined the cost effectiveness of using an mHealth-based screening system to monitor diabetic feet. In a publicly funded health-care system, a single DFU case costs taxpayers $52,360, including costs of admissions, ER and clinic visits, drugs and dressings, home and long-term care [21]. We evaluated the cost-effectiveness of an mHealth for DFUs in a hypothetical cohort of Canadian patients aged 60 years with diabetes using a ten-state Markov cohort model [22]. Given that a history of DFUs is associated with an increased risk for future ulcers, we stratified our analysis into (1) population-wide or (2) targeted screening approaches. Outcomes were expressed in quality-adjusted life years (QALYs), which is a measure of disease burden and reflects both quantity and quality of life lived. A "perfect" year of health is equal to 1 QALY, while death is assigned 0 QALYs. Six months spent suffering from a chronic condition costs 0.5 years $\times$ 1 = 0.5 QALYs. Although the absolute effect of mHealth-based screening on DFU incidence is unknown without clinical data, the potential health benefit associated with screening all diabetics in Canada using an mHealth device was appreciable, ranging from 0.01196 to 0.02369 QALYs per person at a conservative screening effectiveness of 20%–40%. For context, screening for hepatitis C in Canada reported QALY increase of 0.0032–0.0095 per person [23]. However, population-based screening is expensive and would result in incremental costs of $479–$402 per person over 5 years. In contrast, we found that implementing an mHealth strategy following a patient's first DFU had a high probability of being cost-effective while also increasing a patient's quality of life (health benefit of 0.00062–0.00174 QALYs per person). Cost savings were attributed to a reduction in DFU recurrences and complications. As fewer screening devices are required in the high-risk approach, the up-front costs to the health-care system are lower and targeting a group of patients with higher chances of DFU formation eliminates waste.

7.2.1.3 We must reach outside urban centers

The effectiveness and power of an mHealth intervention is underestimated in the previous cost analysis, because it does not capture one of the biggest problems in the treatment of the diabetic foot: variations in access to care. Al Sayah *et al.* [12] found that predictors of poor outcomes included residing in a nonurban location, and there are clear regional differences in amputation rates in the United States, with underserved and rural communities having a +51.3% higher odds of major amputation, +14.9% higher odds of minor amputation and +41.4% higher odds of inpatient death ($p < 0.05$) than their urban diabetic counterparts [24]. These rates are mirrored in northern Canadian Aboriginal communities, where 82% of a cross-sectional cohort of 169 diabetics had diabetic foot complications and 41% were at risk for future ulceration [25].

The advantage to mHealth is the ability to provide equal access to care by overcoming some of the barriers to frequent screening and monitoring like travel distance, time-off-work limitations and limited access to specialists outside of urban hospitals. Telemedicine/mHealth has been used successfully in diabetic populations in the developed world to monitor (and improve) HbA_{1c} levels, increase inpatient understanding of diabetes, and improve cohesion among members of health-care teams [26–29]. Currently, there is mixed evidence on the effectiveness of telemedicine for monitoring DFUs, largely due to the lack of controlled studies in large cohorts [22] and the limited scope of monitoring offered by previous app-based monitoring systems. Moreover, no studies have examined the use of telemedicine for the prevention and/or early detection of DFUs. Several technologies designed to assess wounds have recently been developed, and could potentially compliment a telemedicine-based program [30,31], but so far only take digital pictures of a wound for assessment. A trained wound care clinician uses more than just visual cues when assessing a wound, like its smell, subtleties of the patient's overall health/demeanor and the presence (or absence) of strong pulses in the feet, which are missed when a wound is simply measured and photographed. These are the real barriers to the adoption of an effective mHealth platform: the information that is unconsciously collected by a clinician when making a decision. An effective remote monitoring tool must be able to assess more than just the outward appearance of a wound, and we think we have developed the capability to do just that.

7.3 Our approach

The presence of an ulcer is predated by the vascular changes outlined in the Introduction, and therefore a device that measures local tissue oxygenation (as a proxy for vascular status and perfusion) in the foot would be invaluable in the regular monitoring routine of diabetics. The current standard of care is to monitor the diabetic lower extremity is a visual inspection of the skin for new wounds, monitor for signs of pain, numbness or discomfort in the legs (called claudication) and feel the pulses of the foot. Foot pulses, however, can be present despite severe distal arterial disease and calcification. Ankle brachial indices are frequently normal in a diabetic population as the rigid vessels cannot be compressed once calcified. Therefore, toe pressures are a more reliable way of evaluating ischemia in this patient population. This means that traditional monitoring for perfusion in this patient population is suboptimal but also may not be available to all patients. In addition, the investigative studies performed in vascular laboratories such as the ankle-brachial index, toe pressures and arteriovenous duplex represent the physical perfusion of the limb but do not give physiologic information about the oxygen utilization and offloading to the tissue which may be better indicators of tissue health. In-hospital imaging of vascular status requires large specialized equipment (computed tomography angiography, Duplex ultrasonography, magnetic resonance imaging and the gold standard, digital subtraction angiography) [32] and people to capture and interpret the results. While powerful, these modalities are impractical for use on a routine basis for screening and monitoring (both in terms of allocation of hospital resources and cost) and again bring up the issue of access to care for patients who live outside urban areas (or in low-income countries). Laser Doppler imaging is a lower tech and more portable solution that uses small probes to measure skin perfusion pressure and correlates to wound healing with a sensitivity of 72% and specificity of 88% [33]. Hyperspectral imaging can measure hemoglobin saturation in the skin of patients with diabetes [34], which correlates to wound healing [35]. These are promising technologies in the wound healing area but lack the large-scale clinical trials required for adoption.

For the past decade, our group has focused on using noninvasive near-infrared (NIR) spectroscopy or multispectral imaging to measure oxygenation, perfusion and edema in tissue, albeit with a focus on burn wounds to assess viability [36–38]. NIR spectroscopy can penetrate a variety of tissues and is able to assess perfusion using reflection rather than direct transmission between an emitter and receiver pair [39]. Given its contactless and portable nature, it is a technique well suited to the real-time measurement of skin physiology, and we tested its ability to distinguish viable from nonviable tissue in both a porcine burn model and in a large cohort of human burn patients. Punch biopsies and NIR spectral data were collected from burn sites immediately following burn injury and at 12-h intervals up to 96 h postburn. Biopsies were used to classify burns according to depth and spectra and were analyzed for tissue oxygenation, perfusion and free radical injury. Superficial burns showed high levels of tissue oxygenation compared to their deeper counterparts. Deep injuries (partial and full thickness burns) had higher levels of free radical injury at early time points and over the course of the experiments. This was true for both the porcine and clinical models [40] (Figure 7.1). To better understand the significance of these findings, we used computer modeling to correlate burn depth to spectral data.

7.3.1 Methemoglobin can distinguish viable from nonviable tissue: computer modeling

We constructed artificial neural networks (ANNs) using full NIR spectral data and a two-layer, feed-forward approach to determine if a computer could automatically differentiate viable from nonviable tissue. We created and trained 100 different ANNs to process the NIR spectral data for 12, 24, 48 and 72 h postburn injury. A total of 96 out of the 100 networks we created were able to classify burn depth with an accuracy greater than 91%, using histology and clinical wound healing data as truth. This data confirms our hypothesis that NIR spectral analysis leads to robust classification of burn injury. In an attempt to elucidate the features of the spectra that drive network performance, data was broken down into ranges of 50 nm throughout the spectrum. One hundred networks were again trained on these subspectra and classified. We found that specific ranges of the NIR spectra had more predictive accuracy than others. Particularly, the range between 600 and 650 nm had a very high burn depth diagnostic accuracy (81% of the networks were able to classify burn depth with an accuracy of >86% (Figure 7.2) [40]. This region corresponds to the spectral detection range for a biological marker of free radical injury, methemoglobin (MetHb). In contrast, regions with few spectral characteristics (725–775 and 875–975 nm) performed poorly (only 50% of networks had a classification accuracy of >60%). From these results, we conclude that MetHb is a novel marker sufficient to differentiate viable from nonviable burned tissue noninvasively using NIR spectroscopy [40].

7.3.2 Translating our technology into the diabetic lower extremity

The same values that predict tissue viability in a burn can predict viability in the diabetic lower extremity. Because of the vascular pathologies described earlier, diabetic lower extremity wounds will have localized lower values for oxygenation and perfusion, high levels of free radicals and poor tissue oxygen utilization

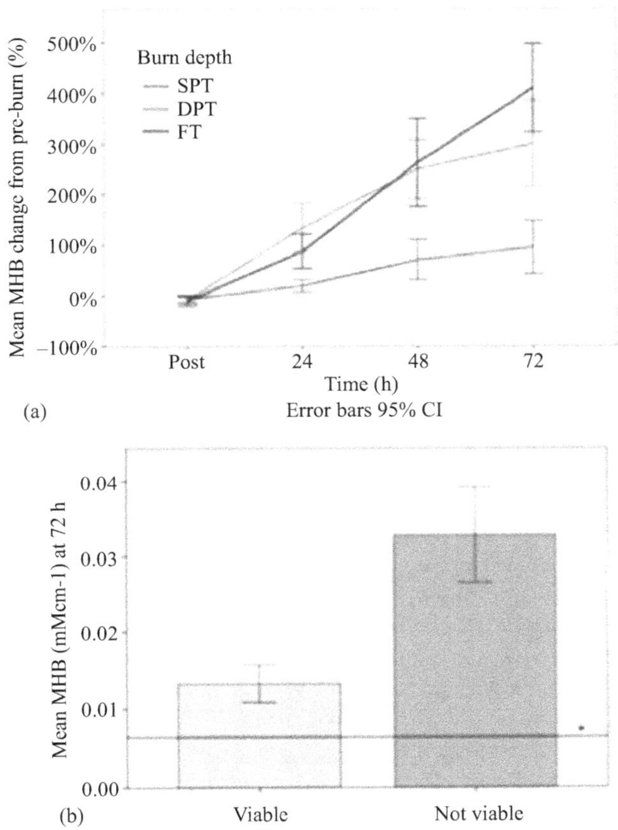

Figure 7.1 Near-infrared evaluation of free radical accumulation (a surrogate measure of tissue damage) in a porcine burn model. (a) Immediately postburn, punch biopsies were taken for histological classification of burns into superficial partial thickness (SPT), deep partial thickness (DPT) and full thickness (FT) burns. NIR imaging quantified free radical accumulation over time and revealed a significant accumulation of free radicals in deep partial thickness and full thickness burns over a 72-h period. Conversely, free radical levels did not rise significantly above baseline in superficial partial thickness burns over the same time frame. Clinically, tissues receiving DPT and FT burns are the equivalent of dead tissue (and require surgical excision), while SPT burns will heal over time. While this difference may not be visible to the naked eye at early time points, NIR imaging can be used to guide clinical decision-making. (b) The results of our porcine study are applicable to human burns. Using the same imaging parameters, we imaged burn patients over time and tracked their clinical outcomes to establish tissue viability. Using NIR, we could predict which tissues were viable as early as 72 h postburn

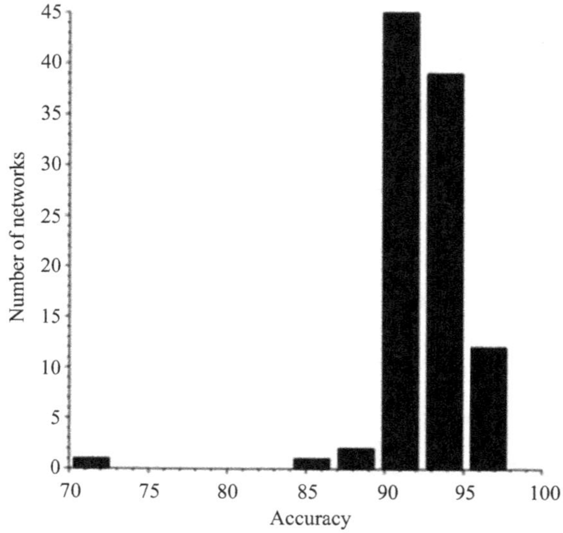

Figure 7.2 Artificial neural networks (ANNs) were built in silico using NIR spectral data to determine if a computer could automatically differentiate viable from nonviable tissue using NIR in our porcine burn model. The majority of networks we created were able to classify burn depth with an accuracy greater than 91%, using histology and clinical wound healing data as truth. We next trained ANNs on spectra broken down into ranges of 50 nm throughout the spectrum and found that specific ranges of the NIR spectra had more predictive accuracy than others. Particularly, the range between 600 and 650 nm (corresponding to the free radical marker MetHb) had a very high burn depth diagnostic accuracy, indicating that spectral data in this range is highly accurate for burn depth determination

compared to non-wounded diabetic limbs. As a result, we can translate our NIR spectroscopy data and expertise into detecting a diabetic foot wound at very early stages using portable, noninvasive light-based technology. Recognizing the issues of treatment burden and access to care on a global scale, we set out to adapt our technology to fit into an mHealth scheme that pairs a smartphone with an imaging device called the MultIspectral MObile tiSsue Assessment (MIMOSA) and accompanying patient–clinician portal.

MIMOSA is a stand-alone class II medical imaging device that collects multispectral images but uses a smartphone app to drive image collection. It is as simple as taking a picture with one's own cellphone, with a small imaging device attached. Patients take a "picture" of their feet daily using MIMOSA/cell-phone combination, and the images are cataloged for review by a wound care clinician remotely. When MIMOSA captures a change in tissue parameters that signals the

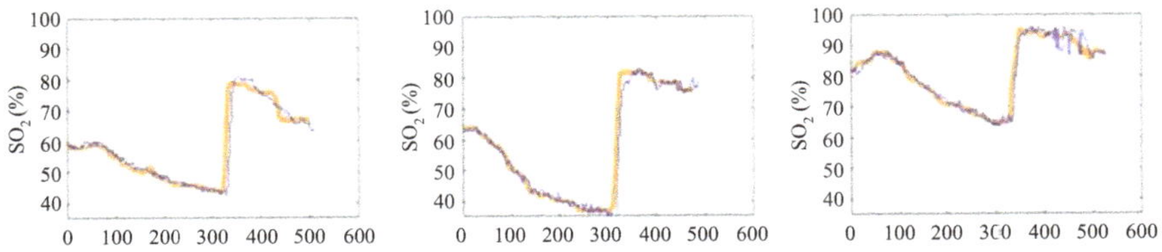

Figure 7.3 Forearm ischemia model of reperfusion. A blood pressure cuff was inflated around the upper arm of three representative subjects (shown in separate graphs) to restrict blood flow to the forearm. Tissue perfusion was recorded at 3-s intervals using the MIMOSA device, and the blood pressure cuff was deflated at 300 s. The imaging data shows a clear decrease in perfusion during the initial stage of the experiment and captures the immediate reperfusion upon cuff deflation. This imaging capability can be used to assess blood flow in a diabetic patient's legs and detect vascular problems preceding wound formation

development of a wound, the patient receives a notification alert and is then seen by a wound care clinician at an early wound stage. Not only does the MIMOSA sound a reminder alert for daily foot checks, it provides an objective measure of foot health remotely, which takes the burden of clinical judgment (and when to seek treatment) off the patient. Since patients are monitored remotely, it extends regular access to care beyond city borders and keeps rural patients in touch with clinical experts. MIMOSA is inexpensive and low tech, such that it can be used in health clinics as part of a diagnostic program in middle- and low-income countries. An 85% of the world is covered by a cell-phone signal, and we hope that by addressing many of the key issues that lead to diabetic foot-ulcer-related amputations we can save limbs and save lives.

We are currently building a large training data set with MIMOSA to construct its artificial intelligence (AI)-based diagnostic algorithms. The device can easily capture tissue perfusion (Figure 7.3), which represents a leap forward from the large bulky devices traditionally used for this purpose clinically. We are in the midst of a large multicenter clinical trial to validate MIMOSA in a heterogeneous patient population with multiple morbidities and anticipate that MIMOSA will be ready for patient use by 2021.

7.4 MIMOSA in practice and overcoming barriers to mHealth adoption

Bringing MIMOSA from the lab to the clinic requires both clinician and patient buy-in. We are currently conducting a large prospective multicenter trial of MIMOSA in the diabetic lower extremity with the aim to further develop the diagnostic algorithms that can ultimately predict wound formation and healing. The physiologic information collected by MIMOSA images will be linked to known outcome measures such as angiography results and pulses. When acquiring such large data sets for training machine learning algorithms, it is imperative to have a "good" training set. The better the quality of the data set the more likely the algorithms can be predictive in the future. Currently, most noninvasive physiologic monitors of tissue health are standalone and provide the measurement of interest at the point of care, but in order to make the technology "smarter" it needs to be paired to known outcome measures. AI in medicine is the future and an adjunct to a health-care provider's workflow. It can help one to create efficiency in triaging patients, efficiency of work and facilitate in diagnosis. It is understood that patients with chronic disease experience high workloads in caring for themselves. Health-care providers are also overburdened, and it can be challenging to convince them that mHealth and AI will not increase their workloads. In addition, billing and reimbursement strategies are not in place to appropriately remunerate physicians and this is a critical "selling" point to break down barriers of technology adoption.

While mHealth is a viable mechanism for monitoring in theory, patients also need to "buy in" to monitoring programs. To determine the feasibility of using mHealth in our patient population, we recently completed both a qualitative and a quantitative survey of foot checking practices at our hospital [20,41]. In one study, 115 patients answered questions describing their foot checking practices and comfort with mobile technology. Most patients were Type II diabetics (59.1%), insulin dependent (79.1%), used a glucometer (93.9%), and were an average age of 54.8 years. Diabetics are often more familiar with health technology due to the need for glucometers in their monitoring routines. Our sample inadvertently consisted of patients who ranked their health as a priority. The vast majority of respondents were nonsmokers (87%), stated that they visit their physician a few times a year (79.1%), and most reported that being in control of their own health is very important to them (mean rating 8.3 out of 10, where 10 is the highest importance). Mobile phone ownership was also widespread (80.4% of respondents) as was glucometer usage (94%). Additionally, 73.1% of patients surveyed would use a device on their phone to help them check their feet (Figure 7.4). While this is encouraging, we acknowledge that our sample is not representative of all diabetics (healthy patients, urban location, widespread cellphone ownership and comfort with technology). For example, we surveyed an older demographic in a second-qualitative study, who expressed considerably more reluctance to adopt mHealth into their monitoring routine [41]. Older patients also expressed a desire to maintain a strong relationship with their doctor and a reluctance to use technology to replace that relationship. One of the respondents in our qualitative survey stated

> *I actually don't do a lot with my phone other than I use it for emails and for phone calls. I am not a techy guy to use my iPhone all the time ... It's a different generation I'm in ... I have no need for it. That's the whole point of technology, it's gotta suit your needs. And it doesn't. I don't need it, so I don't use it.*
>
> 68 year old Male [41]

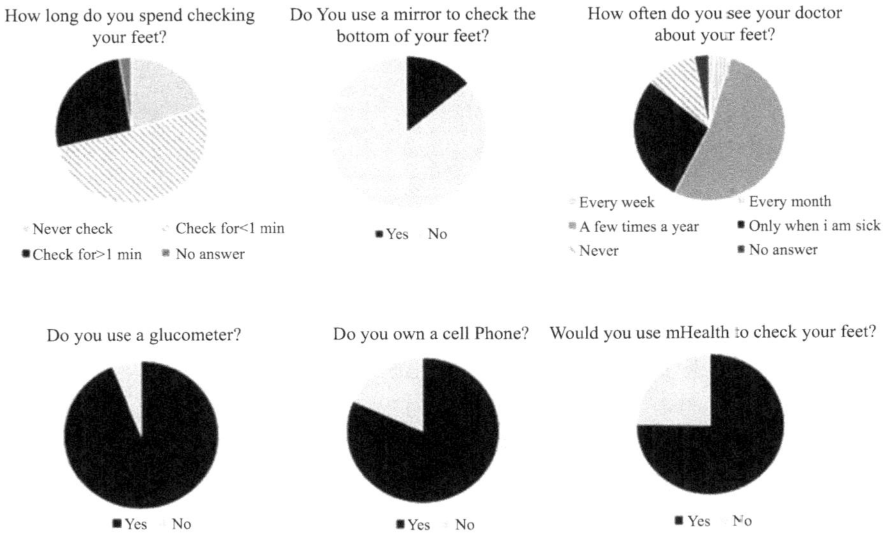

Figure 7.4 Summary of foot checking practices in our patient population. Although our patient population is cell-phone literate and has a strong desire to be involved in their own healthcare, there may be barriers to the adoption of mHealth in older/less affluent populations

This is one of the major barriers we see to the adoption of mobile technology for health delivery- while we can make an app easy to use and accessible to all ages, the invaluable doctor–patient relationship is intangible and hard to replace. Recreating that experience is critical for widespread adoption.

Finally, app burden or paralysis may play a role in boundaries to mHealth adoption strategies by patients. At the time of some of our studies, there were hundreds of apps on Google Play and Apple app stores to help one with glucose management. Very few were related to the diabetic lower extremity and despite estimates that 422 million people worldwide have diabetes (and should be checking their feet), the most highly downloaded app from Google Play had only 500–1,000 installs. Patients may also fail to appreciate the health implications of a DFU and neglect checking their feet in favor of checking their blood glucose regularly. Educational campaigns emphasizing the importance of foot health and efforts to develop strong science for the diagnosis of early-stage DFUs are necessary components of any future mHealth strategies. mHealth platforms are also plagued by the expense of data plans. Although 85% of the world is covered by a cell signal, data plans may not be affordable, and this is one of the big challenges that smartphone platforms face. Also, platforms that require cloud processing would require a Wi-Fi or cell-phone signal that in rural and under-developed countries can be difficult to obtain. Finally, as the patient is the center of one's own care in most mHealth strategies, it is also important that data collection, storage and cloud processing be HIPPA compliant. Privacy and data security are of paramount importance.

7.5 Change is on the horizon

The FDA acknowledges that mHealth is an important part of the future of health care and has a Digital Health Innovation Action Plan. FDA recognized their traditional approach to "medical devices is not suited to the faster iterative design, development and type of validation used for software based medical technologies" and over the past 5 years developed new policies for a more practical approach to digital health. This has been one of the main challenges in the mHealth space: regulatory approval is a long and arduous process, and by the time approval is granted; the technology may be already ready for an update. One of the ways the FDA is trying to expedite approvals is a pre-certification of health technology software developers not the "device." This means the approval sits with the software developers and not the piece of software, if it is deemed relatively low risk. The WHO has affirmed that "mHealth has the potential to transform the face of health service delivery across the globe" and has created a National eHealth roadmap development toolkit as well as data privacy policies to help further the advancement of this technology.

7.6 Conclusions

As the world's population ages, the need for healthcare for chronic conditions is becoming a burden for patients, families and health-care systems. The use of technology in healthcare may offer solutions to these problems but has not been widely adopted due to several key challenges. Despite those challenges, we are confident that mHealth will succeed in revolutionizing healthcare in the next decade, particularly in the monitoring and care of diabetic patients with foot wounds.

References

[1] World Health Organization. *Global Report on Diabetes*. Geneva, Switzerland: World Health Organization; 2016.

[2] Prevention CfDCa. *National Diabetes Statistics Report*; 2017. https://www.cdc.gov/diabetes/pdfs/data/statistics/national-diabetes-statistics-report.pdf2017.

[3] Tamayo T, Rosenbauer J, Wild SH, *et al.* Diabetes in Europe: an update. *Diabetes Res Clin Pract*. 2014;103(2):206–217.

[4] Tran VT, Barnes C, Montori VM, Falissard B, and Ravaud P. Taxonomy of the burden of treatment: a multi-country web-based qualitative study of patients with chronic conditions. *BMC Med*. 2015;13:115.

[5] Strain WD and Paldanius PM. Diabetes, cardiovascular disease and the microcirculation. *Cardiovasc Diabetol*. 2018;17(1):57.
[6] Adler AI, Stevens RJ, Neil A, Stratton IM, Boulton AJ, and Holman RR. UKPDS 59: hyperglycemia and other potentially modifiable risk factors for peripheral vascular disease in type 2 diabetes. *Diabetes Care*. 2002;25 (5):894–899.
[7] Prompers L, Schaper N, Apelqvist J, *et al.* Prediction of outcome in individuals with diabetic foot ulcers: focus on the differences between individuals with and without peripheral arterial disease. The EURODIALE Study. *Diabetologia*. 2008;51(5):747–755.
[8] Smith-Strom H, Iversen MM, Igland J, *et al.* Severity and duration of diabetic foot ulcer (DFU) before seeking care as predictors of healing time: a retrospective cohort study. *PLoS One*. 2017;12(5):e0177176.
[9] Stern JR, Wong CK, Yerovinkina M, *et al.* A meta-analysis of long-term mortality and associated risk factors following lower extremity amputation. *Ann Vasc Surg*. 2017;42:322–327.
[10] Beck J, Greenwood DA, Blanton L, *et al.* National standards for diabetes self-management education and support. *Diabetes Educ*. 2017;2018: 145721718820941.
[11] Riemenschneider H, Saha S, van den Broucke S, *et al.* State of diabetes self-management education in the European union member states and non-EU countries: the Diabetes Literacy Project. *J Diabetes Res*. 2018;2018:1467171.
[12] Al Sayah F, Soprovich A, Qiu W, Edwards AL, and Johnson JA. Diabetic foot disease, self-care and clinical monitoring in adults with type 2 diabetes: the Alberta's Caring for Diabetes (ABCD) Cohort Study. *Can J Diabetes*. 2015;39(Suppl 3):S120–S126.
[13] Debussche X, Besancon S, Balcou-Debussche M, *et al.* Structured peer-led diabetes self-management and support in a low-income country: the ST2EP randomised controlled trial in Mali. *PLoS One*. 2018;13(1):e0191262.
[14] Van Olmen J, Kegels G, Korachais C, *et al.* The effect of text message support on diabetes self-management in developing countries – a randomised trial. *J Clin Transl Endocrinol*. 2017;7:33–41.
[15] Krebs P and Duncan DT. Health app use among US mobile phone owners: a national survey. *JMIR Mhealth Uhealth*. 2015;3(4):e101.
[16] Offringa R, Sheng T, Parks L, Clements M, Kerr D, and Greenfield MS. Digital diabetes management application improves glycemic outcomes in people with type 1 and type 2 diabetes. *J Diabetes Sci Technol*. 2018;12:701–708 1932296817747291.
[17] Rasmussen BS, Froekjaer J, Bjerregaard MR, *et al.* A randomized controlled trial comparing telemedical and standard outpatient monitoring of diabetic foot ulcers. *Diabetes Care*. 2015;38(9):1723–1729.
[18] Armstrong DG, Lavery LA, and Harkless LB. Validation of a diabetic wound classification system. The contribution of depth, infection, and ischemia to risk of amputation. *Diabetes Care*. 1998;21(5):855–859.

[19] Fife CE, Horn SD, Smout RJ, Barrett RS, and Thomson B. A predictive model for diabetic foot ulcer outcome: the wound healing index. *Adv Wound Care (New Rochelle)*. 2016;5(7):279–287.

[20] Wallace D, Perry J, Yu J, Mehta J, Hunter P, and Cross K. Assessing the need for mobile health (mHealth) in monitoring the diabetic lower extremity. *JMIR Mhealth and Uhealth*. 2019;7(4), e11879.

[21] Hopkins RB, Burke N, Harlock J, Jegathisawaran J, and Goeree R. Economic burden of illness associated with diabetic foot ulcers in Canada. *BMC Health Serv Res*. 2015;15:13.

[22] Boodoo C, Perry JA, Leung G, Cross KM, and Isaranuwatchai W. Cost-effectiveness of telemonitoring screening for diabetic foot ulcer: a mathematical model. *CMAJ Open*. 2018;6(4):E486–E494.

[23] Wong WW, Tu HA, Feld JJ, Wong T, and Krahn M. Cost-effectiveness of screening for hepatitis C in Canada. *CMAJ*. 2015;187(3):E110–E121.

[24] Skrepnek GH, Mills JL, Sr., and Armstrong DG. A diabetic emergency one million feet long: disparities and burdens of illness among diabetic foot ulcer cases within emergency departments in the United States, 2006-2010. *PLoS One*. 2015;10(8):e0134914.

[25] Reid KS, Martin BD, Duerksen F, *et al.* Diabetic foot complications in a northern Canadian Aboriginal community. *Foot Ankle Int*. 2006;27 (12):1065–1073.

[26] Siminerio LM, Piatt G, and Zgibor JC. Implementing the chronic care model for improvements in diabetes care and education in a rural primary care practice. *Diabetes Educ*. 2005;31(2):225–234.

[27] Corser W and Xu Y. Facilitating patients' diabetes self-management: a primary care intervention framework. *J Nurs Care Qual*. 2009;24(2):172–178.

[28] Griffith ML, Siminerio L, Payne T, and Krall J. A shared decision-making approach to telemedicine: engaging rural patients in glycemic management. *J Clin Med*. 2016;5(11).

[29] Bonoto BC, de Araujo VE, Godoi IP, *et al.* Efficacy of mobile apps to support the care of patients with diabetes mellitus: a systematic review and meta-analysis of randomized controlled trials. *JMIR Mhealth Uhealth*. 2017;5(3):e4.

[30] Hazenberg CE, van Netten JJ, van Baal SG, and Bus SA. Assessment of signs of foot infection in diabetes patients using photographic foot imaging and infrared thermography. *Diabetes Technol Ther*. 2014;16(6):370–377.

[31] Armstrong DG, Holtz-Neiderer K, Wendel C, Mohler MJ, Kimbriel HR, and Lavery LA. Skin temperature monitoring reduces the risk for diabetic foot ulceration in high-risk patients. *Am J Med*. 2007;120(12):1042–1046.

[32] Brownrigg JR, Schaper NC, and Hinchliffe RJ. Diagnosis and assessment of peripheral arterial disease in the diabetic foot. *Diabet Med*. 2015;32(6):738–747.

[33] Tsai FW, Tulsyan N, Jones DN, Abdel-Al N, Castronuovo JJ, Jr., and Carter SA. Skin perfusion pressure of the foot is a good substitute for toe pressure in the assessment of limb ischemia. *J Vasc Surg*. 2000;32(1):32–36.

[34] Greenman RL, Panasyuk S, Wang X, *et al.* Early changes in the skin microcirculation and muscle metabolism of the diabetic foot. *Lancet.* 2005;366(9498):1711–1717.

[35] Nouvong A, Hoogwerf B, Mohler E, Davis B, Tajaddini A, and Medenilla E. Evaluation of diabetic foot ulcer healing with hyperspectral imaging of oxy-hemoglobin and deoxyhemoglobin. *Diabetes Care.* 2009;32(11):2056–2061.

[36] Cross KM, Leonardi L, Gomez M, *et al.* Noninvasive measurement of edema in partial thickness burn wounds. *J Burn Care Res.* 2009;30(5):807–817.

[37] Cross KM, Leonardi L, Payette JR, *et al.* Clinical utilization of near-infrared spectroscopy devices for burn depth assessment. *Wound Repair Regen.* 2007;15(3):332–340.

[38] Sowa MG, Leonardi L, Payette JR, Fish JS, and Mantsch HH. Near infrared spectroscopic assessment of hemodynamic changes in the early post-burn period. *Burns.* 2001;27(3):241–249.

[39] Seki T, Fujioka M, Fukushima H, *et al.* Regional tissue oxygen saturation measured by near-infrared spectroscopy to assess the depth of burn injuries. *Int J Burns Trauma.* 2014;4(1):40–44.

[40] Leung G, Duta D, Perry J, Leonardi L, Fish J, and Cross K. Rapid tissue viability evaluation using methemoglobin as a biomarker in burns. *Int J Burns Trauma.* 2018;8(5):126–134.

[41] Boodoo C, Perry JA, Hunter PJ, *et al.* Views of patients on using mHealth to monitor and prevent diabetic foot ulcers: qualitative study. *JMIR Diabetes.* 2017;2(2):e22.

Chapter 8

Innovations in medical robotics: surgery, logistics, disinfection, and telepresence

Uri Feldman[1], *Christopher N. Larsen*[2], *Ekaterina Paramonova*[3] and *Daniel Theobald*[3]

Robots are taking on more significant roles in modern healthcare. With their constantly advancing capabilities, robotics can improve medical care. Robotics has the precision to perform the most careful procedures, such as those required for minimally invasive surgery (MIS). Robotics can enhance productivity by allowing people to focus on clinical decision-making tasks rather than on non-value-added tasks, such as in logistics and delivery of supplies. Advances in artificial intelligence (AI) and human–machine interfaces offer opportunities for robots to engage with patients at an emotional level and to provide companionship or service.

A grand vision for medical robotics is one where devices are fully decentralized, connected seamlessly via health informatics systems and networks to provide continuity of patient care across the entire health-care continuum. This chapter provides examples of key areas of innovation and growth in medical robotics. Each section describes the trends, exemplified with cases, design and implementation challenges, and future opportunities.

8.1 The medical robotics landscape

Medical robotics take center stage as health-care facilities modernize to improve outcomes, safety, and cost efficiencies. Robotic systems are present at all stages of the health-care continuum: from registration to surgery and follow-up care, and everything in between, including handling of lab and imaging tests, assisting in treatment, aiding in postoperative recovery, delivering patient education, performing physical therapy and rehabilitation, and facilitating follow-up care at home through telepresence.

[1]Department of Biomedical Engineering, Wentworth Institute, Boston, MA, USA
[2]Vecna Technologies, Inc., Greenbelt, MD, USA
[3]Vecna Robotics, Waltham, MA, USA

Robotics, broadly defined, encompasses actions like speech recognition, natural language processing, image analysis, as well as sensing and actuating capabilities. In this chapter, the focus is primarily on robots that can sense their environment, reason about how to achieve assigned tasks, and perform actions to carry out the plan.

The four application areas covered in this chapter are surgery (Section 8.2), logistics (Section 8.3), disinfection robots (Section 8.4), and telepresence (Section 8.5). The chapter provides an overview of key trends in each area, as well as examples of their use in clinical settings. Each section identifies challenges and opportunities for future development and growth.

Overall, the medical robotics industry worldwide has been sized at between 2.8 and 7.24 billion USD in 2015 and is estimated to reach 20 billion USD by 2023 [1]. This growth has been driven, in large part, by aging demographics and labor shortages. By 2022, 10 percent of the global population will be at least 65 years of age [2]. As the population ages and labor shortages increase, the need for robotic providers and assistants will accelerate.

Participating in this market are over 200 companies across the globe [3]. Surgical robots currently make up the majority of all medical robotics sales, at around 60 percent [4]. Surgical robots are the most expensive type of robotics used in healthcare, averaging about 1.5 million USD each [5]. Surgical robots are prevalent because they can improve the outcomes of many types of surgeries and are making new precision surgeries possible and more effective. Followed in market share are "cyberknife" devices for performing noninvasive radiosurgery in the treatment of cancer. Nonclinical hospital logistics robots are still a relative rarity but are growing in both market penetration and in their capabilities. Disinfection robots have the potential of greatly reducing the number of patients who contract healthcare-acquired infections (HAIs) and nosocomial infections that today occur at a rate of 1 in 25, and of which, 1 in 9 will die from these acquired infections [6].

Overall growth in all these markets should continue to accelerate. The surgical robotics market alone is expected to double in size by 2020 to 6.4 billion USD [7] and double again by 2025 to $12.6 billion [8]. The next fastest growing segment is the medical logistics market, with an estimated 1.9 billion USD value in 2016 [9]. The telepresence market is next, at $1.4 billion in size in 2016 [10]. Disinfection robots are currently not a large market by, estimated at 0.8 billion USD today, or under about 2 percent of the total medical robotics market but are expected to grow rapidly [11].

8.2 Surgery

Robotic systems make it possible to perform surgeries that were previously technically difficult or not even feasible. Despite a 2 million USD price tag, including ongoing service and maintenance costs, plus the lack of additional reimbursements from insurers for robotic procedures, the return on investment for utilizing robots in surgery is nevertheless achieved. Medical robotics offers improved outcomes, higher utilization rates, and the academic prestige and marketing impact of adopting new technologies.

The advantages of surgical robotics are many. For one, they enhance surgical techniques, such as laparoscopy, by providing improved dexterity and control, enhanced usability and ergonomics, and better visualization tools. The most widely adopted applications of robotics in surgery include those which require highly controlled, precise, steady, and repetitive motions. In particular, MIS is one of the most effective applications for robotics in medicine because MIS enables access to surgical locations with great precision and control of delicate actions all while minimizing collateral damage to the surrounding tissues and structures. MIS results in better outcomes and faster recovery times than those with open surgeries. The main specialties that utilize MIS robots are urology, gynecology, and gastroenterology.

Instead of operating on patients through large incisions, in MIS, the miniaturized surgical instruments are inserted through one or more quarter-inch incisions. In addition to the instruments, lights and three-dimensional cameras are inserted to visualize and guide the procedure.

The surgeon controls the instruments and the camera from a console located in the operating room while looking through a stereoscopic high-definition monitor (Figure 8.1). Every movement made with the controls is replicated precisely by the robot. When necessary, the surgeon can adjust the scale of the robot's movement so that motions can be either amplified or diminished. Because of the console's design, the surgeon's eyes and hands are always perfectly aligned with the view of the surgical site, minimizing surgeon fatigue.

8.2.1 Design challenges

The design of surgical robots constitutes a trade-off between size, function, and complexity. The ideal surgical instrument is small, fits through one opening (port), or, ideally, goes through a natural orifice (nose, throat, and bellybutton), and

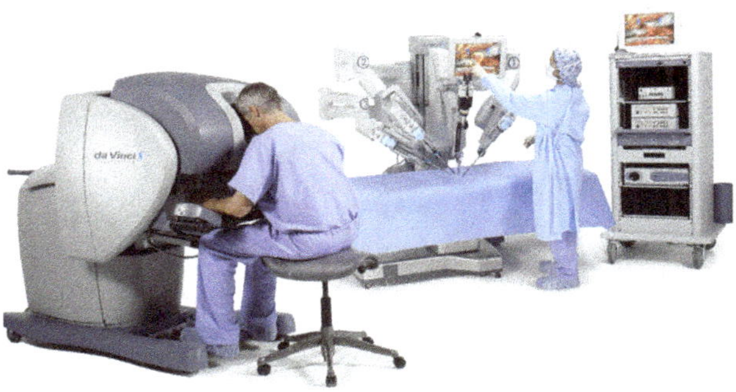

Figure 8.1 da Vinci surgical robot configuration. Robotic apparatus with adjacent remote control console. © 2018 Intuitive Surgical, Inc

performs all tasks precisely, efficiently, and autonomously. Currently, such a system is not attainable. The grand challenges that need to be tackled in the design and implementation of medical robotics include the following [12]:

1. Instrumentation
2. Visualization
3. Sensing
4. Integration
5. Human–machine interaction

8.2.1.1 Instrumentation

The key purpose of robotics in surgery is to perform intricate procedures in confined spaces while executing highly "choreographed" steps such as visualizing, measuring, cutting, suturing, cauterizing, inserting, extracting, draining, and more, all through as few ports as possible. Figure 8.2 shows some of the types of instruments that are attached to robotic arms. From an engineering perspective, utilization of the robotic apparatus necessitates the ability to replace and attach quickly, securely, and safely a myriad of probes and instruments. In practice, multiple ports are needed to provide the access, and visualization needed to perform all the required steps simultaneously and in a synchronized manner.

Innovations in the design of robotic instruments are enabling single-port or single-site techniques (R-LESS) [13]. Surgical robotics manufacturers, such as Intuitive Surgical and Titan Medical, are leading the way in single-port procedures. See Figure 8.3.

8.2.1.2 Visualization

The most common configuration of a surgical robot consists of one or more robotic arms on top of the operating table, with the surgeon sitting at a nearby console, as shown in Figure 8.1. Cameras and lights are inserted through a port to provide continuous real-time visual feedback of all the actions. The fundamental imaging and visualization challenges in surgical robotics are how to render three-

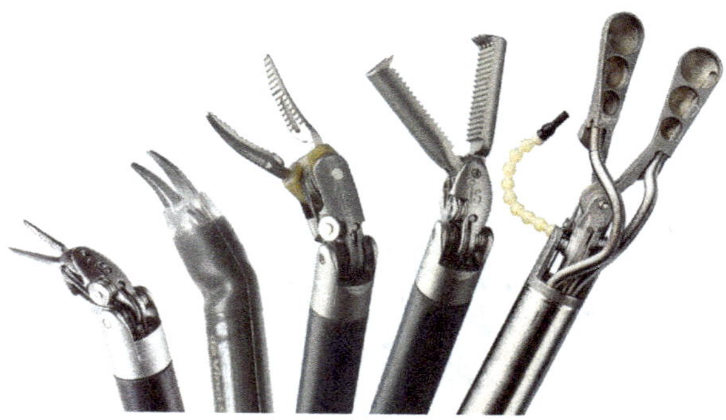

Figure 8.2 Array of instruments for use with the da Vinci system. © 2018 Intuitive Surgical, Inc

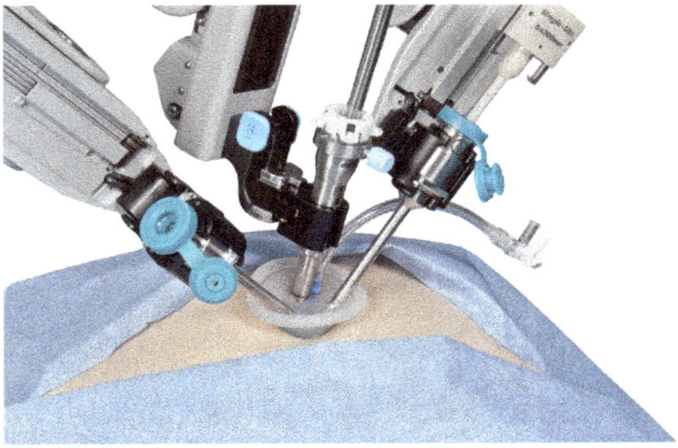

Figure 8.3 da Vinci system with multiple instruments inserted through a single port. © 2018 Intuitive Surgical, Inc

dimensional structures in real-time using, primarily, two-dimensional displays. Visual displays provide the primary means for localization and feedback during a procedure. Effective visualization is essential when operating robotic instruments from a workstation, located either directly adjacent to the patient or remotely, as in a tele-surgery application. For example, in orthopedic procedures, such as knee and shoulder repair, where the joints are somewhat stable in a confined space, the parts are mostly rigid, and the location of the various parts is relatively predictable, two-dimensional displays have sufficed. However, as robotic systems perform ever more complex procedures, in delicate and harder to reach anatomies, there needs to be realistic three-dimensional visualization. MIS is a case where virtual and augmented reality displays could prove valuable.

At the component level, to provide more realistic three-dimensional visualizations of the surgical field, cameras and lights need to be positioned, usually away from where the other instruments and actuators are to provide the right visual perspective. This requirement, in turn, requires the use of additional tips and ports. At an imaging level, accurate three-dimensional positioning as well as tracking of tissues and instruments need to be performed via image processing and analysis methods or through the use of markers, or a combination of these techniques. Registration as well as image fusion methods also need to be applied. One method is to overlay or fuse static pre-operatory CT or MRI scans with the live video streams as the procedure is taking place (Figure 8.4).

8.2.1.3 Sensing

Perhaps one of the most difficult and least developed of all the features of surgical robots is sensing. Sensing is a feedback process where what is happening at the surgical site is interpreted, processed, and adapted to, in real-time. There are two sides to sensing: the response at the interface between instrument and tissue and the response between controls and surgeon.

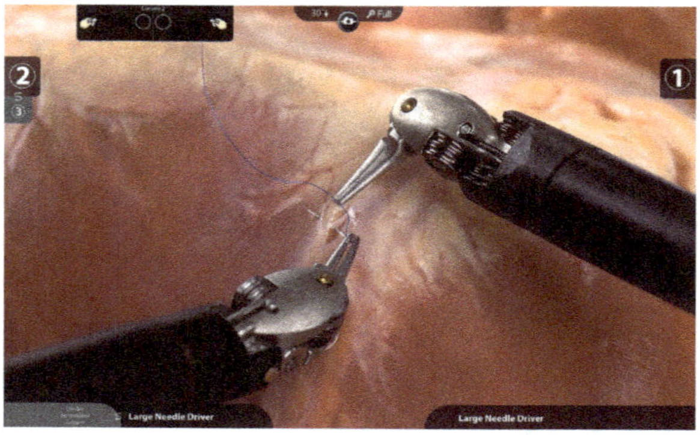

Figure 8.4 Visualization of suturing with robotic instruments. © 2018 Intuitive Surgical, Inc

For example, beating-heart surgery is a very promising alternative to traditional open-heart bypass procedures because of its quicker and much less risky recovery. Accurate and instantaneous tracking of the heart motion is essential for positioning and adjustment of the instruments to move in synchrony with the heart using motion compensation techniques. In addition to motion, when organs, tissues, and fluids are acted on, they tend to change in shape, consistency, and location. It is critical to track these changes and to adapt to them through dynamic placement and coordinated motion of the instruments in the actuator arms. The key is to implement actuators and sensors that recognize subtle changes in the physical behavior of the tissues. The most common sensing methods include the detection of changes in current, resistance, capacitance, vibration, and piezoelectric effects. Optical and machine-vision sensors are used as well.

On the operator side, a key aspect of sensing is to provide haptic feedback to the surgeon through the controls. This tactile feedback is essential to providing the surgeon with the ability to "touch" and "feel" the structures to determine the placement, extent, and duration of the surgical action to be performed on that structure or in its vicinity. Recently released systems from Transenterix and da Vinci have haptic controls that provide tactile feedback (Figure 8.5).

8.2.1.4 Integration

How surgical robots adapt to and enhance the procedures they were designed for is critical. At a procedural level, surgical robots need to be integrated into the operating room as well as into the surgical workflow so as to enhance and not to prolong or complicate the procedures. At an operational level, the robot and its parts must be designed so they are simple to deploy, operate, maintain, and reuse through consecutive procedures. At a systems level, the interactions between the mechanical, electronic, optical, software, and human must be highly synchronized. However, as the design of the instruments and actuators evolves, it becomes more challenging to minimize the mechanics and electronics while preserving the

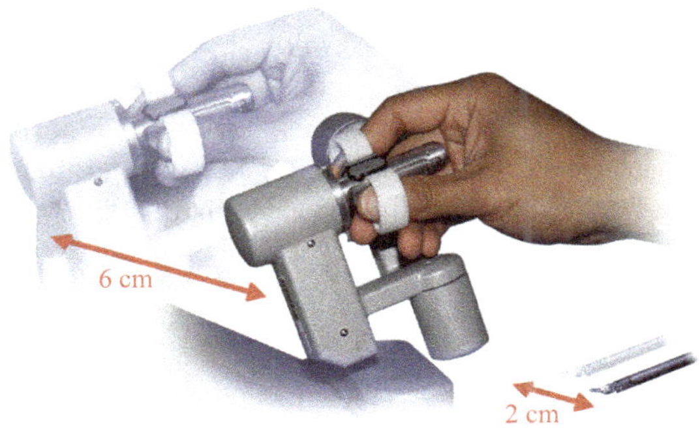

Figure 8.5 Control at console provides haptic feedback. © 2018 Intuitive Surgical, Inc

flexibility, range, weight, and size of the actuators. Another critical aspect that must be taken into consideration from the outset is cleaning or sterilization of all components. Perhaps, self-cleaning methods, such as those described in Section 8.4, could be built into the surgical robots themselves.

8.2.1.5 Human–machine interactions

Control and operation of surgical robotic systems ranges between fully human teleoperated to fully self-guided autonomous operation. Some of the key parameters to consider in the design of an effective human-interface include guidance, positioning, navigation, stabilization, control, range of motion, and actuation. A skilled surgeon knows the insertion angle and depth of placement of an instrument. Surgeons also know the range of the action, such as where to start and finish an incision. A robot is capable of performing highly precise actions, even more precisely than those of a human. It is therefore critical for the system and human operator, or a combination of the two, to understand, plan, and execute the actions in a controlled and highly predictable manner. The mapping of the user interface actions to those of the robotic system is fundamental. The interface needs to take into consideration the imaging, positional, procedural, clinical, and other aspects of the surgery. Instrument and tissue motion need to be synchronized with path planning of how the instruments move. On the safety side, the system must be able to limit certain actions and immediately stop if there are problems.

8.2.2 New directions in surgical robotics

Surgical robots in use today utilize mostly rigid and straight instruments. Continuum robotics (soft-robots) is an emerging category of devices with actuators and manipulators which are not limited by fixed degree of freedom joints. These devices behave more like snakes or other bendable–flexible manipulators. Continuum robotics provides enhanced access and can be deployed along nonlinear paths. These types of structures can be made smaller than conventional actuators and provide access to hard-to-reach or obstructed anatomies.

Microbots are another exciting area of research. These miniature robots are built at a microscale or nanoscale so that they can be inserted into the body in full and navigate to their target destination to execute their actions. Other areas of development include autonomously controlled robots, real-time biopsies using AI, and robotic prosthetics and exoskeletons. The challenges in robot implementation, control, guidance, visualization, sensing, and the robot–human interface still remain.

8.3 Logistics

In addition to the use of robotics for clinical applications, there is a considerable growth in the use of robotics for supporting logistical functions in health-care facilities. As the global population ages and the shortage of health-care providers increases, there is a great need for systems and technologies to perform many of the supporting activities needed in a health-care facility. Medical logistics robotics refers to the use of robots to transport equipment and supplies around the facility. The logistics market is a rapidly growing robotics market, focusing primarily on warehousing and order fulfillment and approaching 100,000 units sold and 1.9 billion USD value in 2016 [10]. Most of these logistical robotic systems are deployed at warehouse distribution centers for major organizations, such as Amazon, FedEx, DHL, Target, WalMart, and the like.

The demand for automated systems that can perform multiple logistical functions in a clinical setting is increasing, as hospital workflows become more automated and employee time becomes more specialized and demanding. A mobile robotic vehicle that can serve as a supply and pharmaceutical storage and delivery platform, as well as a drug dispensing one, will increase hospital productivity and improve cost efficiencies. Most robotic systems in use today are slow and not reliable enough due to their simplistic navigation controls and limited sensing capabilities. A truly effective, safe, and cost-efficient system needs to possess a high level of automation and adaptability so that it can operate in a variety of settings with minimal modifications to existing infrastructure.

In a typical hospital, around 30 percent of a nurse's time is spent on logistics-focused tasks, such as locating and moving equipment and supplies [14]. These types of tasks are ideal for robots to step in and take over. In addition, logistical robots, due to their flexible platform design, have the ability to transport a wide variety of payloads, including pharmaceuticals, laboratory samples, medical devices, medical waste, sharps, secured patient records, hospital administrative documents, patient supplies, and even custom meals.

One illustrative example of the types of constraints encountered in the design of a medical logistics robot is the transport and dispensation of medications and controlled substances. In such instance, drawers holding controlled substances or biomaterials can be secured until they are validated and matched to the correct recipient upon delivery. Currently available medication delivery robots are essentially automated versions of medcarts which perform secure operations but which are wired and tethered to a specific and secure formulary location in the facility.

Additional factors that need to be considered in the design and deployment of robotic medical logistics solutions include sanitation, safety, collision avoidance, secure delivery of protected health records, and identification of biopsy samples and delivery to other departments. These robots also need to be physically robust, capable of cord-free operation in order to roam clinic hallways and doors, yet small enough to navigate through all possible routes, able to call elevators, able to navigate to specific mapped locations while avoiding obstacles, and operate in a finite clinical environment.

8.3.1 Vecna QC Bot

The Vecna QC Bot addresses such needs [15] (Figure 8.6). This robotic platform is capable of performing functions, such as autonomous navigation, visual processing, object avoidance, and even elevator location and activation. QC Bots can be configured to safely move pharmaceuticals, laundry, and small equipment while not violating patient privacy. Vecna designed a wheeled, self-propelled, patient-friendly robotic platform, using minimal infrastructure localization system and an advanced but low-cost vision-based feature extraction system. Signs are placed at important locations in the hospital environment to tell the mobile robot where it is. This vision capability is based on reliable algorithms that can read specially crafted but minimally invasive and low-cost signs. The existing vision capability is highly reliable at detecting door signs.

Coupled with Bluetooth and wireless technology that can be programmed to open up any amenable elevator doors, the QC Bot is capable of multi-floor operation. It is also coupled with low-cost ultrasonic and infrared ranging sensor system, to enable warning-based operation to alert bystanders of the autonomy of the robot, and to stop when something is in the way, or a navigation hazard, such as

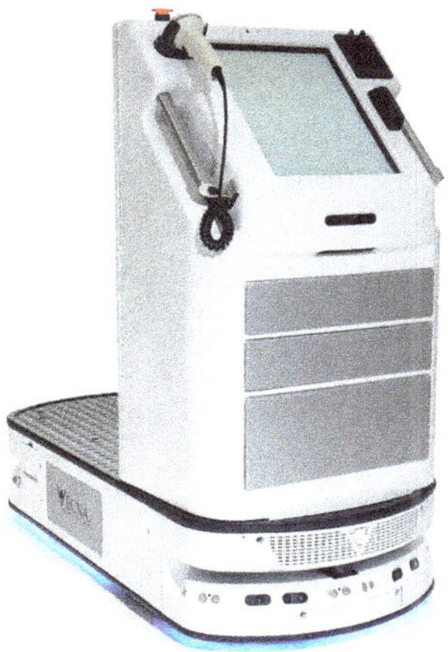

Figure 8.6 Vecna QC Bot

stairs or a glass barrier are encountered. The information from the various sensors is combined in an advanced sensor fusion framework in order to provide optimal localization.

Vecna has also developed vision-based techniques for the extraction of natural features, such as hallway and door frame edges. This also includes the development of vision-based techniques for tracking humans in the vicinity of the robot, to support safe operation, and better human–robot interaction. Last, there is a maneuver-based movement controller. This allows the relatively large, non-uniformly shaped robots to maneuver in tight spaces such as doorways, corners, and elevators. The QC Bot is capable of delivering drugs, medical supplies, patient charts and paperwork, and linens and devices, in a locked or unlocked configuration, using swappable drawers, shelves, or bins.

8.3.2 Aethon TUG

Another hospital robotics system is the Aethon TUG [16]. This robotic system is designed to haul clean or dirty linens, medical waste, or biometrically coded pharmaceuticals and medications or devices, with an associated PIN code so that staff may not remove the package unless authorized. It is designed to free clinical staff from long-range delivery duties, for other human centric tasks. Like the Vecna QC Bot, it has laser-based human and object avoidance systems. Furthermore, TUG can be controlled via a remote tablet-based service and is monitored by the corporate office. Like the QC Bot, the robot uses wireless technology to open elevator doors. One additional feature of the Aethon solution is its ability to respond to fire alarms and evacuate itself from the building, if it can.

8.3.3 Interhospital delivery by drones

Logistics robotics need not only operate inside clinical environments. They are also expanding into the market of flying between hospital locations to rapidly deliver medical supplies. One such example is the Matternet drone system [17]. It operates from a central station to a number of hospital sites within range in Switzerland. To serve as a site for the drone, a Matternet Station is placed on the rooftop of the accepting and sending network node. The station is 2 m across and contains a scanning station with a unique location code. One of the unique features of the drone system is that after landing, the device locks itself in place and swaps out its battery system for a new, charged one, so that critical supplies are not lost to power issues in flight. Further, the drone is a quadrotor robot with a payload bay capable of carrying 1.8 kg to sites within 19.3–22.5 km. The network operates in densely populated areas, broadcasts its location, and performs path optimization calculations in flight.

8.3.4 Challenges

There are several challenges in logistic robots for clinical environments currently. The number of logistics robots, needed at a site, for example, is something of a study at present. How many robots would be needed at a site? Does the site type impact this number? One study has been performed to estimate the number of robots that a particular clinic would need, to replace human porters [18]. This study measured the mean delay time in waiting, and the percent success rate at differing delivery time requirement cutoffs. Adding more robots increased the delivery success rate, if the robots were networked and communicating in a team-deployable fashion. It also reduced the waiting time. However, the model was presented as a tool for hospital management to use based on their sample and package workload, and as a function of their departmental or location budgets.

In the case of multi-robot sites, task allocation and queuing then becomes a complex issue, as does continuous connectivity to a central or distributed system of workload management. The robots may need to hold a hierarchy stating importance for each delivery task, so that the most pressing issues are taken care of first, such as taking chilled or biodegradable biosample deliveries to the pathology or laboratory site, before transporting nonperishables. Nursing personnel can currently queue their workload cognitively by clinical priority. However, establishing this understanding in software represents a large challenge, especially where complex clinical decisions need to be developed to route a path most effectively to the best outcome possible.

Monitoring of logistics robots is still required. Studies corroborate that a successful solution should be monitored 24/7, is low cost, high accuracy, and does not require much maintenance intervention by clinical staff. One prevailing impression is a solution that requires frequent maintenance, and repeated tending is not better than a low-wage worker. The market for such robots will only begin to quickly grow when the price point goes down and automation improves.

Overall, logistics robots are effective in reducing the human workload, taking deliveries via secured means, carrying hazardous or heavy materials, and holding regulated drug compounds securely in drawer systems that have authorization-based security and location-code-based package handling. They can handle the delivery of pharmaceuticals, laboratory specimens, food deliveries to patients, medical or office waste. For the most part, object avoidance, navigation, and security are being addressed. If the more complex issues of fleet optimization and task queuing can be improved, the efficiency and market penetration of these devices will only go up.

8.4 Disinfection robots

Disinfection robots represent a new entrant in the robotics market space. Allied Research Reports suggest a total disinfection market of under $4 billion, but this is largely for water supplies using stationary devices [19]. More specific and reasonable estimates are $80 million market size, or under about 2 percent of the total medical robotics market [9]. Several models are available for clinical settings that can either be passively set in a certain area or autonomously migrate to the site of disinfection. These represent various tiers of functionality, some of which are further described next.

8.4.1 Pathogen disinfection

To understand the disinfection robotic use case fully, and to understand why the current products are designed in the way they are, it will be necessary to view it in the context of the microbiology involved. Described briefly later is the microbiology of disinfection, the operation that the robots are built around, and some details are added as to the underpinnings of the pathogen life cycle, the robotic and human work duty of disinfection, the necessary photonics and biochemistry, and the functional requirements for a robotic disinfection product. The overall basic use case for disinfection robot is to kill pathogens, stopping them either from their ability to (i) transmit their genes, (ii) replicate faithfully by division, or (iii) retain their structural or genetic biological integrity.

Traditionally, disinfection has been done in the past by building services personnel, clinicians, sterilization technicians, or nursing staff, via several means: denaturation of surfaces by ethanol, spray application of chlorhexidine (a disinfectant and antiseptic used for disinfection before surgery and to sterilize surgical instruments), autoclaving, or using alkaline solutions, such as ammonia, or peroxides, phenolics, steam, heat, ethylene oxide, or radiation. These historical methods form a basis of prior art for choosing best what a robot can do, to perform the same functional task.

Disinfection by either heat or solvents is an option but is neither comprehensive nor ideal for robots as tanks of liquid would need to be stored and refilled. In fact, bacteria can be eradicated by many denaturing solvents. However, most viruses are resistant due to their tough protein capsid shell. Many viruses, such as Hepatitis B, enteroviruses, norovirus, sapovirus, adenovirus, rhinovirus, Enterovirus-D68, and others, are even heat stable [20], resistant to ethanol or other solutions, and need to be irradiated, oxidized, or structurally damaged in order to eliminate their threat. Typically, this step is performed by high heat and pressure, chlorhexidine, or irradiation by UV or gamma wavelengths. Among these methods, only UV irradiation is satisfactory. Even fungal spores can be broken apart by UV irradiation [21]. Finally, the ubiquity of nucleic acids polymers as the genetic material for all these pathogens, and the breakage of their chemical structure by UV light make radiative disinfection ideal, especially for robots.

Pathogens are effectively killed by absorption of UV light. In this process, high-energy emissions of light are shed onto all surfaces in a room. UV-C (100–280 nm) is effective in breaking DNA or RNA strands, although it does not occur at the earth's surface and is filtered out by the Earth's ozone layer [22]. Further, UV-C light is strong enough to photocrosslink DNA bases, break the phosphate backbone of the genetic material, or can cleave the sugar-base bonds to mutate the organism's code. All these chemical reactions make it impossible for pathogen genetic information to be stored properly and faithfully and can prevent the nucleotide strand to be duplicated by replicative polymerase enzymes provided by the human host, just as attempting to draw a zipper with bound or missing teeth also renders the device unusable. These natural features of the systems in question reveal robots to be an effective tool in the infection control arsenal of the clinic.

8.4.2 UV disinfection as an ideal robotic occupation

Robotics are an ideal servant for the job of disinfecting health-care facilities, having a vast number of obvious benefits to their use [23]. They are portable, controllable by remote or wireless means, are immune to human pathogens, able to operate in dark, light, cold, or warm climates, at any hour, and in the midst of a wide range of any microbial disease threats to humans and their food or companion animals. The most highly encountered threats in the clinic are viruses, fungi, protists, and bacteria, such as MRSA, *Clostridium difficile*, *Bacillus*, *Staphylococcus*, *Klebsiella*, *Escherichia coli*, *Citrobacter*, *Proteobacteria please check with auth/ed*, and *Pseudomonas*. Being inorganic machines, robots do not carry biological viruses, such as influenza, hepatitis, rhinovirus, papillomavirus, or herpesviruses. They can be sterilized, can be made water impermeable, and they are immutable by radiation that may be harmful to living things. Robots are also not vectors or reservoirs for disease transmission, unlike humans, animals, insects, or liquid vessels. Overall, robots are almost ideal for the purpose of disinfection.

Robots are made to emit UV radiation by the use of incorporating high intensity halogen lamps. The benefits of loading the emission system onto a robot are manyfold. They can sterilize whole rooms, which have multiple surfaces that are permeable or soluble to solvents, inaccessible due to height, or are difficult to clean due to their topology or fabrication delicacy. UV photons are immeasurably light cargo, are controllably emitted, with no physical consequences on the structure of what they impact, except to stimulate oxidation chemistry that can destroy microbes. They leave metals and other substrates mostly untouched. UV light can be focused by a lens or pointed at any surface, in any direction, and in any required intensity or power, as specified. Further, the light beams can easily travel any distance indoors* and reach ceiling surfaces, which otherwise would be too high to be cleaned by health-care staff. The method is also used for sterilization of microbiological fume hoods and has also been applied as a concept to air by stationary units, or to whole rooms, as long as patients and staff are not present, such as after a hazardous event involving quarantine, bleed-out, sepsis or pathogen epidemic cases.

Irradiation, furthermore, represents an open system. Many sterilization operations are performed by closed machinery in the clinic, such as by washers, autoclaves, heat-sterilization units, decontamination units, and hydrogen peroxide vaporizers. However, these are typically stationary units, loaded with implements or waste, and are not typically considered as much robotics as appliances, though they are indeed highly automated with work cycles, sensors, and feedback systems. A more common concept of robotics as defined previously would consider a unit that can operate freely on its environment, in a mobile, intelligent, and unattended way.

The work environment of these robots is dynamic and ever changing, so a mounted device is not practical for the clinic. Because those environments are populated with patients and equipment that move, stationary disinfection devices

*Although irradiation intensity drops as inverse square of the distance.

are not practical, and mobile robotics systems offer significant advantages. These characteristics make UV disinfection robots ideal for the operating rooms, clinics, bathrooms, triage or waiting areas, and storage closets.

8.4.3 Examples of UV sterilizing robots

Several UV disinfection robots have emerged in the market [24]. Power use is heavy in order to create the energy to emit microbe-killing light, so a corded solution is typically used, unless the unit roams freely such as with floor robots. Each solution uses a controlled halogen (Xenon) light emission cycle for continuous or pulse emission. This step is accomplished by controlling power, capacitors, and relay systems using a microcontroller or dedicated operating system that calls pin voltages accordingly.

For the duty cycle, the target room has to first be prepped for sterilization. Drawers should be opened, tubing uncoiled, and beds unmade. All surfaces to be cleaned need to be visible to the light path from the robot. Although this step requires extra manual, human work, the overall process is ultimately faster, because no sterilization chemicals are used and reentry to the room is immediate, requiring no drying time or volatile organics.

For safety, these robots have motion sensors or remote controls that prohibit their operation when a person is nearby, since exposure to UV light may cause skin or retinal damage. This restriction may mean that the work cycle to disinfect a room is tripartite, with a technician operating a cycle, reentering the room to turn devices and equipment, and move the robot to get different irradiation angles to all objects and surfaces in the room.

8.4.3.1 Xenex

One example of a robotic disinfection product is the Xenex robot [25]. The Xenex is purported to clean a room of germs and viruses within 5 min. It uses a high-intensity Xenon lamp emitting a UV-C wavelength band of radiation (200–280 nm), which is emitted from a tower that emerges during operation. The method of operation of the robot is such that the room is first secured, with signage on the door, and a motion-detecting sensor left at the door. In case a person enters the room, the robot shuts down its emissions. The light emitter rotates 360 degrees of rotation within the tower and only leaves spots untouched directly above and below the robot footprint. Sometimes, a second pass is necessary in the room, where objects are turned over, and the footprint of the robot is treated as well by moving it slightly. The Xenex manufacturer claims a 50 percent reduction in hospital-acquired infections. It does not self-propel but does automatically control its emission cycle.

8.4.3.2 Blue Ocean Robotics

Blue Ocean has also developed a UV sterilization robot [26]. The robot is on an AGV platform and was developed in partnership with RoBi-X. It is similar in operation to the Xenex, except that it is directionally and operationally controlled by a tablet app, and the emission bulbs are permanently extended upward. As such, it is somewhat less robust and more top heavy. However, it is also a continuous emission product, unlike the pulsed XENEX. When the duty cycle is called for by the application program, mechanical shields first rotate around the bulbs to allow UV light to be let out. This is in contrast to the XENEX solution of lowering the bulbs into the body of the robot. Blue Ocean uses the RoBi-X partnership model [27] and is headquartered in Odense, Denmark.

8.4.3.3 Skytron—infection prevention technologies

Other devices resembling the Xenex and Blue Ocean models seem to have their capacities stripped down for cost and simplicity. One such example is the IPT3200 from infection prevention technologies. The IPT 3200 claims to be the most powerful UV disinfection method available. It boasts a continuous emission system up to 20 times the energy of the pulsed Xenex, with a result of having fewer placements and room turns needed. Added functionality has been developed to attempt to account for the environmental conditions in which emission will take place. There are sensors that purport to measure the room conditions, such as size, temperature, and humidity, to make the emission session optimal for germicidal activity. The device is an omnidirectional, nonautonomous solution, and such, needs to be wheeled into place and controlled with a remote control. It does not contain shields, except to the center of the robot. In this manner, the device sheds as much energy as possible outward into the room. It is among the least automated mechanically, with fewer moving parts, but has intelligent software design and operation.

8.4.3.4 Steris Pathogon

The Steris Corporation also markets a UV disinfection robot (Figure 8.7). It is similar to others in using a halogen bulb and wheels but has no autonomous mobility. Like the IPT design, all the operational internals are behind the bulb system, so that no shadow is made between the UV emission bulb and the area to be illuminated. The robot has a bulb guard rail and a large plastic shield for transport. Operation is automated and simple. The Pathogon has one user-selectable feature, with the user being able to specify emission from 4 to 25 min depending on the area of treatment required and the germicidal load or pathogen species.

8.4.3.5 UV emitting floor sterilization vacuums

Room disinfection is not the only route to cleaning a clinical bay or area. Other robots focus their effort only on the floor. These devices navigate the flat floor surface, mapping out their path or performing object avoidance maneuvers. For example, the iTouchless corporation claims that their robotic vacuum cleaner "has a ... stronger 1.2 kPa motor, quieter (<50 dB) operation, automatic return to and charging at charging station when the battery is low, 5 pre-set cleaning modes, anti-fall and anti-collision sensors, an extra-large 900 ml dustbin that requires less frequent emptying, low-profile design (less than 4" height), and a remote control that offers one-button control." Other product offerings include the Rollibot (Model BL618) and Sharper Image.

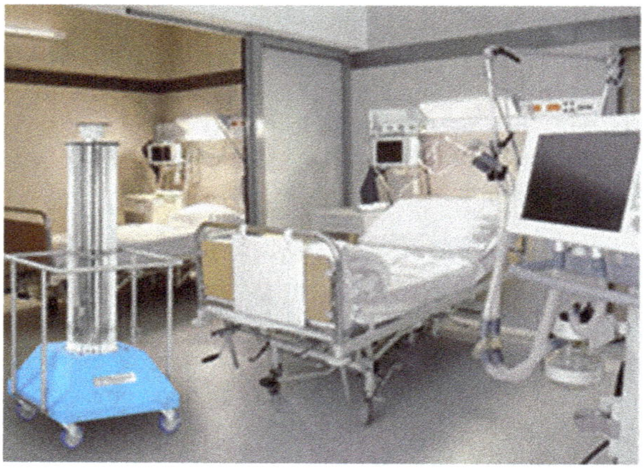

Figure 8.7 Steris Pathogon disinfection setup

Such a robotic UV-emitting vacuum device is useful for dried or cleaned biological spill hazard areas, but not for cleaning raised surfaces that are touched by hands and patients, such as doorknobs, device buttons, bedrails, or lavatories. Furthermore, due to the size of the robot, it cannot operate within 25.4 cm of any floor standing furniture or leg, thus making a margin of untreated area around every object on the floor.

8.4.4 Challenges

The main downside to UV-based sterilization robots is their indiscriminate operation. The entire area in a light beam path is irradiated; the whole room is exposed, whether contaminated or not. As UV photons are capable of breaking carbon–carbon bonds in various configurations, organic materials such as vinyl, wood, or paintings may over time become bleached or worn as if by sunlight, aging prematurely.

One possible improvement to this downside scenario would involve a two-step robotics work cycle of detection, followed by eradication. If the robots were capable of finding microbial contamination first, they could be programmed to work only on those areas. For example, if a room could be exhaustively scanned via light spectrometry by the robot, at 190–230 nm wavelength[†] and the spatial positions mapped by point cloud, those same positions could also be irradiated by the robot. This work cycle however represents both a technical barrier and an expense. It is unclear if the market would bear that cost and the additional complexity. The same procedure could be performed by a floor robot, searching for fluorescence emitted by *Pseudomonas*, for example, and then irradiating the area only after detection.

[†]The absorption of the protein amide bond present in all life.

The second downside to UV-based disinfection robots is their ability to irradiate only what they can "see" or reach mechanically. Light only travels in a straight line, so shadows are always going to be present in a three-dimensional world. Presumably a combination of methods or passes would be ideal in overcoming this shortfall, for example, turning around objects, repeating the disinfection cycle, or coupling work with robotic floor, air, and water sterilization methods. A mobile robot that can sense shadows would be able to move itself in order to minimize the untreated areas.

Overall UV-emitting disinfection robots are serving a valuable purpose, to eliminate pathogens from the clinical environment, thus lowering the number of HAIs and other cases, such as MRSA and sepsis, reducing insurance costs, and lowering hospital-associated morbidity and mortality.

8.5 Telepresence

There are many options for using telepresence or telerobotics in the clinical space. Telepresence devices offer specialists and physicians the opportunity, for example, to reach patients with rare disorders who are not in concentrated urban areas with large facilities that specialize in pediatrics, geriatrics, radiology, endocrinology, neurology, or any other specialties. By enabling a remote presence solution, any specialist can eliminate the travel time and deliver faster care to more persons. Remote diagnostics can be coupled with telepresence solutions. These devices can also facilitate telehealth delivery in a pandemic situation when social distancing is imperative.

Many marketed products exist in the telepresence space, which is estimated to be about $1.4 billion in size in 2016 [10]. Later we describe examples of marketed products that can provide telepresence, catalyze telemedicine, act as a concierge, companion, or kiosk solution. Each section includes a discussion of their features, limitations, and growth potential.

Robotics can also offer customer service and support setting for staffing required for working with patients, by virtue of acting as a kiosk, administrative assistant, or way-finding companion. While logistics-oriented robots focus on getting materials from one location to another, with minimal interaction with patients, customer service medical robots are in fact built to interact with a human patient for emotional support, such as companionship for operational support, such as getting from the lobby to the examination room. Recent advancements in AI allow robots to be able to quickly learn about the needs of the patients and its surroundings and adapt as necessary.

Telepresence is also key in military and natural disaster situations, for example, casualty extraction (CASEVAC). Battlefield Extraction Assist Robot (BEAR™), for example, is designed to remove wounded soldiers from combat. In the stead of another person being sent out to retrieve a downed soldier, the robot is sent instead. This solution is especially useful for hazardous environments, radiological or chemical hazards, such as in the case of chemical weapons. The BEAR is remote-control operated and can be sent to the casualty, with the protected user at a distance location. This functionality is also useful for the extraction of civilian casualties, such as after natural disasters like hurricanes, earthquakes, and radiological disasters.

In all these cases, the ability of the robot platform to serve as an informational extension of a subject matter expert or professional is the key. The ability to send the consciousness to a site without the physical person is the central element. Whether on the battlefield, clinic, home, school, or in public, a telepresence robot that focuses on videoconferencing, image and sound, information, and felt presence, is an important product that can amplify the utility of persons with useful skills, such as in the clinic or military theater.

8.5.1 Telepresence

8.5.1.1 Double Robotics

Double makes a balancing robot with audio–video capability, which targets telecommuters in the office, school, clinic, or at events. Backed by the YCombinator startup accelerator in 2012, Double Robotics began shipping in May 2013. The founders include David Cann, a designer and iOS developer, and Marc DeVidts, an electrical/embedded system engineer. The company is located in Burlingame, California.

Doubles are widely distributed worldwide, on Amazon, and on the Apple store. However, the buyer must supply their own iPad to sit at the top of the robot. The company has found the original iPad audio/video to be lacking, so they have recently added speaker and camera accessories for better performance. The Double 2 promises better stability as it is a balancing robot that tended to fall down, and now slightly faster speeds. The remote user can use any Windows, Apple, or Android device as starting point for operational control. It is believed that Double is the market's leader by volume, as a result of its lower price point, iPad branding, and wide distribution.

8.5.1.2 Suitable Technologies

Suitable Technologies makes a telepresence robot called the Beam (Figure 8.8). Suitable is a spinout of the robotic research company Willow Garage, who are the inventors of the Robot Operating System (ROS) [28]. Willow Garage developed a prototype they called Texai for use by a remote developer so that the person could be with the development team. The prototype was featured on an episode of "The Big Bang Theory" television show (the Shelbot). Texai was the first introduction of the capability of telepresence, to many people in the USA. ROS is an open-standard platform. As stated on the group's documentation, ROS was developed at multiple institutions and for multiple robots, including many institutions who received PR2 robots from Willow Garage. Although it would have been far simpler for all contributors to place their code on the same servers, over the years, the federated model has emerged as one of the great strengths of the ROS ecosystem. Any group

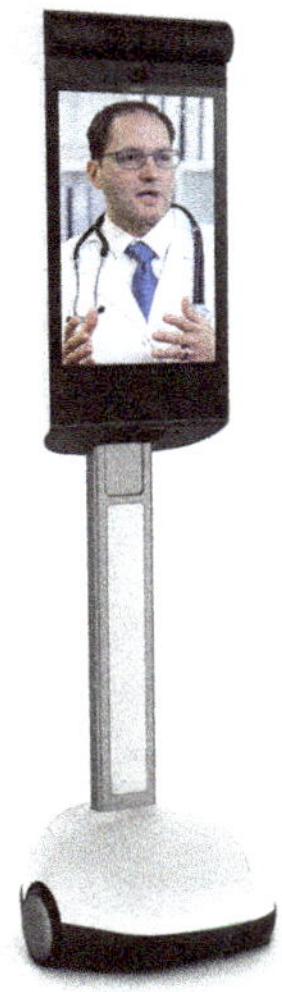

Figure 8.8 Suitable Technologies sample

can benefit from specific technical feedback and improvements, like all open-source software projects.

Suitable was funded by the CEO, Scott Hassan. Scott was the founder of eGroups (now Yahoo! Groups) and was a key software architect and developer of Google, Alexa Internet, and the Stanford Digital Library. The first product was called Beam, the second was Beam Pro, followed by the Beam+. The Beam Pro was seen at public events, as the very large screen is inviting. The Beam+ is new and sales data is unknown, but it is targeted at the home given its feature set and shorter battery life. However, the list of developments is large, with a 17-in. screen size, Wi-Fi connectivity, front-mounted loudspeaker, three times zoom capability, suspension system, LIDAR-assisted driving, and an app for control.

Later is shown the newest model, the Beam Pro2. It claims a more immersive experience, enhanced functionality, clearer connections, and easier operation. A much larger Gorilla glass screen and LCD touch operation has improved the usability, as well as larger wide frequency speakers, adjustable height, 12 mega-pixel camera with low-latency video processing, a digital microphone array, and improved battery life. Stability is increased by moving up to six wheels.

8.5.1.3 iRobot AVA500 and RP-Vita

iRobot has the only fully autonomous telepresence robot (Figure 8.9). Much of its development was driven by InTouch health who had a remotely driven robot supporting medical devices for hospitals. InTouch drove the autonomous driving given the push back from customers on the first-generation implementation. iRobot developed the autonomous base sold to InTouch and added as the top half (screen,

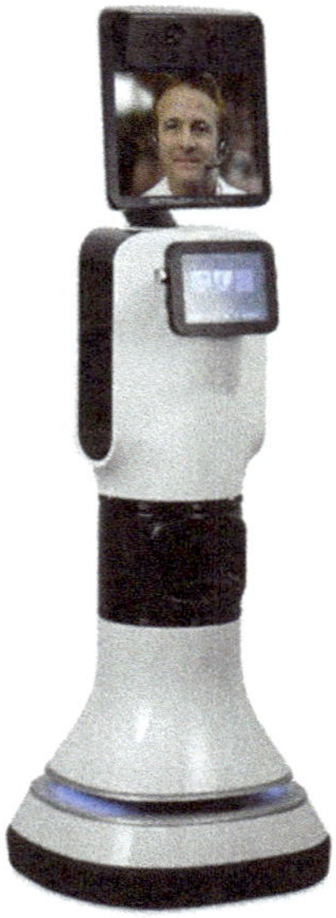

Figure 8.9 iRobot AVA500 and RP-Vita

camera, and devices). iRobot's product, the AVA500, uses a Cisco desktop telepresence appliance as the top half. The iRobot product can raise and lower the top half by a foot. The founder of iRobot is a believer in telepresence robot solutions—the AVA is his fifth attempt at delivering a product. iRobot is known to be working as a next-generation product that is rumored to be half the price of the AVA500.

8.5.1.4 InTouch Health

InTouch Health provides technology-enabled services to health-care providers for the delivery of high-quality clinical solutions. InTouch Health started with only their robotic telepresence product but have branched into a large multi-platform organization that "*Empowers healthcare systems to deploy telehealth applications across their own enterprise, and into other care sites, such as non-affiliated hospitals, rehab centers, long-term care, clinics and homes. InTouch Health also offers physician services to assist healthcare systems in meeting their telehealth demands, and to address physician shortages*." At $150,000 or $5,000 a month, the robot is not a big seller but is the top of the line benchmark with excellent usability, video quality, camera control, medical device integration, and EMRs. InTouch devices are FDA approved.

8.5.1.5 Vecna VGo

The Vecna V-1000 VGo is a small, feature-rich robot that has a set of advantages (Figure 8.10). Overall, the VGo has the advantages of having a friendly design,

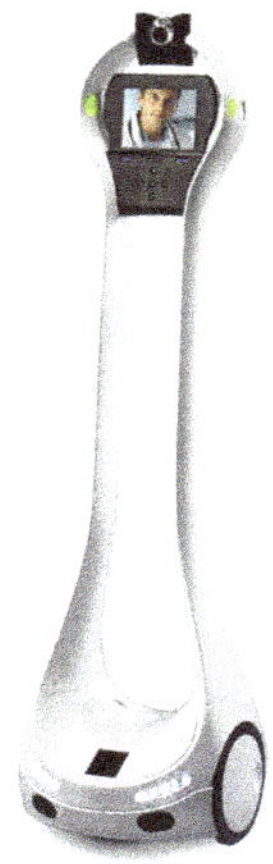

Figure 8.10 Vecna VGo

simple setup, strong feature set at reasonable price, the lightest weight at 8.2 kg, a battery life of 15 h, and a tilting high-resolution camera.

The VGo enables remote students to attend class, remote physician visits, patient monitoring, care of the elderly, videoconferencing, and full telepresence in a low cost, semiautomated platform that can find its way to a charging dock with a programmatic routine.

Other telepresence robots are now being seen in the press, but they are not yet available. One is the robot Pepper which, at $10,000, is too expensive for the home but is beginning to promote its autonomous interactivity.

Other telepresence robots include offerings from Anybots, Mantaro, Revolve Robotics, Awabot, Telerob, Kongsberg, QinetiQ, and Inbot Technology.

These telepresence robots meet the need of getting communication between parties to occur when a person or party cannot physically be there. However, all of these telepresence solutions do not fully address market needs. Specifically, they do not offer cost-effective solutions to navigate autonomously, as the cheapest solution today is $60,000. Also, they do not deliver hospital-specific applications except for video telepresence. They also do not offer an open platform to allow for easy integration with proven software applications.

8.5.2 Customer service

Arriving at a hospital facility, patients need to check in, perhaps fill out some paper, go to their appointment room, and finally complete follow-up tasks. Typically, nurses or hospital staff have to work with patients at every step along the way, which is not ideal for either party, as these tasks are an inefficient use of staff time and cause long wait times and discomfort for patients. The long wait times and difficulty of taking frequent vital readings can put patients, particularly in emergency situations, at risk of not receiving the attention that they need in-time. Robotic solutions, namely, kiosks, can offer a better solution. However, these solutions are far from ideal; they require a good visual user interface, robust functionality behind the screen, and effective navigation, if it is mobile.

8.5.2.1 Advanced Kiosks

As a 15-year-old company in the space of kiosks for various industries, Advanced Kiosks [29] has been developing mobile and stationary kiosk solutions for industries from education to government, retail, and hospital applications. One of the advances of Advanced Kiosks is in data security—Wi-Fi connections pose data privacy concerns, while 4G technology offers increased protection via encryption.

8.5.2.2 LifeBot Triage

One of the most important applications of kiosk systems are emergency rooms. First of all, not all patients who arrive at the emergency room need immediate care—some of them need less urgent care than others. But the priorities can only be assigned after getting additional information from the patient about their condition and taking the patient's vitals. Correctly assigning priorities can help one to get the patients who are in the most critical conditions the help they need sooner while reducing the wait time for all others. In 2010, a team from Vanderbilt University envisioned the LifeBot Triage concept as a system that combines kiosks, mobile robots that can check patient vitals, and a supervisor robot that interfaces with nurses. Today, its focus is more on the software solution part of it, providing nurses a guided interface for assessing and triaging patients [30].

8.5.2.3 Vecna Kiosks

Vecna offers a series of kiosks, from freestanding to tabletop and wall-mount options. These products offer self-service registration, bill payment, private communication with providers, and viewing results. The solution also offers a queueing feature to manage the flow of patients and information. By checking in at the kiosk, the patient is able to identify their appointment. Integration with payment services and insurance is also currently under further development (Figures 8.11 and 8.12).

8.5.3 Challenges

Both telepresence and kiosk robotics applications have several challenges that stem from integrating with either the human or IT infrastructure environment in which they are deployed. Human interaction needs to be at the same physical height as the patient, whether they are standing, sitting, or in bed. Second, the lag time on video and audio needs to be minimal, even if the location of deployment is rural or distant. The goal of this design focus is to prevent the system from inhibiting the interaction, such as between patient and caregiver or physician. If the application is stationary and freestanding, integration to the site or venue needs to occur seamlessly. This may require tedious security clearances, reviews, or certifications so that the kiosk system can engage the information systems at the site. Patient security and HIPAA regulations also need to be tended to. If the patients are not

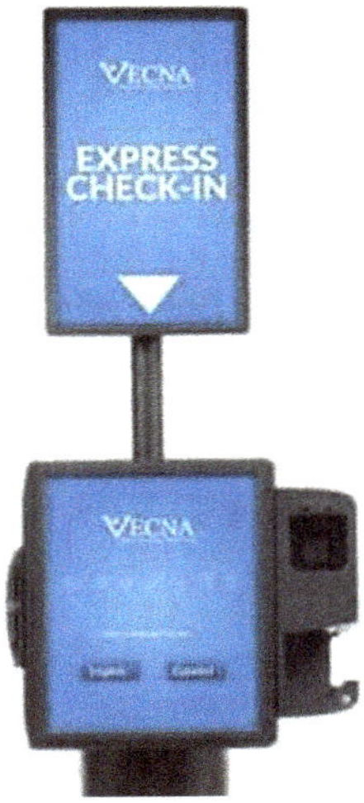

Figure 8.11 Vecna Kiosk check-in terminal

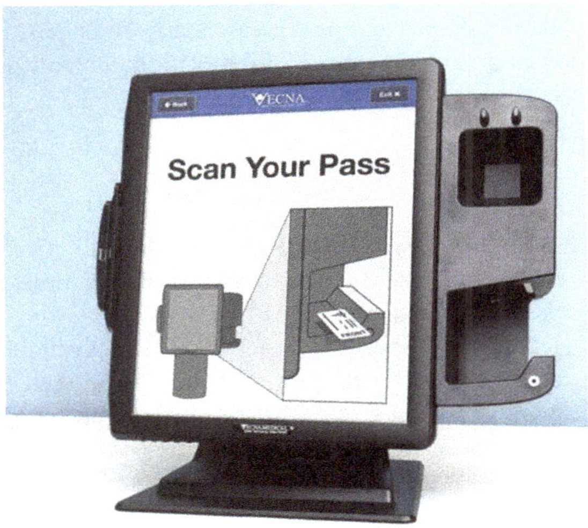

Figure 8.12 Vecna Kiosk scanning terminal

sure that the telepresence robot or kiosk has a secure connection, they are reluctant to use it. Concurrent with this is the need in any encounter or session to inform the patients about their rights, gather approval or signatures, and proceed with the sharing of personal or sensitive information. In most cases, no existing model of concierge, kiosk, or telepresence robot has all of these bases covered. While most robots can find their power dock and self-charge, or identify a network and communications protocol, several other issues exist surrounding the human interaction that are important to manage as well.

8.6 Conclusion

Medical robotics is quickly becoming important enablers of improved outcomes, safety, as well as operational efficiencies in modern healthcare. The application areas covered in this chapter highlighted the impact and growing importance of robots in clinical settings. Other robotics applications that exist, but were not covered here, include exoskeletons, smart prostheses and bionics, therapy robots, assistive robots, cleaning, pill delivery and dispensation, and robotic nurses.

Some of the recent technology advancements that have enabled this progress include AI needed for patient service systems and medical companions, fine-motor nanoscaled robots that allow for highly precise autonomous surgeries, and autonomous driving systems that unlock more automated logistics transportation solutions.

The medical robotics market is quickly growing. North America is one of the largest markets for medical robotics applications, with nearly 50 percent of global demand for medical robotics in 2013 [31]. As these technologies become increasingly tested, improved, and accepted in the market, patients can expect increased quality of care, while physicians and health-care staff can benefit from a reduction of wasted time and resources. The impact of innovation in medical robotics will be felt widely for years to come.

References

[1] Credence Research. "The Global Robotics Market". Credence Research. Available from: https://www.credenceresearch.com/press/global-medical-robotics-market [Accessed Apr 2018].

[2] Tractica. "Healthcare Robotics". Tractica. 2016. Available from: https://www.tractica.com/research/healthcare-robotics/ [Accessed April 2018].

[3] IFR. "Considerable Increase of Medical Robots and Logistic Systems." International Federation of Robotics (IFR). 2013. Available from: https://ifr.org/ifr-press-releases/news/considerable-increase-of-medical-robots-and-logistic-systems [Accessed April 2018].

[4] GVR. "Global Medical Robotics Systems Markets." Grand View Research (GVR). 2015. Available from: https://www.grandviewresearch.com/press-release/global-medical-robotic-systems-market [Accessed April 2018].

[5] Robotics Tomorrow. "The Most Important Robots in Medicine". Robotics Tomorrow. 2017. Available from: https://www.roboticstomorrow.com/article/2017/06/the-most-important-robots-in-medicine/10201/ [Accessed April 2018].

[6] He, W., Goodkind, D., and Kowal, P. "An Aging World: 2015." US Census Bureau. P95/16-1. March 2016. Available from: https://www.census.gov/content/dam/Census/library/publications/2016/demo/p95-16-1.pdf] [Accessed April 2018].

[7] Bogg, W. "Robotic-Assisted Surgery: More Expensive, But not Always More Effective." Thomson Reuters. 24 October 2017. Available from: https://www.reuters.com/article/us-health-surgery-robots/robotic-assisted-surgery-more-expensive-but-not-always-more-effective-idUSKBN1CT2U1 [Accessed April 2018].
[8] PR Newswire. "Global Surgical Robotics Market to Reach $12.6 Billion 2025." PR Newswire. 23 January 2018. Available from: https://www.prnewswire.com/news-releases/global-surgical-robotics-market-to-reach-126-billion-2025-300587080.html, [Accessed April 2018].
[9] Tractica. "Warehousing and Logistics Robots." Tractica. 2017. Available from: https://www.tractica.com/research/warehousing-and-logistics-robots/ [Accessed April 2018].
[10] Wintergreen Research. "Telepresence Robots". Wintergreen Research. 28 March 2018. Available from: http://www.wintergreenresearch.com/telepresence-robots [Accessed April 2018].
[11] OR Today Magazine. "Market Analysis: Disinfection Robot Market on the Rise." OR Today Magazine. 1 October 2016. Available from: http://ortoday.com/market-analysis-disinfection-robot-market-on-the-rise/ [Accessed April 2018].
[12] Burgner-Kahrs, J., Rucker, D. C., and Choset, H. Continuum robots for medical applications: a survey. IEEE Trans Rob. 2015;31(6):1261–1280.
[13] Nelson, R. J., Chavali, J. S. S., Yerram, N., Babbar, P., and Kaouk, J. H. Current status of robotic single-port surgery. Urol Ann. 2017;9(3):217–222. Available from: http://doi.org/10.4103/UA.UA_51_17 [Accessed April 2018].
[14] Ackerman, E. Diligent robotics bringing autonomous mobile manipulation to hospitals. IEEE Spectr. 2018. Available from: https://spectrum.ieee.org/automaton/robotics/industrial-robots/diligent-robotics-bringing-autonomous-mobile-manipulation-to-hospitals [Accessed April 2018].
[15] Castellanos, S. Vecna technologies' QC Bot shuttles supplies around hospitals. Boston Bus J. 2014. Available from: https://www.bizjournals.com/boston/blog/techflash/2014/09/watch-howvecna-technologies-qc-bot-will-shuttle.html [Accessed April 2018].
[16] "Aethon TUG". 2018. Available from: http://www.aethon.com/tug/tughealthcare/ [Accessed April 2018].
[17] "Matternet Drones". 20 September 2017. Available from: https://mttr.net/images/Matternet_Press_Release_09.20.2017.pdf [Accessed April 2018].
[18] Jeon, S and Lee, J. "A simulator for performance analysis of multiple robots for hospital delivery." 2016 13th International Conference on Ubiquitous Robots and Ambient Intelligence (URAI), 19–22 August 2016.
[19] Allied Market Research. "UV Disinfection Equipment Market". Allied Market Research. 2018. Available from: https://www.alliedmarketresearch.com/press-release/uv-disinfection-equipment-market.html [Accessed April 2018].
[20] Song, X. X., Ju, L. W., Wei, G. R., and Jiang, Q. W. Heat impact upon the infectivity of hepatitis B virus in serum. Zhonghua Yu Fang Yi Xue Za Zhi. 2011;45(8):723–726. PubMed PMID: 22169694.

[21] Setlow, P. Spore resistance properties. Microbiol Spectr. 2014;2(5). doi:10.1128/microbiolspec.TBS-0003-2012. Review. PubMed PMID: 26104355.

[22] Yang, J. H., Wu, U. I., Tai, H. M., and Sheng, W. H. Effectiveness of an ultraviolet-C disinfection system for reduction of healthcare-associated pathogens. J Microbiol Immunol Infect. 2017. pii: S1684-1182(17)30200-1. doi: 10.1016/j.jmii.2017.08.017. PubMed PMID: 28951015.

[23] Fleming, M., Patrick, A., Gryskevicz, M., *et al.* Deployment of a touchless ultraviolet light robot for terminal room disinfection: The importance of audit and feedback. Am J Infect Control. 2018;46(2):241–243. doi: 10.1016/j.ajic.2017.09.027. Epub 2017 Nov 3. PubMed PMID: 29103637.

[24] Lee, J. and Rice, S. The robot will clean up now. Rival technologies sans data compete for a growing market. *Mod Healthc.* 2015;45(2):20–21. PubMed PMID: 25671888.

[25] Xenex. "UV Disinfection Robot". 2018. Available from: https://www.xenex.com/ [Accessed April 2018].

[26] Blue-Ocean Robotics. 2018. Available from: https://blue-ocean-robotics.com/ [Accessed April 2018].

[27] Steris Pathogon System. 2018. Available from: https://www.steris.com/healthcare/products/ultraviolet-disinfection/ and https://www.steris.com/onbDocs/V422/1307/692420.pdf\ [Accessed April 2018].

[28] Robot Operating System, ROS. 2018. Available from: http://www.ros.org/about-ros/ [Accessed April 2018].

[29] Advanced Kiosks. 2018. Available from: https://advancedkiosks.com/ [Accessed April 2018].

[30] Research News @Vanderbilt. "Developing Robots for the Hospital Emergency Room." Research News @Vanderbilt. 6 December 2010. Available from: https://news.vanderbilt.edu/2010/12/06/developing-robots-for-the-hospital-emergency-room/ [Accessed April 2018].

[31] Bio IT World. "Medical Robotic Systems Market To 2020 – Industry Size, Growth Prospects: Grand View Research, Inc." Bio IT World. Available from: http://www.bio-itworld.com/Press-Release/Medical-Robotic-Systems-Market-To-2020—Industry-Size,-Growth-Prospects–Grand-View-Research,-Inc-/ [Accessed April 2018].

Chapter 9

New reality for surgical training and assessment using immersive technologies

Justin Barad, M.D.[1] *and Jennifer McCaney, Ph.D.*[2]

As medical technology leapfrogs the historical boundaries of size, scale and accessibility, and surgical techniques evolve, operating room teams must adapt to managing a complex bundle of open, minimally invasive, and robotic-assisted procedures. Renewed interest in operative performance and the link between surgical proficiency and medical errors directly impacts patient outcomes and the long-term trend toward demonstrating value-based care for an increasing number of surgical procedures. Surgical residency training programs, simulation platforms, performance measurement tools, and standards for assessment are facing increased scrutiny as national education boards pilot new mechanisms to address the rising gaps in training and competency. The development of virtual reality (VR) platforms that integrate technical and nontechnical skills with team training in a low-cost, low-risk, scalable delivery environment is representative of how technology can be leveraged to empower and educate the next generation of surgeons globally.

9.1 History of surgical training

Surgery is derived from the Greek cheiros, or *hand*, and ergon, *work*. As such, the role of the early surgeon has evolved from one that manually assuages the pain of acute and life-threatening injuries, such as amputations at the bedside to the modern surgeon, *in situ* behind a robotic console, performing elective procedures still with one's hands' through a virtual interface. Evidence of surgical procedures exists as far back as 3000 B.C.; however, until the discovery of anesthesia and application of antiseptic techniques in the mid-1800s, elective surgery was rarely performed. As time has passed, surgery has evolved and with this new era of medicine, a cadre of

[1]Osso VR Inc., San Francisco, CA, USA
[2]Department of Medicine, Division of Pulmonary and Critical Care Medicine, David Geffen School of Medicine at University of California Los Angeles, Los Angeles, CA, USA

life-saving procedures, medical device technologies, and adjuvant therapies has been ushered in. In 2012, an estimated 312M surgeries* were completed worldwide, representing an increase of 38% from 2004 [1]. The American College of Surgeons recognizes 14 different surgical specialties that are further divided into dozens of subspecialties; each often needs to know how to perform hundreds of procedures. The cognitive, technical, and nontechnical skills required to master these professions are not innate and require a lengthy period of training and supervision and continue to be a challenge as a surgeon ventures out into practice. Furthermore, the vast amount of medical knowledge is increasing at an exponential rate. In 1950, it is estimated that the doubling time of medical information was 50 years; in 1980, it was 7 years; and in 2010, 3.5 years. In 2020, that rate is projected to drop to 0.2 years, or 73 days [2]. Assuming a combined medical school and surgical training tenure of 9 years, students entering medical school in fall 2020 will experience 45 doublings over the course of their training. While the emergence of artificial intelligence and the application of computer-assisted diagnosis, treatment, and management of disease will likely play a role in mediating the exponential growth of medical information, technology will likely play a central role in clinical education.

9.1.1 Origins of residency training

In the late 1800s, surgical training was startlingly informal. Practicing surgeons were either self-taught or were trained through loosely structured and sometimes never-ending apprenticeship programs. In the 1890s, William Halsted, the surgeon-in-chief at the newly established Johns Hopkins Hospital, rapidly rose to become a global leader in medicine and one of the fathers of modern surgery. Inspired by the rigor and structure of his European counterparts, Halsted instituted a system of graduated responsibility and is credited for the birth of the modern residency training program [3]. Halsted's model was built upon a type of apprenticeship in which residents would follow attending surgeons and observe both their cognitive and technical work (Figure 9.1). As residents progressed in the program, they were given greater and greater responsibility at points, performing some if not all of many procedures. In Halsted's original incarnation, residents would compete with each other to move up the pyramid, ultimately rising to the top to become house surgeon, what is now known as the chief resident. At that time, it was designed so that not all residents would make it through the program, in contrast to modern surgical training programs, where virtually all residents successfully complete their program.

Since that time residency has seen a few changes that took place relatively early on. Almost all residents make it through to graduation. A match system was implemented to try and promote fair access and distribution of trainees around the country. And most recently in 2003, the 80-h workweek was implemented, limiting

*Surgeries are defined as operations performed in an operating theater that require general anesthesia or profound sedation to control pain.

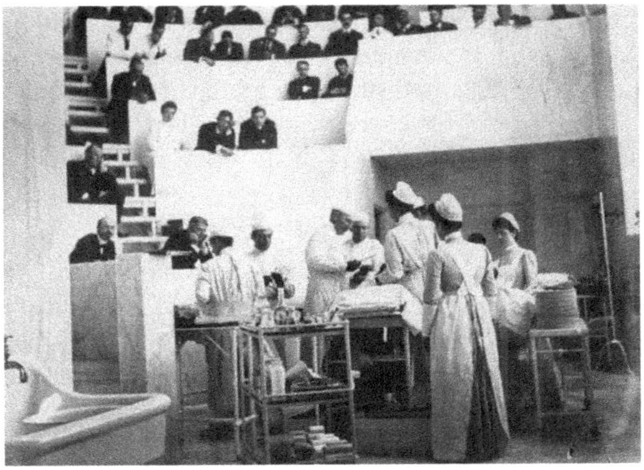

Figure 9.1 Architect of the modern surgical residency program, William Halsted operating in the surgical amphitheater [4]. Reprinted with permission from the Johns Hopkins Alan Mason Chesney Medical Archives

the time residents had to train in the hopes of decreasing the risks to patients associated with resident fatigue.

9.1.2 Modern surgical training and licensure

While surgical residency training has undergone minor evolutions over the years, it remains at its core relatively unchanged since its inception. The structure of the modern surgical residency program consists typically of an intern year followed by 4 years of training as a resident. Additional time can be spent through the addition of research years and subspecialization through fellowship training, which can add anywhere from 1 to 3 years. An increasing number of surgical trainees are seeking fellowship training, with orthopedic surgery and general surgery topping the list of add-on fellowships at 87.4% and 71.2%, respectively [5]. While written and oral board exams are held at the end of the residency, these exams assess medical knowledge versus operative skill or autonomy, and it is not necessarily required to pass them to be able to practice surgery. Increased rates of surgical subspecialization and debate on the correlation of minimum case requirements to surgical competency have led to an international trend to develop a more generalizable assessment of a trainee's ability to manage defined tasks versus individual case assessments [6].

A common adage associated with residency training is "see one, do one, teach one." While not taken 100% literally, residents are often asked to perform procedures or operations that they have seen very few times or sometimes never at all. While supervision is encouraged, it is not necessarily required. This is interesting considering 28%–42% of residents do not feel ready to safely perform various procedures alone for the first time, and a frequent cause of medical mistakes are inadequate knowledge, experience, and/or supervision. The exposure to real-world clinical cases is largely random and is based on the patients coming to a particular teaching hospital and what procedures the attending surgeon chooses to perform. This leads to a somewhat random distribution of experience among residents in the same program and can result in some residents never having performed certain critical procedures during their training [7].

9.1.3 Link to health-care outcomes

An increasing body of evidence suggests a link between surgical volume and outcomes. While technology has greatly advanced healthcare, medical errors are cited as the third leading cause of death in the United States, and it is hypothesized that medical errors are also underreported in other nations, such as the United Kingdom and Canada [8]. The absence of ICD10 codes or data capture for medical error consequently leads to a lack of data in the field; however, the root causes may range from human factors, such as poor judgment, communication breakdowns, and the lack of training and skill proficiency to technological factors, such as diagnostic errors or device failures. Specific challenges associated with minimally invasive and robotic surgery procedures present a unique set of training and implementation hurdles due to the degree of technical mastery. The emergence of the field of surgical data science is anticipated to provide a link between surgical performance and outcomes through tools that provide decision support, predictive monitoring, and technology-enabled surgical training [9]. Immersive training platforms, such as VR simulators, have the potential to close the loop on objective measures of technical skill and correlate to actionable information collected in the patient-care process, such as patient data and outcomes across a larger dataset.

9.2 Emerging industry trends

Modern medicine has entered an era of vast technological advancement, further accelerated by the integration of data and analytics into the diagnosis, treatment, and prevention of conditions that were previously inoperable. As technology becomes integrated across the continuum of care, driven by advances in sensors, robotics, materials science, and artificial intelligence, an increasing number of medical devices with inherently complex procedures and procedure-specific skills are entering the market. Historically, the discovery of new technologies and subsequent commercialization of novel medical devices have led to great advancements in patient care and outcomes. For example, the invention of the transistor in 1947 facilitated the core technology that paved the way for the invention of the first battery-operated wearable pacemaker by Earl E. Baaken, founder of Medtronic, Inc in 1957. Furthermore, the invention of the fully implantable pacemaker by Wilson Greatbatch in 1960, licensed to Medtronic in 1961, spurred a new surgical procedure, enabling cardiac surgeons to pace the heart's rhythm via leads connected to an implanted synchronization device. Today, pacemaker implantation is one of the most common types of heart surgery, and every year, over one million pacemakers are implanted worldwide to treat patients suffering from conduction disorders, arrhythmias, and heart failure [10]. Advances in minimally invasive and robotic surgery are steering the next generation of surgical procedures toward an operating interface that displaces the surgeon directly from the bedside of the patient and poses new technical challenges and complexity.

9.2.1 Increasing number of medical devices and surgical procedures

Within the surgical medical device market, leading segments include cardiology, orthopedics, and general and plastic surgery, while neurology represents the fastest growing sector [11]. Medical device complexity is often correlated to the designated regulatory pathway through which the US Food and Drug Administration (FDA) grants market approval. While the sophistication of a particular device is difficult to quantify, factors, such as the user complexity, which is a combined measure of both the skill to use a device safely and correctly and of the operation of the device in that manner, are directly correlated to the rigor of the associated device training [12]. Typically, the lowest risk devices, Class I, do not pose any significant safety risk and are external to the body. In the amphitheater of the operating room, most medical devices are typically designated Class II or Class III and gain market entry through a 510(k) clearance, *de novo*, or premarket approval (PMA) pathway. These higher risk devices generally constitute implantable or other tools that interface directly with the body. In 2018, the FDA continued to follow an upward trend with 106 approvals of novel medical devices, setting a new record for approvals novel medical devices, including 510(k), *de novo*, and PMA pathways [13]. This represents a 4× increase in novel device approvals since 2009. Additionally, the establishment of innovative regulatory channels, such as the Breakthrough Device Program, which was introduced by the FDA in 2015 (initially the Expedited Access Pathway) to facilitate the review of highly novel devices that treat or diagnose life-threatening or irreversibly debilitating conditions has ushered in 112 designations and 9 breakthrough device approvals in 2018 alone [13]. Evolving regulatory guidance and novel pathways in parallel with an increasing number of medical device approvals and decreasing number of days to decision represent two levers through which the historical barriers to medical device commercialization are easing. The downstream effect on the practice of surgery represents an increasing burden of education on surgical trainees, practicing surgeons and clinical staff, and the sales and marketing teams of medical device manufacturers that oversee the commercial launch of these complex new technologies.

The technical complexity presented by the physical design of medical devices and the number of components and tools required during the surgical procedure in part can also drive the user complexity. As devices and the associated procedures become more complex, the training paradigms associated with these devices and supporting technology become a rate-limiting step as the learning curve growth steeper. At the end of a 5-year residency, general surgery trainees are expected to

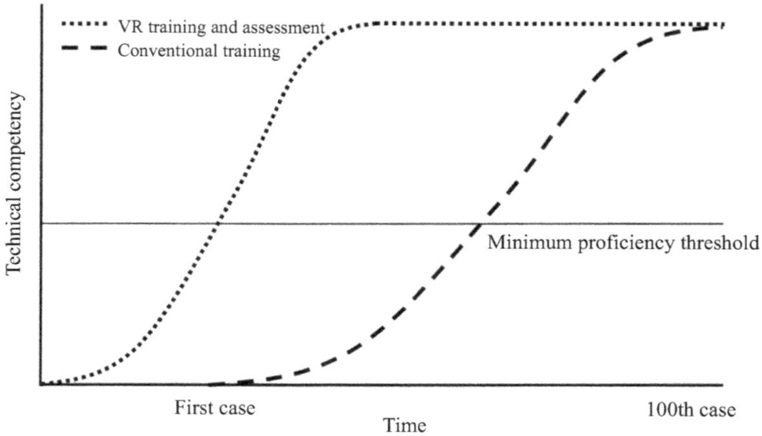

Figure 9.2 Surgical training case competency curve shows potential efficiencies of VR simulation platforms versus traditional training methods

know 121 critical procedures [7]. The skills required for minimally invasive and open surgical procedures have shown limited transferability to robotic-assisted surgery, and as the suite of clinical applications for robotic-assisted surgeries expands from gynecology and urology to general surgery, so will the training burden [14]. Figure 9.2 demonstrates the projected case competency curve for medical devices and the potential of how VR simulation can lead to increased training proficiency and cases to surgical competency. Further challenges in surgical education are addressed in the following section. In addition to physician training on new devices, nurses and other operating room staff are central to the procedure implementation and device deployment and require training methodologies that are accessible and cost-effective.

9.2.2 Looming physician and specialist shortage

Over the past 60 years, a cascading series of government measures to forecast physician supply and demand have prompted subsequent reforms, resulting in both the stimulus and restriction of clinical trainees. Beginning in 1963, with the passage of the Health Professions Education Assistance Act, US medical schools underwent significant growth, and the number of graduates between 1965 and 1980 grew from 7,409 to 15,135. Further measures in the 1990s sought to counteract a perceived physician surplus through restrictions on the ratio of generalists to specialists, the number of international trainees, and the number of residency slots secured by federal funding. However, the dynamic shift of physician supply and demand has acutely driven a looming physician shortage, and the American Association of Medical Colleges (AAMC) predicts a shortage of between 40,800 and 104,900 physicians by 2030. The AAMC attributes three primary factors leading to a physician shortage, including an aging population, declining physician work hours, and impending physician retirements [15]. Additional factors, such as increased access to care in the United States, facilitated by the Affordable Care Act (ACA) in 2010 have driven the number of newly insured to over 20 million in 2014. Currently, there are over one million active physicians in the United States, of which ~15% are classified within a surgical specialty [16]. In 2012, there were an estimated 18,000 general surgeons, a ratio of 5.8 general surgeons per 100,000; however, it is estimated that there should be approximately 7.5 general surgeons per 100,000 people. While the number of general surgery residency slots has risen, the increases are not sufficient to keep up with the aging and steadily rising population and will be acutely felt in rural areas. By 2032, the AAMC estimates a deficit of between 14,300 and 23,400 surgeons [15]. The aging population and rise in obesity in developed nations, such as the United States, where total joint replacements are forecasted to see a 171% and 189% growth in hip and knee placements, respectively, by 2030 will place an additional burden on specialties, such as orthopedic surgery [17]. In a field where there are few nonsurgical options for advanced osteoarthritis and with 10-year revision rates hovering at 12%, objective measures and ongoing training for both new trainees and practicing surgical professionals are needed [18].

Certain specialties will acutely face the effect of the supply demand shortage, including cardiothoracic surgery, urology, ophthalmology, neurosurgery, orthopedic surgery, and plastic surgery, which are all expected to reach workforce deficits of 20% or greater by 2025 [19]. Increased efficiencies in the deployment of care through automation, mobile health, remote monitoring, and telehealth may potentially mitigate the effect of a physician shortage; however, the deployment and distribution of highly specialized surgical specialties will require training technologies that can close the gap on the cases to competency for new procedures.

9.2.3 Global education and democratization of access to training

While the market for medical technology approaches maturity in developed nations, the rate of growth of medical devices in emerging markets is expected to increase, which will drive annual industry growth of 5% over a 5-year horizon [20]. By 2022, emerging markets are expected to make up one-third of the global medtech market, up from less than 25% of the market 5 years earlier [21]. Upon further examination of the annual global surgical volume, only 1 in every 20 procedures is performed in very-low-expenditure nations as defined by the World Health Organization, despite these countries representing well over one-third of the population [1]. Even greater growth compared to the average global surgical rate of 38% was reported in low and very-low-expenditure nations, which experienced estimated increases in the surgical rate of 69% and 115%, respectively, between 2004 and 2012 [1]. Globally, the demand and access to medical devices in emerging economies will approach an inflection point where access is limited by the current supply of surgical trainees and the high cost of training. The shortfall will be acutely felt in these areas and will be compounded by the limited training and education available; however, scaling surgical training tools through technology platforms, such as video-based instruction and VR, have the potential to address gaps in access and cost.

9.2.4 Transition to value-based care

The advent of value-based care is largely driven by the ACA and enabled by government programs to implement electronic medical records over the past 10 years. The aggregation of patient data alongside billing and claims information creates the opportunity to link outcomes to payment, thereby moving away from the traditional fee for service model, where reimbursement is delivered on per-procedure basis. There is an ongoing transition to bundled payments for Medicare-based reimbursement of in-hospital procedures. In addition to optimizing surgical training, it is inherent that health systems explore new ways in which surgeons and other professional clinical staff can maintain the competency of skill as the margin for medical error erodes their bottom line. Additionally, the relatively static, and declining level of reimbursement by Medicare for most procedures creates additional pressure for health systems and providers to demonstrate a return on value through improved outcomes and decreased cost.

9.3 State of surgical education

9.3.1 Current approaches to surgical training

Both trainees and practicing surgeons employ a variety of training methods when learning new procedures and technologies. Following medical school training, many physicians choose to pursue a medical specialty in the form of a residency, which can range from 3 to 7 years in length. Surgical specialties are a minimum of 5 years duration, over which trainees master complex skills and procedures, followed by the option to pursue fellowship training in various specialties. Internationally, the duration, structure, and specialty-specific training guidelines can differ between surgical training programs, but, a broad consensus in the medical community supports the need to identify new methodologies and metrics [22].

9.3.2 Current challenges of surgical training

In the context of the evolving health-care landscape, increasing complexity of medical devices and associated procedures, rising utilization of medical technology globally, and an impending shortage of physicians, a review of the current surgical training methodologies elucidates several challenges. A rising number of surgeons are pursuing additional fellowship training, suggesting a trend of emerging deficits in current surgical resident training programs. The lack of empirical data to quantify training gaps makes it difficult to point to the impetus for this trend; however, it is hypothesized that the passage of work-hour restrictions and rules surrounding resident autonomy have hampered the apprenticeship model pioneered by William Halsted and led to a decline in the readiness level of residents for independent

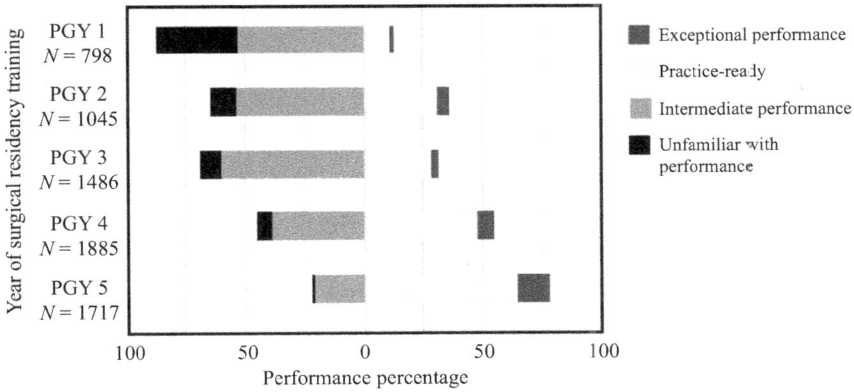

Figure 9.3 Distribution of operative performance of general surgery residents by postgraduate year (PGY). Surgical competence is considered achieved for ratings (exceptional performance and practice ready). Reprinted and adapted with permission of Wolters Kluwer Health, Inc

practice [23]. A prospective multi-institutional study across 14 general surgery programs investigating resident operative performance reported that 77.1% of final-year trainees (PGY5) were rated at competent across 5 of the most frequent out of 132 core procedures as defined by the American Board of Surgery (ABS) (Figure 9.3), while nearly 50% of trainees were rated below competency for a set of 85 noncore procedures [24]. While a predictive probability model raises core procedure competency to an estimated 90.5% at the end of year-5 training, it does not account for the occurrence of multiple procedures in the same case, patient complexity, or the startingly high number trainees unprepared for clinical practice [24]. In addition to competency, the demonstration of surgical autonomy is an important metric for independent practice. In the second study of surgical independence in general surgery, resident trainees reported similar expectations of autonomy between attendings and residents, but a significant gap between observed and expected autonomy was reported for the ten most common procedures across 1,467 operative cases [25].

Surgical residencies face several training challenges, including work-hour restrictions, inadequate simulation resources, limited and typically untimely access to cadavers, lack of standardized, objective-based measurement tools of proficiency, and minimal integration of soft skills and team training. Surgical competence simulations are conducted through both low-fidelity (e.g., step-by-step surgical technique guides, synthetic bench models) and high-fidelity (e.g., cadavers, virtual simulators) models, as well as situational environments, such as patient encounters and live clinical experience [26]. The optimal stimulation environment should be able to accurately assess and improve a trainee's skills. Each of these is addressed later with an emphasis on how emerging trends are driving the need for new paradigms in surgical training.

9.3.2.1 Shift in work-hours

As discussed earlier, the Accreditation Council for Graduate Medical Education (ACGME) passed a measure to reduce the number of residency duty hours for all training programs, as well as restrictions around consecutive on-call shifts and time off between shifts. Previously, residents had been working on average 110 h per week; however, while studies have shown that trainees under the new guidelines reported lower burnout and improved quality of life, it is unclear how to measure the direct effect on the quality of patient care [27]. Work-hour restrictions coupled with increased time spent on nonclinical administrative tasks, such as charting, have reduced the amount of time the trainees can spend apprenticing with expert surgeons in the operating rooms. In addition to the implementation of residency work-hour restrictions, the ABS began increasing the minimum number of total operative procedures required for general surgery training, from 750 in 2009 to 850 in 2017. The challenge for current trainees then becomes a balance between meeting case quotas, gaining operative experience, and also demonstrating competency, particularly given the acute shortcoming across both core and noncore procedures demonstrated in Figure 9.3.

9.3.2.2 Drawbacks of cadavers as simulation resources

Outside of live patients, surgeons rely on cadavers and live animals for practice and simulation. Even today these forms of training are seen as a gold standard that allow for near-perfect fidelity; however, there are a number of limitations to these modes of training. Cadavers can be relatively expensive, ranging from $1,300 to $2,300 per Anatomical Gift Association of Illinois. In certain regions, cadaver availability is limited or due to local taboos is not used. Cadavers often require specialized labs and staffing, although carefully prepared hotel ballrooms are also commonly used [28]. While low, cadaver labs not only carry some risks due to the handling of biologic tissues but also common risks associated with surgical procedures, such as that posed by sharp instruments and power tools. A frequently identified shortcoming of cadavers is that they will rarely have the pathology of the real-world equivalent. For example, when practicing knee replacements most cadavers do not have knee arthritis. Pathology can drastically change the anatomy and approach required for a successful procedure, and this cannot be reliably reproduced in a cadaver model. Another problem with cadaver training is typically there is no formal or standardized assessment that takes place, so it is unclear if the trainee was successful or if he/she has met some type of learning outcome/goal. Live animal training has some advantages over cadaver training; however, it only has limited use cases—commonly for practice in laparoscopic techniques. The tissue quality is much more similar, and availability is generally not an issue. Two of the biggest drawbacks of cadaveric and live animal training are the lack of reusability and the lack of access. Spaced repetition is the foundation of learning theory but given that cadavers and live animals are single use and are not easily accessible, it is difficult to practice any procedure more than once or over a period of time. Furthermore, access to cadaver models is often not synchronized with operating schedules and patient cases as they present. Often, long periods of time can lapse between cadaver training and presentation of patient cases or the release of new devices.

9.3.2.3 Lack of assessment tools and standardization

Methods for currently measuring surgical skill include questionnaires and surveys, video recording, motion tracking and analysis, and directly measured quantitative metrics, such as suture closure time and the length of task. Current questionnaire and survey-based methods to measure proficiency rely on the most commonly used Objective Structured Assessments of Technical Skills. For example, the emergence of new technologies, such as motion tracking and analysis, is enabling the shift of robotic simulator assessment tools, such as the Global Evaluative Assessment of Robotic Skills scale from human evaluators to objective measures that are predictive of skill acquisition and readiness to operate [29]. These same models can be incorporated into VR training platforms and spur the marriage of surgical readiness with objective assessment metrics without the need for high-cost surgical simulation platforms.

9.3.2.4 Lack of integration of soft skills (nontechnical skills) and team training

The importance of nontechnical skills in surgical training, such as teamwork, leadership, situational awareness, and communication, is high on the spectrum of surgical skills that instill confidence in trainee readiness for the operative setting [30]. Given these interpersonal and decision-making skills are often cited as sources of perioperative error in adverse events, it is critical to incorporate team coordination and training into current paradigms in order to improve patient outcomes [31]. A review of surgical malpractice claims showed that of cases involving communication breakdowns, 92% were due to verbal miscommunication, which included factors such as status asymmetry, ambiguity around responsibilities, handoffs, and transfers, and attending surgeons were identified as the most common team member in these exchanges [32]. Workshop-based training programs, such as the one-off cadaver-based hotel ballroom sessions, involve only a handful of trainees, and typically just the surgeon. While these sessions are effective in improving trainee skills and knowledge, other members of the surgical team and the role of the team are not amply addressed through this paradigm, particularly when it comes to new technology that requires changes in procedure workflow.

9.3.3 Changing role of the surgeon of future

As minimally invasive and robotic surgery methods evolve, surgeons of tomorrow will evolve into specialists who will require an understanding of the evolving disease pathophysiology revealed by the increased knowledge base in an era of precision medicine, such as genomics and metabolics. The additional education and training burden will require a balance of skill sets and an ability to execute treatment plans in the context of a vast array of data. As competency-based training programs gain acceptance, decreasing emphasis will be placed on the length of training and number of cases and shift to the demonstration of specific competencies, such as medical knowledge, technical expertise, leadership, communication, collaboration in a team setting, patient advocacy, and health-care administration [33]. Furthermore, the transition to value-based care and outcome-based payment models places an additional emphasis on reducing medical errors through preoperative and postoperative planning, as well as surgical training and execution. The surgical trainee has a suite of tools for skill development, which are discussed in more detail in the following section.

9.4 Emerging approaches in surgical simulation

The rapidly growing training and assessment challenges facing surgeons, surgical teams, and trainees are not new. Around the mid-twentieth century, it was recognized that allowing residents to learn and practice during active procedures potentially places patients at risk as well as leads to increased operating times and a higher cost burden. Thus, the ability to experiment and refine cognitive, technical, and nontechnical skills repeatedly in a risk-free environment could be quite valuable, in other words: simulation. Simulation through VR offers the trainee a tailored and self-directed learning experience that is tunable to different learning paces and styles in a risk-free environment [34]. Another advantage of virtual simulation is the platform allows trainees an unlimited number of scenarios, whereby they can achieve spaced-repetition learning.

9.4.1 First generation of simulators

Anesthesiologists led the charge in the development of the field of modern simulation. They needed a way to better prepare for occasional high stakes situations, dubbed “low frequency, high urgency events.” Subsequently, several pioneers created sophisticated electromechanical mannequins that simulated human physiology and could be practiced upon with relatively high fidelity that gained significant popularity in the 1980s. General surgery was not far behind. With endoscopy gaining widespread popularity and robotics just around the corner, general surgeons needed more efficient ways to train and evaluate this new set of cognitive, psychomotor, and visuospatial skills. This led to the development of a wide variety of simulator platforms (see Figure 8.2). Recently simulation has seen greater adoption within residency training and is increasingly becoming a mandatory component. In 2004, the Society of American Gastrointestinal and Endoscopic Surgeons launched the Fundamentals of Laparoscopic Surgery (FLS), a tool to assess the knowledge and skills needed for basic laparoscopic procedures. FLS became mandated by the ABOS in 2009 to qualify for board certification. In 2014, the American Board of Orthopaedic Surgery (ABOS) additionally added the need to complete the Flexible Endoscopy Curriculum, a stepwise approach to teaching endoscopic skills which incorporates simulation as well in the Fundamentals of

Endoscopic Surgery component. In 2013, the ABOS mandated simulation training for first-year residents to prove practice for basic operative skills.

Surgical simulation platforms

Reality-based (RB) simulation

These are physical simulators consisting of components, such as rubber pegs and rings, that are low cost, are relatively portable, have high instrument fidelity, and provide passive haptic feedback. The drawbacks include the need for manual assessment and lack of clinical context. In orthopedics, plastic bones called "sawbones" are a very popular form of physical simulation.

Computer-based simulation

The computer-based simulation consists of an input device and monitor in which a user can see the targets and results of one's actions. Some varieties will synthesize haptic feedback using grounded kinesthetic haptics. A classic example is the LapMentor from Simbionix. Advantages include automated assessment, high variety of procedures, and clinical scenarios. Disadvantages include typically high cost ($100k–200k for some models), maintenance and support issues, and typical lack of portability.

Hybrid simulators

These simulators seek to combine the advantages of reality and computer-based simulation. Typically, there is a physical component that can provide passive haptic feedback and a simulated visual component to provide a variety of tasks and clinical scenarios. A classic hybrid simulator in the orthopedic space is the VirtaMed arthroscopy simulator.

9.4.2 Haptic feedback in surgical simulation

Surgeons have three senses to work from: visual, somesthesis, and touch. The field of study relating to the sense of touch is described as "haptics." The simulation of haptic feedback can be grossly broken into two categories: kinesthetic and cutaneous. Kinesthetic haptics can be broken down into force, motion, and compliance. The simulation of grounded kinesthetic force feedback is frequently found in the form of a haptic stylus like 3D System's Touch Haptic Device. This type of haptics has been studied extensively in the literature, mainly as applied to laparoscopic simulation, and interestingly has been shown to either have no effect (in one case a negative effect and in some cases a statistically significant but not necessarily meaningful effect) cases leading to less skill transfer when compared to no simulation at all [35–37]. In one study, the majority of participants preferred a simulator without kinesthetic force feedback saying it felt "more realistic" and that they performed better [36]. The theory why kinesthetic force feedback does not seem to have beneficial effects and is less preferable to users is possibly related to the concept of the "uncanny valley"—which is the psychological effect in the brain that leaves us feeling put off when we experience something that is nearly but not completely realistic. Kinesthetic haptics can be prohibitively expensive, adding tens of thousands of dollars to the cost of a simulator and due to the mechanical nature of the device, often breakdown frequently requiring high levels of maintenance and support. Cutaneous haptics involves the simulation of light touch, vibration, and temperature. Cutaneous haptics is seeing interest within the field of surgical robotics with some studies showing a positive effect on task performance [38]. Cutaneous haptics are low cost and require little to no maintenance. Another interesting area phenomenon within simulation is the concept of tactile memory [35]. This involves allowing the brain to "fill in the gaps" creating the sense of touch when there is none. This may explain why anecdotally many first-time users of non-haptic robotic systems like the da Vinci® Surgical System initially think there is some level of haptic feedback.

9.5 Immersive technology

Immersive technology is an umbrella term for augmented reality (AR), VR, and mixed reality platforms that enable the visualization and/or manipulation of a virtual environment highly representative of a real-world setting. The concept of immersive VR has been of interest in the consumer and enterprise spaces over the years, driven by demand from the gaming and entertainment industries alongside a growing interest in the education sector. However, the high cost of the technology has historically been too expensive or clunky in order to see widespread adoption. Continued advances in the software and hardware components of immersive technology, such as sensors, processors, and other semiconductor components, will drive costs down and enable increased adoption.

9.5.1 Evolution and adoption of virtual reality technology

The immersive technology revolution was spurred by the launch of a 2012 crowdfunding campaign for a new generation of VR technology: the Oculus Rift. This novel breed of VR technology harnessed recent advances in graphics processing units (GPUs), mobile phone displays, and motion tracking technology to create a lower cost VR headset that solved many of the issues plaguing prior attempts. When a user dons a VR headset, he/she is completely immersed in a fully simulated space. Each eye sees a slightly different perspective allowing for natural stereoscopic vision. If the experience is designed correctly, a sense of "presence" is conveyed, in which the brain perceives the simulation as if it was really happening. Following the release of early developer kit in 2013 and 2014, the commercial release of the Oculus Rift in 2016 led to an explosion of interest in immersive technologies and the release of a wide variety of hardware peripherals and software platforms (Figure 9.4). Eventually, the introduction of touch controllers alongside

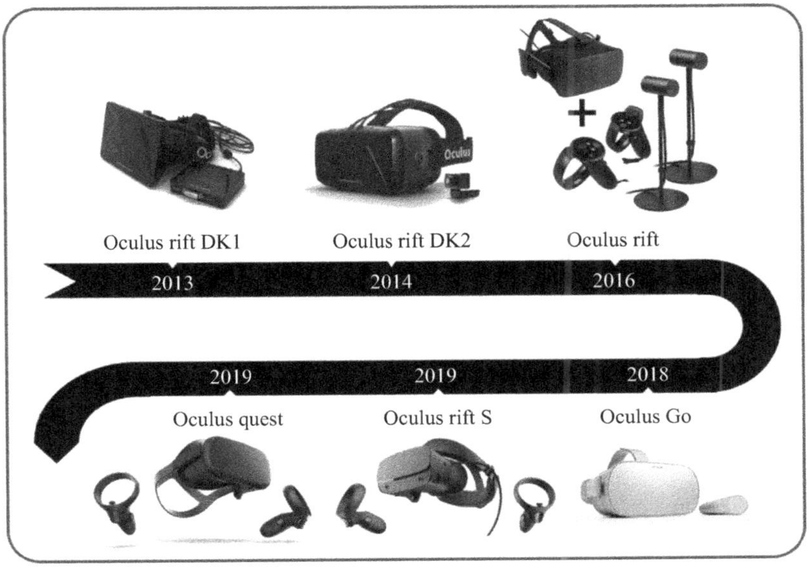

Figure 9.4 Timeline of modern virtual reality platform product launch

the Oculus Rift and the HTC Vive allowed the user to accurately track the position of their hands, enabling interaction with the virtual worlds.

Widespread commercial adoption of early modern VR platforms was somewhat limited due to a phenomenon commonly called "VR Sickness." Almost all users after a period of time would experience significant nausea when using VR, which would limit the amount of time they could spend. For the general population, this led to the perception that all VR caused motion sickness and decreased their interest in using future VR experiences. The source of VR sickness is mainly a disconnect between the vestibular and visual systems of the brain and can easily be avoided. This could be caused by a lack of positional tracking for head motion, poor performance, or certain design elements, which for the most part have been eliminated with modern systems. The incidence of VR sickness (also called "cybersickness") is anywhere from 40% to 70% of users as shared by Kinesiology Service, University of Minnesota. VR head-mounted displays (HMDs) have rapidly evolved since the release of the first consumer version of the Oculus Rift. Each category of HMD contains advantages and disadvantages, and it is helpful to understand the subtle differences as the technology has evolved (Table 9.1).

9.5.1.1 Tethered headsets

Tethered headsets are the classic form factor of VR headsets, which include the Oculus Rift and HTC Vive. The term tethered comes from the requirement of a wired connection to a computer. Since these headsets can be paired with powerful graphics cards, they are currently the most powerful and high-fidelity of available

Table 9.1 Technical evolution of virtual reality platforms

	Oculus Rift DK1	**Oculus Rift DK2**	**Oculus Rift**	**Oculus Go**	**Oculus Rift S**	**Oculus Quest**
Consumer grade	No	No	Yes	Yes	Yes	Yes
Tethered	Yes	Yes	Yes	No	Yes	No
Memory or other?	–	–	–	32–64 GB	–	64–128 GB
Resolution	1,280 × 800	1,920 × 1,080	2,160 × 1,200	2,560 × 1,440	2,560 × 1,440	2,880 × 1,600
Motion tracking	3DOF	6DOF	6DOF	3DOF	6DOF	6DOF
HMD weight (oz)	13.4	15.5	16.6	16.5	16.6	20.1
MSRP[a]	$300[b]	$350[b]	$599[b]	$199–$249	$399[b]	$399–$499

[a]Manufacturer retail suggested price at the time of publication.
[b]Does not include estimated cost of external PC needed to operate system.

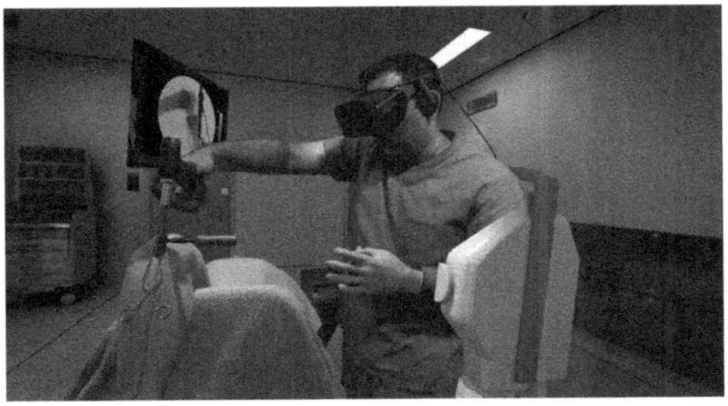

Figure 9.5 VR simulation of tibial nail procedure using the Oculus Rift. Image courtesy of OssoVR

HMDs. Tethered headsets allow for what is described as 6DOF tracking, meaning that they can track both head rotation and position, which allows user to move around a virtual space. Tethered headsets require a tracking system in order to detect their position in 3D space. For the Oculus Rift, this takes the form of IR cameras that detect IR LEDs on the headset. For the HTC Vive, IR "base stations" emit lasers that are detected by sensors on the headset. Newer generations of tethered headsets carry onboard cameras that perform "inside-out" tracking, obviating the need for external tracking systems. Currently, the price of tethered VR can be relatively low, with the Oculus Rift S costing around $399 at the time of publication. Figure 9.5 shows a rendering of a virtual operative environment where the user is participating in a training module for an orthopedic surgical procedure that is commonly replicated using a synthetic bench top model.

9.5.1.2 Wireless headsets

One of the major downsides of tethered VR is a limited tracking area for exploring a virtual space and a decreased "presence" due to the headset cable interfering with the overall experience. To address this issue, there are some adapters that allow for the wireless transmission of the visual and motion data from the headset to and from the virtual workstation. The most popular wireless headset adapter is the TPCast system, which works to make the HTC Vive effectively wireless.

9.5.1.3 Mobile headsets

Since modern immersive technology is based on mobile devices, phones themselves can actually be modified to function as AR headsets. This led to an explosion of popularity with the release of Google Cardboard, a $25 piece of cardboard that can make almost any mobile phone into an AR headset. This form of VR currently has rotational tracking (3DOF) only and does not allow for hand tracking. The phones primarily used for Google Cardboard were not optimized for VR leading to relatively low-quality experiences mainly limited to 360-degree photos and videos. Samsung Gear VR saw a more focused approach to mobile VR. Only specific VR compatible phones would work, which allowed for higher quality experiences and games. Unfortunately, with the Gear VR there was still only rotational tracking. The cost of entry for the Samsung Gear was relatively high as well, unless the user already owned a compatible phone.

9.5.1.4 Standalone headsets

Standalone headsets are a single device that does not require a phone or computer for use. Standalone headsets come in 3DOF varieties (like the Oculus Go) which start at $200, and 6DOF versions with hand tracking like the Oculus Quest, ranging from $400 and up. The Oculus Go, while high quality, still suffers from many of the mobile headset drawbacks, mainly being limited to 3DOF. The Oculus Quest, which was released in May 2019, is seen as a promising contender for VR mass adoption, as it requires minimal setup, has almost unlimited tracking volume, and deep presence with no wires detracting from the experience. One of the main drawbacks of standalone headsets is the limited processing power when compared with tethered solutions, leading to less sophisticated simulations and experiences and a limited battery life.

9.5.2 Applications of immersive technology in healthcare

VR in healthcare has seen a variety of applications and use cases develop in a short period of time. Some of these use cases have shown remarkably positive evidence of efficacy and are seeing relatively rapid adoption across the areas of surgical planning and visualization, medical education, surgical training, rehabilitation, and therapeutic administration. For example, instructional and didactic-based lectures in medical education have progressed to computer-based anatomical representations and simulation of both anatomy, organ function, and even valuation of physiological pathways through molecular interactions. Beyond the capability of traditional tools, VR can be used as a bridge to teach complex clinical concepts in a more straightforward and intuitive manner. For example, pediatric cardiologists at Stanford's Lucile Packard Children's Hospital created "The Stanford Virtual Heart," an immersive VR platform, which allows users to explore congenital heart abnormalities in a highly interactive way. The content is geared toward medical students and residents; however, it can be used for patient education as well to help families understand these complex conditions. VR can be utilized for a wide variety of rehabilitation, including postoperative physical therapy, and neuro-rehabilitation poststroke. The current markets for VR and AR technologies are indicative of the potential use cases for fully immersive technology healthcare.

The advent of AR and VR in surgical planning and visualization is an extension of current technological attempts to guide, navigate, and operate with the assistance of imaging-based tools. In preparation for a case, surgeons, interventionalists, and radiologists often study two dimensional representations of three-dimensional scans, such as ultrasound, computed tomography scans, fluoroscopy, magnetic resonance imaging, positron emission tomography. In the preoperative arena, virtual models of these anatomical images make it relatively straightforward to allow the user to naturally view patient-specific renderings in a 3D immersive space and manipulate it in novel ways. Surgical Theater and Echopixel are examples of companies utilizing this approach for neurosurgery and cardiology. Applications in radiotherapy can also utilize surgical preparation and planning by constructing VR models that enable the targeted mapping of high-intensity radiation to tumors and minimize the exposure of healthy tissue. The utility of AR during image-guided procedures enables surgeons to projection medical images onto live video stream or through the console of robotic-assisted surgical systems in tandem with haptic feedback. The Stryker Mako system for robotic-assisted orthopedic surgery is an example of VR and haptic feedback combined on one immersive technology platform.

9.5.3 Immersive technology for surgical training and assessment

Over the past few years, VR technology has improved rapidly and shows no sign of slowing. The limitations of current surgical training paradigms discussed in Section 9.3.2 are indicative of a need for disruption in the space. In addition to resident work hour restrictions and the failure to demonstrate competency and autonomy of surgical trainees, there are minimal training opportunities for surgeons in practice. The trends toward increasing device complexity and rising number of new device approvals raised in Section 9.2.1 leave surgeons in practice with inadequate time and resources, leading to risky usage of more complex technologies. In addition, "lower volume" surgeons have been shown to have worse outcomes than "higher volume" surgeons due to less practice[†]. As surgeon shortages loom, demonstration and maintenance of competency will be critical to reigning in medical errors and delivering value-based outcomes.

One method which has been successfully utilized in attempts to address the recognized problem of too few and undertrained surgeons is the use of VR for surgical training. VR simulation allows surgeons to become familiar with instruments, equipment, and procedures before performing certain surgeries on patients (Figure 9.6). While not new, the VR technology evolution reviewed in Section 9.5.1 highlights changes in the hardware marketplace that have made the next generation of simulators possible. These changes include increased GPUs processing power, the widespread availability and affordability of high quality OLED screens, advances in motion sensors, improvements in tracking technology, and a greater understanding of the technical and design requirements of a tolerable VR experience that does not lead to VR sickness (see footnote 2). These advances allow for a new and disruptive surgical simulation platform that provides a much more scalable, affordable, immersive, and effective solution over prior generations. The benefits of VR simulation platforms also extend beyond surgical training into the realm of medical device development. Virtual simulations of device prototypes can easily be transferred into immersive scenarios, allowing the surgeon, engineer,

[†]Data used in this section is from the Small Business Innovation Research (SBIR.gov).

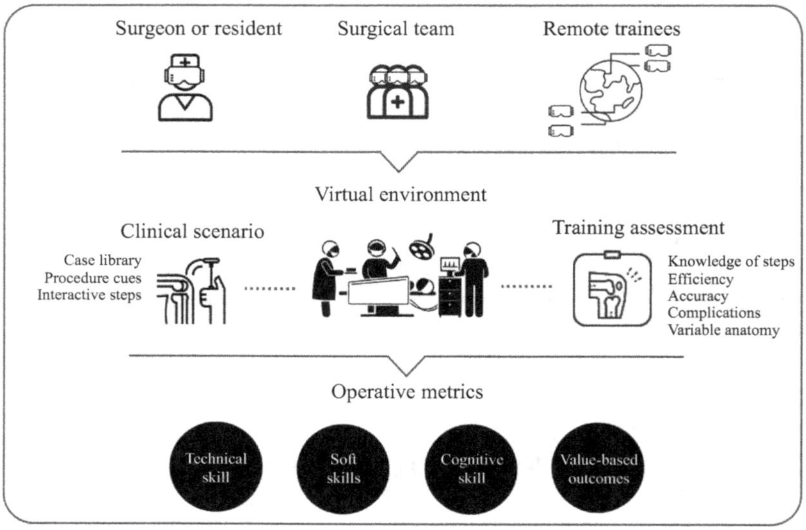

Figure 9.6 Immersive surgical training multiplexes the traditional simulation process across trainees, independent of timing, location, and staff and provides objective metrics for technical, cognitive, and soft skills that can be linked to value-based outcomes through surgical data science implementation

and clinician to test deployment and design in a low-risk, geographically independent, virtual environment.

Training with VR simulators has been shown to improve surgeon performance over time, and these skills have been shown to be transferable to improving performance in the operating room. In fact, it was shown that a VR "warm up" significantly improves the performance of laparoscopic colectomies in swine models by trainee surgeons (see footnote 2). This benefit of pre-procedural "warm-up" training with VR simulators has similarly been shown for cholecystectomies as well (see footnote 2). A study on percutaneous spinal fixation simulation with VR and haptics found significant performance accuracy improvement between needle placement attempts, supporting the efficacy of AR and haptics as a learning tool (see footnote 2). Recently, Osso VR has developed a VR platform specifically for use in orthopedic surgery training. A study comparing the transferability of skills gained in OssoVR's training program simulating tibial nail fixation to a standard guide in a cohort of VR platform-trained medical students doubled surgical performance on a Global Assessment Scale compared with traditional training g method (Figure 9.7; [39]).

VR simulation addresses many of the challenges of training a global surgical workforce that is at the frontier of medical device technology. The ease of accessibility and steadily declining cost of high-quality, untethered VR headsets

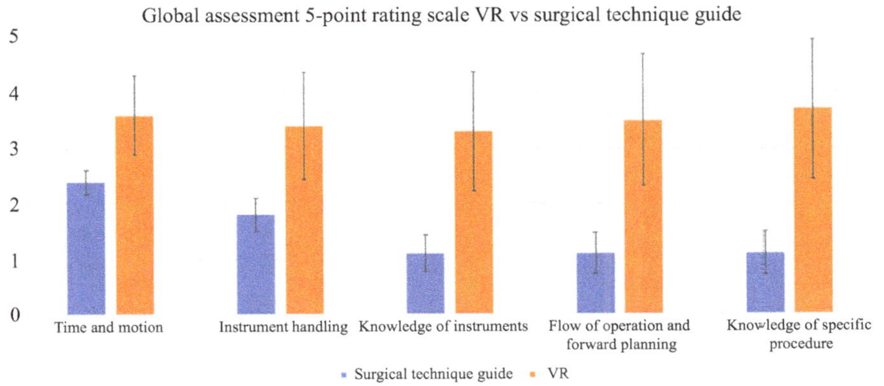

Figure 9.7 Surgical training assessment using immersive technology platform. Image courtesy of OssoVR

breakdown the hierarchy of the Halstedian pyramid and place high-quality surgical training in the hands of many, from surgeons to trainees to the entire surgical team. In addition to clinical users, medical device sales staff can deploy an interactive suite of tools to educate, train, and collect feedback that accelerates the adoption of novel medical technology. Successful utilization of VR in surgical training has led to the wide-spread adoption of such systems in general surgery training programs, with at least one program mandating that residents undergo VR training before performing any live surgery. However, the adoption of new training methodologies means little if proficiency increases cannot be accurately measured, and the remaining challenge for VR surgical training and assessment needs to be proven by longitudinal studies that link VR simulation to gains in technical proficiency, communication, cognition, and ultimately, outcomes.

9.5.4 Future directions and barriers to adoption

Over the past few years, VR technology has improved rapidly and shows no sign of slowing. We will likely see continued improvements in visual fidelity such as resolution, pixel fill, field of view, optics/sweet spot, eye tracking, foveated rendering, performance, and audio. For the reasons listed earlier in this chapter, surgical training and assessment are proving to be major areas of focus for immersive technologies. Early studies are showing greater effects than those of simulation technologies of the past and in most cases is less than 1% the cost of simulation. Combine this with the ease of accessibility, the wide variety of applications under development, and the portability, it is hard to deny the promise of this new form factor for simulation. Osso VR's early-stage surgical training platform is currently being used by "early adopter" residency programs across US medical schools, such as Harvard University, University of California Los Angeles, University of California San Francisco, Vanderbilt University, Columbia University, University of Pittsburgh, University of Florida, and Johns Hopkins University as well as by medical device manufacturers, such as Johnson & Johnson, Zimmer Biomet, and

Smith & Nephew, among others. Furthermore, governing bodies, such as the American Board of Orthopaedic Surgeons, American Academy of Orthopaedic Surgeons, Association of American Medical Colleges, and ACGME, are more likely to accelerate integration of simulation into their curriculums with the ability to assess surgeon proficiency.

Commonly perceived drawbacks of this mode of simulation include the lack of kinesthetic haptics, the slight learning curve for the hand tracking controllers, and the relative lack of individual finger tracking. While there are a variety of haptic and non-haptic gloves and finger-tracking controllers on the market, they do not yet have the widespread traction than the standard VR controllers.

Finally, the device industry stands to benefit on a ubiquitous scale due to the lack of scalable and affordable surgical training options—a critically unmet need. This underscores the imminent demand for the adoption of higher value immersive technologies in healthcare.

References

[1] T. G. Weiser, A. B. Haynes, G. Molina *et al.*, "Size and distribution of the global volume of surgery in 2012," *Bull. World Health Organ.*, vol. 94, no. 3, pp. 201–209F, 2016.

[2] P. Densen, "Challenges and opportunities facing medical education," *Trans. Am. Clin. Climatol. Assoc.*, vol. 122, no. 319, pp. 48–58, 2011.

[3] B. N. Carter, "The fruition of Halsted's concept of surgical training," *Surgery*, vol. 32, no. 3, pp. 518–27, 1952.

[4] "William Halsted and others operating in surgical amphitheater." The Alan Mason Chesney Medical Archives, Johns Hopkins Medical Institutions.

[5] A. H. Daniels and C. W. DiGiovanni, "Is subspecialty fellowship training emerging as a necessary component of contemporary orthopaedic surgery education?," *J. Grad. Med. Educ.*, vol. 6, no. 2, pp. 218–21, 2014.

[6] E. J. Elsey, G. Griffiths, J. West, and D. J. Humes, "Changing autonomy in operative experience through UK general surgery training: a national cohort study," *Ann. Surg.*, vol. 269, no. 3, pp. 399–406, 2019.

[7] R. H. Bell, T. W. Biester, A. Tabuenca *et al.*, "Operative experience of residents in US general surgery programs: a gap between expectation and experience," *Ann. Surg.*, vol. 249, no. 5, pp. 719–24, 2009.

[8] M. A. Makary and M. Daniel, "Medical error-the third leading cause of death in the US," *BMJ*, vol. 353, p. i2139, 2016.

[9] L. Maier-Hein, S. S. Vedula, S. Speidel *et al.*, "Surgical data science for next-generation interventions," *Nat. Biomed. Eng.*, vol. 1, no. 9, pp. 691–696, 2017.

[10] O. Aquilina, "A brief history of cardiac pacing," *Images Paediatr. Cardiol.*, vol. 8, no. 2, pp. 17–81, 2006.

[11] EvaluatePharma, "World Preview 2018, Outlook to 2024," 11th Edition, p. 47, 2018.

[12] J. W. Senders, "On the complexity of medical devices and systems," *Qual. Saf. Health Care*, vol. 15, no. Suppl 1, pp. i41–i43, 2006.

[13] FDA, "Statement From FDA Commissioner Scott Gottlieb, M.D., and Jeff Shuren, M.D., Director of the Center for Devices and Radiological Health, on a record year for device innovation," FDA, 2019. [Online]. Available: https://www.fda.gov/news-events/press-announcements/statement-fda-commissioner-scott-gottlieb-md-and-jeff-shuren-md-director-center-devices-and-1. [Accessed: 28-Jan-2019].

[14] K. F. Kowalewski, M. W. Schmidt, T. Proctor *et al.*, "Skills in minimally invasive and open surgery show limited transferability to robotic surgery: results from a prospective study," *Surg. Endosc.*, vol. 32, no. 4, pp. 1656–1667, 2018.

[15] T. Dall, T. West, R. Chakrabarti, and W. Iacobucci, "The complexities of physician supply and demand: projections from 2013 to 2025 final report Association of American Medical Colleges," *Assoc. Am. Med. Coll.*, pp. 1–68, 2015.

[16] AAMC, "Active Physicians in the Largest Specialties," AAMC, 2017. [Online]. Available: https://www.aamc.org/data/workforce/reports/492556/1-1-chart.html. [Accessed: 17-Jul-2019].

[17] American Academy of Orthopaedic Surgeons, "Projected Volume of Primary and Revision Total Joint Replacement in the U.S. 2030 to 2060," American Academy of Orthopaedic Surgeons, 2018. [Online]. Available: https://aaos-annualmeeting-presskit.org/2018/research-news/sloan_tjr/. [Accessed: 06-Oct-2019].

[18] G. Labek, M. Thaler, W. Janda, M. Agreiter, and B. Stöckl, "Revision rates after total joint replacement," *J. Bone Joint Surg. Br.*, vol. 93-B, no. 3, pp. 293–297, 2011.

[19] H. Workforce, "National and Regional Projections of Supply and Demand for Surgical Specialty Practitioners: 2013-2025 The National Center for Health Workforce Analysis (the National Center) informs public and private-sector decision-making on the U.S. National and Regional,", pp. 2013–2025, 2016.

[20] V. Laxmi, "Medical Devices: Technologies and Global Markets," BCC Publishing, 2018.

[21] S. Dora, D. Khanna, Y. Luo, L. Poon, and C. Schweizer, "Medtech May Be Emerging Markets' Next New Thing," Boston Consulting Group, epub. March 2, 2017.

[22] R. S. Haluck and T. M. Krummel, "Computers and virtual reality for surgical education in the 21st century," *Arch. Surg.*, vol. 135, no. 7, pp. 786–792, 2000.

[23] S. G. Mattar, A. A. Alseidi, D. B. Jones *et al.*, "General surgery residency inadequately prepares trainees for fellowship," *Ann. Surg.*, vol. 258, no. 3, pp. 440–449, 2013.

[24] B. C. George *et al.*, "Readiness of US general surgery residents for independent practice," *Ann. Surg.*, 2017.

[25] S. L. Meyerson, E. N. Teitelbaum, B. C. George, M. C. Schuller, D. A. DaRosa, and J. P. Fryer, "Defining the autonomy gap: when expectations do not meet reality in the operating room," *J. Surg. Educ.*, vol. 71, no. 6, pp. e64–e72.

[26] D. Manthey and M. Fitch, "Stages of competency for medical procedures," *Clin. Teach.*, vol. 9, no. 5, pp. 317–319, 2012.

[27] M. M. Hutter, K. C. Kellogg, C. M. Ferguson, W. M. Abbott, and A. L. Warshaw, "The impact of the 80-hour resident workweek on surgical residents and attending surgeons," *Ann. Surg.*, vol. 243, no. 6, pp. 864–871, 2006.

[28] E. Culliford, "Cadavers in the ballroom: Doctors practice their craft in America's favorite hotels," Reuters, epub. December 15, 2017.

[29] A. K. Dubin, D. Julian, A. Tanaka, P. Mattingly, and R. Smith, "A model for predicting the GEARS score from virtual reality surgical simulator metrics," *Surg. Endosc.*, vol. 32, no. 8, pp. 3576–3581, 2018.

[30] K. A. Barsness, "Trends in technical and team simulations: Challenging the status Quo of surgical training," *Semin. Pediatr. Surg.*, vol. 24, no. 3, pp. 130–133, 2015.

[31] D. Woods, E. Thomas, J. Holl, S. Altman, and T. Brennan, "Adverse events and preventable adverse events in children," *Pediatrics*, vol. 115, no. 1, pp. 155–60, 2005.

[32] C. C. Greenberg, S. E. Regenbogen, D. M. Studdert *et al.*, "Patterns of communication breakdowns resulting in injury to surgical patients," *J. Am. Coll. Surg.*, vol. 204, no. 4, pp. 533–540, 2007.

[33] M. Louridas, P. Szasz, S. de Montbrun, K. A. Harris, and T. P. Grantcharov, "International assessment practices along the continuum of surgical training," *Am. J. Surg.*, vol. 212, no. 2, pp. 354–360, 2016.

[34] G. S. Ruthenbeck and K. J. Reynolds, "Virtual reality for medical training: the state-of-the-art," *J. Simul.*, vol. 9, no. 1, pp. 16–26, 2015.

[35] M. W. Salkini, C. R. Doarn, N. Kiehl, T. J. Broderick, J. F. Donovan, and K. Gaitonde, "The role of haptic feedback in laparoscopic training using the LapMentor II," *J. Endourol.*, vol. 24, no. 1, pp. 99–102, 2010.

[36] M. Zhou, S. Tse, A. Derevianko, D. B. Jones, S. D. Schwaitzberg, and C. G. L. Cao, "Effect of haptic feedback in laparoscopic surgery skill acquisition," *Surg. Endosc.*, vol. 26, no. 4, pp. 1128–34, 2012.

[37] C. Våpenstad, E. F. Hofstad, L. E. Bø *et al.*, "Lack of transfer of skills after virtual reality simulator training with haptic feedback," *Minim. Invasive Ther. Allied Technol.*, vol. 26, no. 6, pp. 346–354, 2017.

[38] C. Pacchierotti, D. Prattichizzo, and K. J. Kuchenbecker, "Cutaneous feedback of fingertip deformation and vibration for palpation in robotic surgery," *IEEE Trans. Biomed. Eng.*, vol. 63, no. 2, pp. 278–87, 2016.

[39] G. Blumstein, B. Zukotynski, N. Cevallos *et al.*, "Randomized trial of a virtual reality tool to teach surgical technique for tibial shaft fracture intramedullary nailing," *J Surg. Educ.*, vol. 77, no. 4, pp. 969–977, 2020.

Chapter 10

Applications of blockchain in healthcare

Ron Urwongse, MISM, M.B.A.[1] *and*
Kyle Culver, M.S., M.B.A.[2]

Since 2016, interest in blockchain has emerged across all sectors of healthcare. This interest has been expressed in the form of collaborative initiatives led by notable organizations within the healthcare industry. Some showed promising results, but none has yet achieved scale in adoption and economic sustainability to be considered an unqualified success. After reading this chapter, the reader will be able to describe what blockchain is and the new business models it can enable. In addition, the reader will have a framework to consider blockchain for a use case and to understand the potential barriers to adoption. Finally, the chapter will review multiple use cases being considered across diverse healthcare sectors, the early industry experiments exploring how blockchain can be used, and what ideal end states could look like. Please note that this chapter has been authored with a focus on healthcare in the United States, and as a result, most examples will be presented with a US perspective.

10.1 Introduction to blockchain

10.1.1 How blockchain works

In 2019, if someone were asked, 'What is the Internet?', one would likely speak about the value it creates, the business models it enables, and the digital experiences inextricably linked to our modern lives. However, in 1994 when the Internet was still an emergent phenomenon, the question 'What is the Internet?' would have elicited a more technical explanation because the transformative change the Internet would unleash on the world was still years away. Blockchain in 2019 is analogous to the Internet in 1994. It is an emerging technology that has found a starting point with niche use cases. The media is learning how to talk about the technology, and the market disruption that could result has not yet been deeply examined by most business leaders. How blockchain disrupts any industry segment

[1]Urwongse: CAQH, Washington DC, USA
[2]Culver: Humana, Louisville, KY, USA

or company is in question, but the scenarios most conducive to disruption are important for healthcare leaders to consider. This chapter describes the technology and its capabilities to help the reader appreciate the benefits offered by blockchain, while avoiding the granular details that would be relevant to a technical audience looking to tactically implement such solutions.

The Internet is a layered collection of technologies with physical networks and TCP/IP as a foundation, HTTP and other transport protocols as a middle layer, and web sites and mobile apps as the top human-facing layer. Similarly, blockchain is a collection of technologies that revolve around a structure of data blocks linked by cryptographic hashes and replicated across a decentralized network. The cryptographic hashes prevent tampering with historic blocks in the chain, making it apparent to all participants in the network if the data has been tampered. Participants must come to a consensus for each new data block added. This consensus paired with how the data is chained together makes it difficult for any one participant to add incorrect data or tamper with historical data. These features of the unique blockchain data structure drive transparency, accessibility, and trust among the network of participants.

The value of a blockchain solution is driven by network effects as the value of a decentralized network increases as the number of participants increases. This is because as the number of participants increases, the number of potential transactions that can occur within the network increases. This makes the overall network more valuable as it grows. In a traditional blockchain model, all participants have equal access to the data (i.e., they all have a copy of it) and are all able to verify the integrity of the data, building collective trust in the data and the network.

Another component included in the blockchain technology stack is smart contracts. These are self-executing contracts between two or more parties that do not require the oversight of a centralized authority or intermediary. This extends blockchain from just a store of data to a distributed and transparent computation mechanism. The logic of these smart contracts is visible to all in the network and can be inspected and verified, further increasing the trust and reliability, not only of the data, but also of the logic that processes the data. This method is different from a system with a central authority in which data is shared or a transaction executed, while the underlying business logic for the transaction is hidden.

For instance, in the current banking system, people use banks and the automated clearinghouse network to process payments and validate that funds are available. Alice can write a check to both Bob and Charlie without enough funds in her account to cover both. The banks verify those transactions and manage which check is processed, which one fails with the overdraft penalty to Alice. In a decentralized solution, as seen in Figure 10.1, all the logic and business rules of that transaction are determined by the network, and the decentralized community agrees on which transaction succeeds and which one fails as there is only $10 to go around. In the example presented, one of the transactions will be successfully written to the blockchain and the other will fail. Alice cannot pay both Bob and Charlie, and the community decides how the rule is applied, not the banks. Having

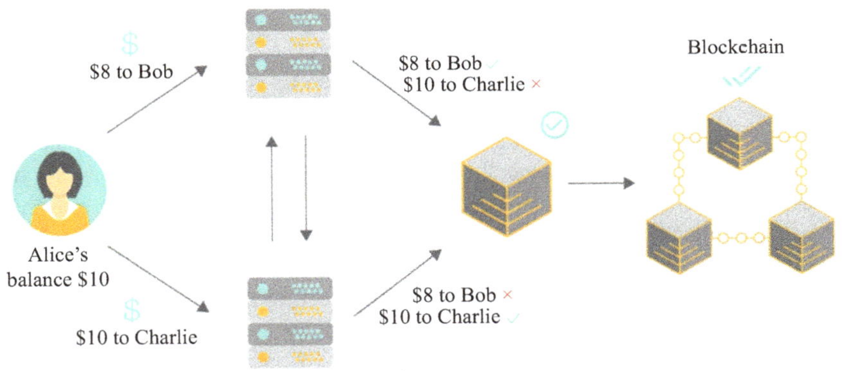

Figure 10.1 Double spend example (Image credit: Joe Gilbert)

direct access to the data and the system logic allows participants to transact directly with each other and to reduce the friction points that are symptomatic of centralized intermediaries, such as rent-seeking behaviour. This decentralization creates both opportunities and challenges that will be discussed in more depth later.

The trade-offs that need to be considered in these open solutions are privacy, confidentiality, and security. If patients' data is made available to multiple parties on a blockchain, how is data privacy protected? If a business has a unique contract with another stakeholder that provides a competitive advantage, how is that kept confidential? These are all issues to consider when determining the right mix of blockchain and traditional technologies to deploy as part of a solution. For example, there are emerging models where data is stored locally or 'off-chain' and the blockchain itself is used primarily for verification and transaction purposes. There are also methods by which blockchains can be used to prove the knowledge of data, without revealing the data itself. Most solutions will rely on a blend of centralized and decentralized technologies to help address the concerns of privacy, confidentiality, and security.

10.1.2 Reducing the need for intermediaries

Blockchain-powered solutions can reduce the need for intermediaries, as well as the costs and overhead they impose upon a network of participants. In addition, the transparency of blockchain solutions can increase the trust of participants in a network and in their transactions. This trust enables new models of collaboration among competitive organizations that were difficult to realize previously or required the formation of trusted intermediaries.

Intermediaries in healthcare exist to provide platforms that enable organizations to collaborate or exchange data and to streamline the sharing of data among their disparate systems. There are clearinghouses that focus on claims submissions and payments, health information exchanges, and emergent clearinghouses for provider data use cases. While the organizations may not necessarily trust each other, they have enough trust in the intermediary to transact through it with the other parties. The intermediary is a connection hub, acts as a referee, and often takes some nominal fee from participants who use its infrastructure. Blockchain technologies can enable the creation of decentralized autonomous utilities that more efficiently enable collaboration among untrusting parties in contrast to a centralized intermediary. A deeper exploration for why organizations may not trust each other occurs in a following section, but the issue boils down to not wanting to be taken advantage of by other organizations when collaborating. As was aptly captured by the 1980s British music duo Eurythmics, 'Some of them want to use you. Some of them want to get used by you'. Decentralization creates the opportunity for all participants to have a stake in, contribute to, and use a shared utility that can mitigate the distrust organizations have towards each other or a notional intermediary for an emergent use case.

10.1.3 Enabling improved interactions in healthcare

Amazon is the dominant online retailer with 47 per cent of total US online retail sales and 5 per cent of the total US retail market [1]. In the brick-and-mortar world, Sears and Kmart stores are shuttering weekly, and while Walmart earns a respectable hundreds of billions of dollars in annual revenue, its growth is modest compared to Amazon. Imagine a scenario where the top US brick-and-mortar retailers Sears, Target, and Walmart joined forces in 1995 to build a shared, web marketplace that allowed customers to shop across the offerings of each retailer. In addition, these retailers could lease online space to smaller retailers and manufacturers just as Amazon is currently doing with its Marketplace offering. If the founding retailers had the will and foresight to collaborate in 1995, they could have established the 'everything store' that Amazon would eventually become. This would have allowed them to compete against each other within the jointly owned marketplace instead of collectively being disrupted by Amazon. The ownership of the utility could have been managed in a mutually agreeable way with 'smart contracts' to dynamically manage the proceeds of the jointly owned, online 'everything store'. Alas, the retailers chose to compete against each other, opening an opportunity for Amazon to create a platform that serves as the online retail 'utility', capturing the lion's share of online retail revenue. While it is unlikely Sears, Target, and Walmart could have foreseen the quick rise to dominance of Amazon, it is nevertheless useful to consider how incumbents in other industries can collaborate on blockchain to streamline work that is redundant across their organizations and fend off would-be disruptors.

Direct business-to-business (B2B) interaction between parties via a blockchain utility could be more efficient and flexible when compared to centralized intermediaries in terms of reducing rent-seeking behaviour and adapting to the changing interests of participants. In the healthcare industry, there are significant opportunities for these types of blockchain-based utilities. Automated teller machines have been available since the 1970s, providing customers with access to banking services [2]. This same level of access to healthcare data is not yet available to US patients 50 years later. Every day, patients receive care, and healthcare administrators are not equipped with the information to discuss with the patient the exact cost of care at the point of service. Technology has existed for decades that could address these issues, but organizational constraints and limited interoperability make it challenging to realize these benefits. Blockchain is a different type of technical approach because it enables collaboration, shared ownership, and could potentially remove the barriers that block people from having ideal experiences with the healthcare system. By facilitating collaboration in non-competitive areas, blockchain could channel industry attention to compete where they should: on quality of care, cost of care, and access to care.

10.1.4 Reducing administrative costs in healthcare

In the US healthcare system, clearinghouses are entrenched intermediaries, providing the connection between health insurance companies (payers) and doctors and other healthcare professionals that provide care (providers). Today, a payer normally handles adjudicating medical claims. The payer has a contract with a member for coverage and a contract with a provider for the payment associated with the services rendered and/or value created. Providers work with multiple payers, who have different processes and interaction points that can create significant costs to the overall system. These costs are referred to as Billing and Insurance Related (BIR) cost, and in 2018, these costs were estimated to reach $315B (billion) annually [3]. Blockchain will not remove all these costs; however, reducing the friction of accessing adjudication logic and duplicative B2B processes would result in efficiency improvements. This specific use case will be discussed in more detail later, but the takeaway is that sharing logic via smart contracts in blockchain is a new capability that could streamline transactions. Other use cases that can benefit from smart contracts are focused on the pharmaceutical supply chain and provider credentialing. These utilities could drive down costs resulting from shared friction points by enabling collaboration and encouraging competition.

10.1.5 Barriers to adoption

Blockchain technologies were first deployed with Bitcoin in 2009, and as of 2019, they are still nascent as they relate to enterprise applications outside of cryptocurrencies. Many public implementations cannot handle the scale, specifically transaction processing speed, required for enterprise adoption. Various pilot efforts are still proving their ability to address industry-wide enterprise use cases. Advances are occurring at a rapid pace among technology companies, and these advances paired with lessons from the first wave of pilots will inform design decisions for future efforts. One of these decisions entails how the network of participants determine agreement on the next block of data to add, which is referred to as a consensus algorithm. There are different types of consensus approaches, including proof-of-work, proof-of-stake, and proof-of-elapsed time. Each has a trade-off, and decisions on selecting an appropriate consensus algorithm should be informed by the use case. These choices have implications on the security, efficiency, and scalability of the overall solution. For example, should data be stored on a blockchain, or off a blockchain? What identity management capabilities should complement a blockchain? As these technologies mature, reference implementations will provide repeatable models for selecting technologies to solve specific business problems. Currently, the technology decisions early adopters are making are risky, and the uncertainty dissuades many would-be adopters.

Blockchain solutions drive increased value as the network of participants expands. Establishing a critical mass early in the life cycle of a solution is important, since the most influential factor that will bring in new participants is the current base of participants with whom they can transact. A blockchain initiative that lingers for too long without a growing base of participants may never achieve momentum to scale. Creating a minimum viable network is more difficult than creating a minimum viable product, a term of art used by entrepreneurs to describe the first version of a product launched. For a B2B solution, creating a minimal viable network requires finding early adopters that value the future potential of collaboration over any perceived competitive risk. Collaborating with competitors requires a culture shift, and an understanding that some business functions can be considered non-competitive and that it is acceptable to work on these areas with competitors. It is important to identify key stakeholders within these companies, who can strongly represent both the interests of their employers and the interests of the collaborative. Finding key individuals within an organization who have the optimism, business context, technical aptitude, influence and political savvy to walk this tightrope remains the challenge. Maintaining a collaborative culture through the unforeseen compromises and trade-offs that participants will have to make will also be a challenge as there will be internal pressures and temptations to prioritize the near-term interests of individual organizations over the long-term success of a new alliance.

Collaborating with multiple parties requires governance and clear expectation setting. Public blockchain implementations, such as Bitcoin and Ethereum, attempt to codify this governance which comes with trade-offs to scalability and efficiency. For instance, public implementations require a 'cost' to fully participate and cost requires computation which results in significant energy costs. Private or permissioned blockchain implementations can shift governance to more familiar legal agreements that parties sign before being allowed to participate. These barriers are traditional but are nonetheless barriers to collaboration. Governance needs to outline the technical and business aspects of participation which include frameworks for architecture decisions, how the group will manage the need to rollback changes, and the requirement for uptime and other service level agreements. Business-related governance decisions will also need to include how to remove a bad actor, the process to determine who should be included in the network, intellectual property ownership, and the scope of appropriate data and use cases for the blockchain platform. Getting these governance decisions right will ensure that organizations trust the collaborative and are willing to come to the table to collaborate.

Aligning on a business model that makes the interactions equitable for all stakeholders and ensures that long-term sustainability is another barrier. One of the most interesting aspects of Bitcoin is how it rewards its stakeholders for participation. Storing transactions in a stakeholder's block is rewarded with cryptocurrency, motivating more people to store transactions and expanding the network footprint as a result. Understanding the motives of stakeholders using a decentralized solution is key to defining a business model that incentivizes the right behaviour and that appeals to all stakeholders. Because these solutions are decentralized, each participant will have the ability to interact equally with each other, which levels the playing field, though this can be an uncomfortable position for dominant incumbents. Like financial markets, the potential implications of incentives on these new solutions and industries they disrupt can be difficult to predict. Historical examples are in short supply as decentralized solutions are still emerging, and no wide-scale market disruption to intermediaries has yet occurred.

10.2 When is it appropriate to use blockchain?

10.2.1 Industries are searching for the "killer app" for blockchain

In 2015, the *Economist* published its October cover dubbing blockchain as 'the trust machine', and entrepreneurs and technologists began aggressively exploring how they could leverage blockchain for applications beyond cryptocurrency [4]. Two years later in 2017, venture investment into blockchain companies increased to over $1B, and then in 2018, the investment spiked to over $5.5B [5]. As Bitcoin and alternative cryptocurrencies climbed in price, healthcare industry's attention began to focus on the underlying technology. The value of cryptocurrencies has since decreased, and the investments are also settling back to 2017 levels [6]. Leaders in industries ranging from financial services to consumer retail to healthcare are exploring the technology to inform their point of view on blockchain, resulting in a range of proofs-of-concept and industry consortia. Amid the 'hype-cycle', it is important to understand how the fundamentals of the technology make it suitable to solve use cases meeting specific criteria. It is important to understand the capabilities offered by blockchain to determine how blockchain may be applied to address current business problems or enable a new opportunity.

10.2.2 Framework for determining the fit of blockchain to a specific problem

A popular criticism of blockchain solutions is after breaking down the technical components, it becomes apparent a solution could have been implemented using traditional database, networking, or security technologies [7]. In these cases, blockchain itself does not add novel benefits to the solution. The most cynical critics accuse entrepreneurs of applying the blockchain label to their start-ups to attract publicity and increase market valuations.

Table 10.1 Criteria for appropriate blockchain use cases

Criteria	Description
Multiple sources of truth	A decentralized database is needed only when there are multiple sources of truth. If only one real-world entity is a source of truth, then a centralized database is enough
Distrust of centralized authority	Blockchain solutions are most suitable when participants are unable to trust a centralized authority to facilitate the transactions among them
Willingness to collaborate	Participants need to be willing to convene to agree on priority use cases and a governance framework to establish and manage the solution collaboratively
Verifiability and traceability are important	The verifiability and traceability features of blockchain support on-going trust among participants for the collaborative solution, which give them the ability to inspect the data and system logic to verify its integrity
Market-level business case	The problem to be solved needs to be one large enough to justify a shift in how the organizations do business and how they interact with each other. This bar lowers over time as technology becomes proven, more economical, and as blockchain demonstrations succeed and scale

While these scenarios are common, there are specific cases where blockchain can provide unique benefits. It is important to understand when blockchain makes sense, and what its differentiating capabilities are that make it suitable to solve particular types of problems. Understanding this will provide a common framework for business decision makers and technologists alike to determine whether to explore and leverage blockchain.

The following are the critical criteria a use case or problem must meet for blockchain to be a suitable technical approach over more traditional technologies. While some of these criteria are more 'litmus test' style questions, others require in-depth analysis and are subject to judgment (Table 10.1).

10.2.2.1 Multiple sources of truth

If there is only one writer for a database, then by default, any party willing to consume from that database trusts the one writer of the database [8]. A non-healthcare example of this would be the US Social Security Administration's (SSA) service to verify Social Security numbers (SSNs). The SSA is the sole writer of SSNs and is the most trustworthy source of these identifiers [9]. In terms of an SSN registry, there is no need for multiple writers for this database, and no need for this database to be implemented in a distributed model. A healthcare example would be the National Plan and Provider Enumeration System (NPPES), operated by the US Centers for Medicare and Medicaid Services (CMS), which assigns unique national provider identifiers (NPIs) to healthcare providers. Similar to SSA, there is a sole writer of NPIs, and no need for a distributed database for the NPI registry itself [10]. All consumers of both SSA and NPPES will trust the identifiers they issue, since SSA and NPPES are the sole authorities of their identifiers. In these cases, a blockchain to verify SSNs or NPIs would be unnecessary because a sole authority exists to verify each. Borrowing from an upcoming example, healthcare provider credentialing is a use case where there are multiple writers: there are hundreds of license boards and over 170 medical schools in the United States, so there are multiple writers and authorities of the data leveraged in this use case [11].

10.2.2.2 Distrust of centralized authority

If stakeholders are willing to trust a centralized third party to manage the data, then a distributed database (i.e., blockchain) is not necessary [12]. A centralized database controlled by the third party, or even one of the incumbent stakeholders, is acceptable and more efficient to build and manage, although choosing a centralized authority may result in trade-offs in terms of openness, verifiability, and any costs imposed by the intermediary on the participants.

There is often debate, for specific use cases, whether a trusted centralized entity can or will practically emerge. For example, Surescripts emerged as the de facto standard platform for e-prescriptions in the United States in an odd alliance of pharmacy benefit managers and pharmacy associations after years of discussion, pressure from healthcare providers, and government incentives to promote e-prescription among physicians [13]. This demonstrates that with the right confluence of factors and time, centralized trust can be established among competitors. There are, however, more examples when alliances could not be forged, or when collaborations were abandoned prematurely. Likewise, critics will argue centralized entities could begin to exhibit economic rent-seeking behaviour, and opportunities to adapt to the evolving needs of participants may not be addressed as they would in a more collaborative arrangement.

Trust is elusive for multiple reasons when attempting to establish industry alliances. Actors may believe there is a winner-take-all (or winner-take-most) scenario and may want to be the dominant player or believe other actors may want to become the dominant player then seek economic rents from other stakeholders. Some actors may believe other actors are more nefarious, and any emergent centralized authority has a risk of tampering with data in the platform or creating some unfair advantage over their competitors. Notice how most organizations do not believe themselves to be the one feared. From an inertia perspective, many actors may simply feel that the benefits of collaboration do not outweigh the overhead costs and risks of collaboration. A company can continue to transact inefficiently rather than risk any of the aforementioned outcomes or incur the cost of changing how they operate.

Centralization is difficult when a significant proportion of stakeholders views the use case as competitive and, thus, is unwilling to participate in a centralized platform. However, if a critical mass of parties agrees a use case is non-competitive and is willing to trust a centralized entity, then the overhead of alignment can be streamlined. It may then be more efficient to deploy a centralized solution than build a distributed system and establish the governance necessary to manage such a system. Decision-making, development, and maintenance would be centralized and could be executed in a more economical fashion than with a blockchain approach.

However, blockchain-driven decentralization is the best fit in a medium-trust environment. A low-trust environment is not conducive, because if stakeholders cannot come to the table and agree on foundational exchange standards and governance, then a distributed platform will not emerge. Stakeholders must be willing to compromise at least, while retaining some governance stake when a new alliance is established. They would be willing to collectively decide which functions they deem non-competitive and should be managed on a shared utility, and those they deem competitive and should remain within respective companies.

10.2.2.3 Willingness to collaborate

Stakeholders need to trust each other enough to convene and establish a governance framework in the context of a non-public, permissioned blockchain. Key steps to establishing an alliance include prioritizing use cases, deciding on data exchange standards, and determining business and funding models. Investing in these initial steps is resource-intensive for any one organization and getting key players around a specific use case to come together and to align is a nontrivial endeavour. Outside of healthcare, blockchain initiatives demonstrate how important the will to collaborate is. TradeLens, which is a joint venture between IBM and shipping giant Maersk, demonstrates how a culture of competition and distrust can handicap a blockchain collaboration out of the gate [14]. Maersk's competitors decided to opt out of TradeLens when they discovered Maersk and IBM would retain ownership of the intellectual property [15]. On the other hand, IBM and Walmart's Food Trust initiative shows how a higher level of trust supports blockchain adoption. To date, Food Trust counts multiple marquee participants, including Carrefour, Smithfield, TopCo, and Albertsons in addition to Walmart [16].

As of 2019, there are early examples of blockchain consortia pursuing initiatives within healthcare. The Hyperledger Healthcare Working Group convenes interested stakeholders to identify use cases and open-source software opportunities, with subgroups meeting to discuss patient use cases, payer use cases, and general interoperability [17]. The Synaptic Health Alliance convenes health plans and other healthcare organizations around the provider directory problem. ProCredEx brings together various healthcare organizations around the credentialing use case [18]. Other non-blockchain consortia within healthcare include CAQH, WEDI, and Sequoia Project, which demonstrates that distributed governance among competitors can scale a solution through work group and rule-making processes. It will be interesting to observe how incumbent consortia will play a role in emergent blockchain consortia. Organizations within healthcare are willing to collaborate with each other; however, the governance framework needs to be designed to attract influential, market-moving participants.

10.2.2.4 Verifiability, traceability of transactions is important

Use cases that require verifiability and traceability in the context of multiple writers are a good match for blockchain. Immutable transactions in blockchain allow for complete traceability and transparency [19]. This allows participants to verify the integrity of the database and ensures that it is tamper resistant. In addition, blockchain can present the complete history or life cycle of an asset, allowing participants to know how other participants interacted with the asset over time [20]. These benefits may come at the cost of system performance, storage, and computing resources. Electronic medical records are a good match for blockchain given the high level of audit and access control requirements. In addition, supply chain use cases such as IBM Food Trust as well as pharmaceutical supply chain use cases are an excellent fit for verifiability and traceability criteria.

10.2.2.5 Market-level business case

Is there any industry problem that cannot be solved by individual actors, or where there is some fundamental market failure when the behaviour of independent actors is preventing a larger problem from being solved? Did that problem pre-exist blockchain technology, and is blockchain providing a novel method to align and collaborate? Blockchain can be a good fit when the threat of market failure is well understood, and individual actors are willing to set aside their differences to collaborate. If a critical mass of stakeholders can agree on the magnitude of the problem and are willing to make the upfront investment to establish a governance framework, then there may be an opportunity for blockchain to help solve the problem at hand. Many of the use cases described in the following sections are related to such market failure scenarios.

10.3 Introduction to blockchain solution models

This section defines four high-level categories for blockchain solutions in the healthcare industry: shared audit trail, public data exchange, multi-party workflow, and protected data exchange. These categories are ordered by risk and complexity with shared audit trail being the lowest risk and least complex, and protected data exchange being the highest risk and most complex. After introducing these categories, examples of each will be discussed in more detail. These categories are meant to help the reader understand overall risk and complexity as well as the capabilities of these emerging technologies. A solution could potentially span categories, and new capabilities may emerge that result in new solution models. The users of these solutions can also be referred to as participants of the decentralized network (Table 10.2).

10.3.1 Shared audit trail

Use cases that fall into the shared audit trail category focus on sharing information with the group for the sole benefit of transparency. There are many reasons this may provide value to the overall group; however, the most common is to ensure that data has not been tampered with over the course of time. One of the capabilities that are heavily utilized in distributed ledger technologies is a one-way cryptographic hash. This capability allows for the creation of a digital fingerprint, called a hash or digest, which uniquely identifies a dataset. Contents of an entire book or database can be 'hashed' to create a unique fingerprint, should one character be

Table 10.2 Blockchain solution models

Category	Description
Shared audit trail	Participants share data with an entire network so audit can be performed, and accessibility is equal across participants
Public data exchange	Participants exchange public, non-sensitive data assets and the value associated with those assets
Multi-party workflow	Participants utilize the solution for inter-company workflows, handing off data and assets along a process and ensuring transparency throughout
Protected data exchange	Participants exchange personally identifiable information (PII) or protected health information (PHI) and the value associated, ensuring privacy and security through the transaction

changed then the hash or fingerprint would be drastically different. There are many ways to generate a one-way cryptographic hash, but the strength is that the same data will always provide the same fingerprint and the hash cannot be reverse engineered to reproduce the dataset. This feature allows participants to share hashes with each other; and should participants need to prove that data has not been altered, they can reproduce the hash with the dataset, and the network of participants can validate dataset matches what was shared earlier. An example of how this could prove valuable is 'hashing' official documents, then everyone can later verify that the hash is the same and the documents were not altered or manipulated. Proof-of-existence is a blockchain solution that is a digital notary service for documents to prove that information existed at a certain date. The country of Estonia also uses this technique for healthcare records and goes as far as to print the hash in a newspaper so it can be verified later that the health data stored has not been altered.

10.3.2 Public data exchange

Public data exchange use cases target improving the efficiency of information dissemination. Even though data is publicly accessible and not protected, it is often acquired at some cost, so these use cases need to leverage a business model that ensures the cost of data acquisition, and exchange is covered by some means. An example of this would be the provider directory data use case, where health plans are charged with maintaining correct service addresses and the phone numbers to make an appointment for each provider in their network. This data is surprisingly fluid and expensive to maintain, so some health plans are collaborating through the Synaptic Health Alliance to crowd source this curation work. There are other examples of data that is public and not perceived as a competitive advantage where collaboration can occur.

10.3.3 Multiparty workflow

Improving administrative processes normally fall into the multi-party workflow categorization. One of the best fit use cases gaining traction in this space targets the pharmacy supply chain. Regulations have been put in place with the Drug Supply

Chain Security Act (DSCSA) that pressure the industry to enable clear visibility into the drug supply chain as it moves across manufacturing, distribution, wholesaler, pharmacy distribution, pharmacies, hospitals to patients. Using a blockchain solution, these stakeholders can share information about each step in the process to provide an audit trail as well as account for these drugs through the multiple companies involved in the process. Medical claims are another use case that falls into this process as it requires the health plan (payer), healthcare professional (provider), patient, and potentially other parties to successfully adjudicate the claim and determine accurate cost share.

10.3.4 Protected data exchange

Protected data exchange is like public data exchange; however, the information is sensitive and requires privacy and security to protect patient data and comply with US regulations such as Health Insurance Portability and Accountability Act (HIPAA) Privacy Rule and the HITECH Act [21]. Patient identity matching and validating consent for data exchange and usage are high barriers to use cases in this category. There are significant opportunities for use cases that can overcome these barriers as interoperability issues are a significant driver for costs with conservative estimates at $30B per year in the United States [22]. Enabling patients to steward their own data and democratizing that data so it can be accessible across the industry require these types of barriers to be addressed. Patients can benefit from medical record portability to help reduce the need for the still prevalent fax machine, which remains a common tool for exchanging information within healthcare. Fax is a channel of communication that prevails despite there being more modern technologies because incentives are not aligned to promote greater interoperability, and these incentives need to flow to the right parties.

10.4 Healthcare provider data use cases

10.4.1 Industry focus on provider data use cases

While blockchain has been considered across many use cases within healthcare, provider data use cases have emerged as a popular target of blockchain. Two of the major multi-company initiatives gaining traction focus on provider data. Provider data issues are certainly market-level, big-ticket opportunities. Many have also identified provider data as a good initial use case as it is less sensitive from a privacy standpoint than patient data, and applying a nascent technology to this use case seems less risky. Finally, administrative processes related to provider data use cases have become more complicated and costlier over time; thus, there is a willingness to try something new and work differently to solve these challenges.

10.4.2 What is healthcare provider data?

Data about healthcare providers is used to accomplish many core functions within healthcare. Health insurance plans use this data to enrol providers into their networks, pay claims, communicate provider availability, and to address an emerging wave of US regulatory requirements. Health systems, hospitals, and other provider organizations use provider data to perform similar functions such as onboarding providers, verifying credentials, and otherwise managing providers. Regulatory bodies such as the US CMS and individual state Medicaids also perform similar functions with the data. Many of these organizations have their own siloed systems for capturing, storing, and validating this data.

10.4.3 What are the current challenges with provider data?

One of the biggest challenges of healthcare provider data is that it is sourced from multiple individuals and organizations. This includes the practitioners themselves, the schools and institutions where degrees and residencies were completed, licensing and specialty boards, and current and previous employers. These represent information silos that require either the provider be the collector and conduit of information or the consuming organization to obtain the information from multiple sources with the provider's authorization. This process of connecting silos incurs unnecessary cost throughout the industry and presents opportunities for data misalignment between different organizations.

The quality, reliability, and timeliness of information have an impact on business performance dimensions such as regulatory compliance, patient safety, and administrative costs. Lack of a single source of truth and challenges with accuracy, timeliness, and quality have plagued provider data, resulting in excessive complexity. The intractability of the problem, the intrinsic nature of decentralized sources of truth, the need for trust and transparency result in provider data use cases being perceived as a suitable opportunity for decentralized technologies.

10.4.4 How blockchain could be a good fit for provider data use cases

The following section is an exploration of blockchain applications within two provider data use cases, provider directory and credentialing. These use cases represent leading industry efforts to demonstrate how blockchain technology can be applied, anticipate challenges to be faced and potential new business models that may emerge.

10.5 Healthcare provider directories

10.5.1 Provider directory use case

A health insurance plan's provider directory is a tool to assist a member of that plan to search for a healthcare provider who is covered by the plan (in-network), who is qualified to address their health issue, and who is conveniently located near the member. These are maintained by health plans so their members can access information (e.g., phone numbers, addresses, and hours) about in-network doctors and make appointments with them. Maintaining the accuracy of provider directory information is surprisingly difficult because a provider may work at multiple locations and for different companies. These additional dimensions of data can result in a single doctor having eight or more directory records, and large health plans may need to manage millions of directory records to support hundreds of thousands of providers. This complexity paired with the fact that providers change employers, move states, retire, and pass away leads to a dataset with 50 per cent of the records requiring an update every 180 days [23].

Across healthcare in the United States, $2.1B is spent annually maintaining provider data, and 75 per cent of cost is duplicative [24]. This duplication comes from multiple companies managing data independently and providers submitting data redundantly. Directory data is only a small slice of the overall provider data needed to support the many functions across healthcare (i.e., other provider data supports claims payments, credentialing, and value-based care). One of the interesting aspects of provider directory data is the information that is mostly public data. For instance, a health plan knowing Dr Jane accepts appointments at 123 Market Street and the best number to call for an appointment is 867-5309 is not a competitive advantage or a confidential secret. A health plan is more likely to compete on the breadth of their provider network, their reimbursement rates to providers, or the premiums they charge to customers rather than accurate directory data. While the data is public and non-competitive, it is difficult to maintain and aggregate into an accurate online directory. The inefficiencies are understandable given that a doctor can be contracted with 12 health plans, and each of those health plans is accountable for maintaining an accurate directory. Health plans use a combination of techniques: direct phone calls, faxes, their own web portal, and emails to request and receive directory updates This redundancy in directory data submission is burdensome to the provider and has serious implications on directory data quality.

CMS began to audit the provider directories of health plans that participate in Medicare starting in 2016. A 2016 audit of 54 Medicare Advantage Organizations (MAO) by CMS found 45 per cent of the entries had at least one error. These errors result in delays in care, surprise bills, and can have negative impacts on access to care and patient health outcomes. To combat this data quality issue, CMS announced on-going audits and a maximum fine of $25,000 per beneficiary per day [23].

Despite this steep penalty, the CMS audit results in 2017 found that quality had actually declined and 52 per cent of entries had at least one error [23]. There are some cases of health plans that have been able to improve their directory accuracy within specific markets through different interventions. However, CMS audit results indicate that the challenge of maintaining accurate provider directory persists for most health plans, and most interventions attempted to improve directory accuracy have fallen short.

Because health plans have not considered directories a competitive asset, they viewed them merely as a secondary use of provider data and did not manage them with rigorous quality control processes. Likewise, providers knew that health plans were not paying much heed to directory data submitted, and little effort was taken to improve the quality of data submitted. For example, many provider groups submit all affiliated locations for every provider, regardless of how often a provider practiced at that location. This is a large factor in the inaccuracies identified in an average health plan's directory.

Because MAOs are held accountable by CMS for accurate provider directory data, the onus is on them to ensure the data is accurate, and they have processes to scalably identify and correct inaccurate data. Healthcare providers also have a hand in improving health plan provider directories as many directory errors can be traced upstream to providers. Why are providers submitting inaccurate data? Reasons include lack of a high-quality data within their own organization, misaligned understanding of directory data quality, and lack of incentives to submit accurate data to health plans. In other cases, provider organizations contract third parties: payer enrolment vendors and credentialing contractors. These third parties have narrow responsibilities, and accurate directory data may not be part of their defined scope of work. Making meaningful progress on data quality issues and streamlining the currently burdensome process will require collaboration among all relevant parties and new solution concepts since currently available approaches have not yet proven successful.

10.5.2 Proposed solution

A blockchain-powered solution could enable crowdsourcing of provider directory management activities. A crowdsourcing approach is attractive since multiple parties, including the health plans, providers, and third parties, have fragments of accurate provider data they could contribute and piece together accurate provider directories. Similar crowdsourcing approaches have been used to create a reliable and ever-expanding web encyclopaedia in Wikipedia. Collaboration could drastically reduce duplication of efforts, accelerate the dissemination of data, and improve the overall quality of directory data. If a critical mass of health plans adopts a shared solution, providers would be able to broadcast their information to impacted stakeholders faster and through a unified channel. Because health plans have not converged upon a single solution, frustrated providers are forced to update information across many channels such as fax, phone, email, and health plan portals. Providers also receive quarterly outreach, mandated by CMS, from each contracted health plan. A blockchain solution could share the outreaches across health plans, keeping them compliant with the regulations, and minimizing the amount of outreach healthcare providers and their staff must receive.

10.5.3 Incentive alignment

Because there is a cost in collecting and maintaining directory data, sharing this data altruistically among competitors is not sustainable in the long run. Appealing to various organizations' mission to increase and improve access to care may result in some long-term participation. However, concern about free riders not contributing enough to the utility may drive participants away. This could be addressed by establishing a dynamic market where firms can price directory data assets to be consumed by other participants. For example, a verified phone number for Dr Jane, which can be used by patients to make appointments, could be put up for sale to health plans that need to publish an accurate phone number for Dr Jane. That phone number would be available for some nominal credits which could be purchased outright with cash or could be obtained by contributing a verified phone number for Dr Jane. Also, a recently verified phone number could sell for a higher number of credits than one verified 3 years ago. A bounty system could also motivate participants to contribute to the utility. This would allow a company to post a bounty for a specific directory data asset and offer to pay any organization able to deliver the asset. An example is outlined in Figure 10.2. Automation and machine learning controls could also be overlaid on this utility to create a self-improving directory ecosystem to the benefit of all participants.

10.5.4 Why this makes sense for blockchain

Crowdsourcing the collection of provider directory data and managing the exchange of assets that cost healthcare organizations real hours and dollars to obtain will require trust among participants and trust in the exchange platform. Blockchain technologies add a level of transparency that allows participating firms to inspect the exchange rules as well as the actual transactions with the exchange and to observe whether all the participants and the exchange itself are playing by the established rules. This trust will establish a level playing field that allows for constructive competition and maximizes value to the industry at large.

Participants in such a collaborative utility will compete on the efficiency by which they are collecting and verifying data, which may result in taking advantage of accurate data where it exists today instead of making costly phone calls. It may also result in sharing some of the value created by such a utility with the providers and their constellation of third-party vendors, which will motivate them to align on a mutual definition of quality and submit data in a timely fashion.

The transparency of a distributed ledger provides an audit trail that can be used to understand the provenance and lineage of the data. For instance, participants may need to know when any company learns that Dr Jane has changed her phone number. The metadata around these changes becomes important when trying to determine if the data is credible. Over time, different sources of information may prove more reliable than others, and context such as when the change was captured, who captured the change, and how it was captured can help the utility understand the reliability of the data. An example of this would be a lab services company sharing reliable address data collected from when they pick up samples at provider offices. The Synaptic Health Alliance is developing a blockchain-powered solution for the provider directory use case that leverages many of the above-mentioned concepts. Aetna, Ascension, Humana, Quest Diagnostics, Optum, Multiplan, and United Healthcare are the founding members of the Synaptic Health Alliance.

Actors	Step 1	Step 2	Step 3	Step 4
Buyer humana	*Shares truth* −2 Coins			*Pays rewards* −72 Coins
Seller vendor A	*Reads truth* Free	*Proposes update* −2 Coins *Pays escrow* −20 Coins		*Collects reward* +50 Coins *Retrieves escrow* +20 Coins
Validator vendor B			*Validates record* −2 Coins	*Collects reward* +20 Coins
Miner	*Records action* +2 Coins	*Records action* +2 Coins	*Records action* +2 Coins	*Records action* +2 Coins

Steps in a successful flow

1. **Buyer** (Humana) shares latest provider demographics (Truth) as well as a reward for (A) the firm who finds an issue or suggests an update (Seller) and (B) the firm who validates the proposed update. this information is shared with participants via 'writing to the shared ledger' so there is no minimal cost paid to the miner for supporting the infrastructure.
2. **Seller** finds the data quality issue and proposes an update. This seller could be anyone seeking the reward. note that the validation cost would be put into escrow, and in the event, the update is incorrect that cost would be paid by the seller.
3. **Validator** reviews the proposed update and decides if the record does in fact require an update and then the reward is paid by the buyer. The validator could be the subscriber (Humana) or some set of trusted third parties looking to obtain the reward. This part of the process would likely be automated as the process matured.
4. **Buyer** pays the validator and seller for their contributions to the process. The buyer then has an opportunity to share an updated provider demographics (Truth) as a new standing offer to restart the process for a future update when made available.

Figure 10.2 Example bounty workflow (Image credit: Emily Braun)

10.6 Healthcare provider credentialing

10.6.1 What is healthcare provider credentialing?

Credentialing is the process by which health plans, hospitals, and other healthcare organizations verify the qualifications of licensed healthcare professionals and assess their background and legitimacy. Credential misrepresentation and provider disciplinary actions occur frequently enough, and this reality necessitates the continued safeguards that robust credentialing affords. In 2017 alone, state medical licensing board in the United States took 8,813 disciplinary actions against physicians with 1,615 actions, including license probation, revocation, or suspension [25]. One important aspect of credentialing is 'primary source verification' that requires the healthcare organization to verify the provider's credentials before contracting with them or employing them. This is a routine function and is a budgeted role in many large healthcare organizations. In smaller practices, an administrator may play this role part-time.

10.6.2 What are the challenges in healthcare provider credentialing?

The typical provider has on average 12 contractual relationships with health insurance plans, and there are hundreds of millions of required verifications annually across all providers in the United States [26]. The increased number of contractual relationships and non-physician provider types entering these relationships results in the burden of credentialing being greater than ever. In particular, from the provider's perspective, much of the work is redundant. There is duplicative data entry, repeated verification work, and the repetitive submission of this data to multiple organizations. There is also a lack of economic incentive alignment between verifiers and primary sources. Primary sources have an effective monopoly on verifying data associated with their organization, and either charge fees to verify or simply rely on an inefficient process to verify credentials, which results in delays to provider credentialing and deferred revenue.

10.6.3 Blockchain solution concepts for provider credentialing

Since 2016, the notion of leveraging blockchain to address credentialing challenges has been proposed by technologists and entrepreneurs (Figure 10.3). The European Commission's Joint Research Centre even claims that blockchain 'will accelerate the end of a paper-based system for certificates' and that self-verifying credentials will minimize the need for institutions to verify [27]. Emergent solution concepts share characteristics: they utilize an immutable, distributed ledger to write and digitally sign credentials to formalize their provenance; they have some form of identity management around practitioners and primary sources; they establish traceability of transactions related to verifying credentials; and they persist and reuse both the capture and verification of credentials to avoid redundant work. This core solution concept fits with a decentralized, blockchain approach: multiple writers

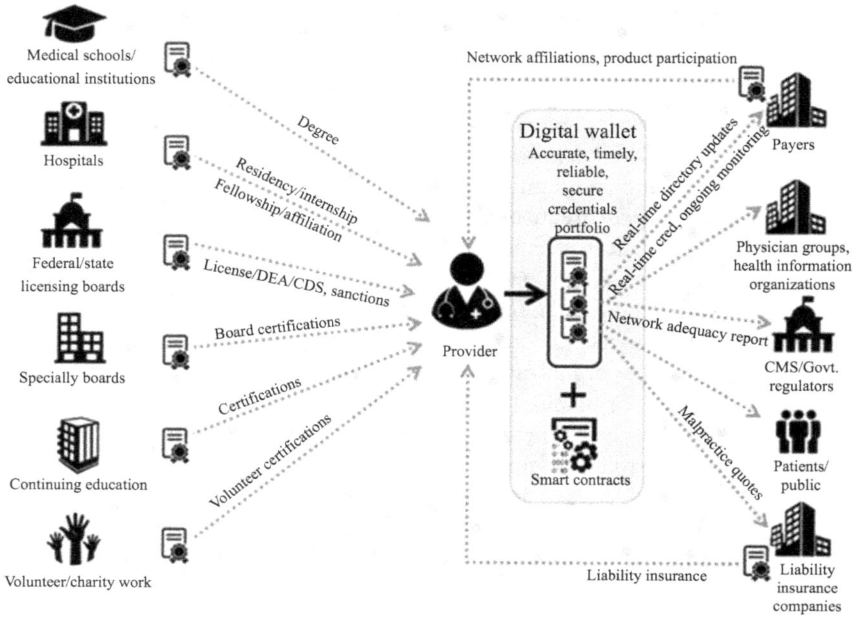

Figure 10.3 Blockchain credentialing solution concept (Image credit: John Koshy)

(i.e., hundreds of license boards, thousands of provider organizations, medical schools, etc.), no centralized authority for verification, and traceability of transactions are required per credentialing guidelines. The economic burden of credentialing is great, but is there a critical mass of organizations across the industry willing to put their differences aside to collaborate on a decentralized approach?

10.6.4 Early entrepreneurial activity and proofs-of-concept

There are multiple organizations exploring opportunities and forming alliances to address healthcare credentialing utilizing blockchain-based solutions. These companies are in various stages of development and adoption, and their efforts will help determine the effectiveness of blockchain in solving long-standing problems within healthcare credentialing.

ProCredEx has set out to build a 'trust layer' within the credentialing ecosystem. Their solution enables an authorized member of the exchange to observe the life cycle of a verified credential. This includes the source of the verification, the method used (e.g., electronically from the primary source or manually with the primary source), the identity and credentials of the organization and individual(s) associated with the verification, the outcome of the verification, and all redundant duplicate verifications found across other members of the exchange [28]. In addition, ProCredEx wants to build a marketplace for reusable verified credentials to minimize the redundancy of data collection, credential verification, and dissemination [28]. A core component of the solution utilizes a high-performance permissioned blockchain. ProCredEx is positioning itself to complement the existing credentialing ecosystem rather than disrupt it. They are constructing a marketplace for those with verified credential assets to list these for sale and provide a trust layer to ensure there is sufficient transparency on how data elements were collected and verified before they are used [28]. They are working with an early adopter 'design' cohort, including WellCare, Anthem's National Government Services subsidiary, Spectrum Health, Texas Hospital Association, Accenture, HealthLink Dimensions, and Hardenbergh Group [28]. This solution is focused on maturing scalable proofs-of-concept that will be submitted for peer review before reviewing with regulatory and accreditation bodies.

BlocHealth is solving the same problem of breaking through credentialing data silos but is taking a different approach. They are opting for a public blockchain straightaway and are focusing almost exclusively on the individual practitioner experience [29]. The use case focuses on upstream work of employment applications and initial credential submissions. Like ProCredEx, they want to use blockchain to enhance the traceability and transparency of credential data assets and increase automation through verification reuse [29]. The focus is building out an optimal user experience for the provider who is submitting the data, developing a smart application that collects the data needed from the practitioner, and generating the appropriate applications for those organizations that require it. Once collected, the provider credentials will persist on an immutable distributed ledger where they can be reused for future verifications, and where they will be portable beyond BlocHealth's solution [29].

Learning Machine is a company utilizing the Blockcerts open standard to write professional credentials to a blockchain and make them available via a mobile wallet [30]. They worked with the Federation of State Medical Boards to develop a workflow for institutions to issue Medical Education and Graduate Medical Education certificates to physicians and allow the physicians to share a verifiable certificate with third parties [25].

10.6.5 Minimal viable network

As is the case for new platforms that seek to address two-sided market problems, gaining a critical mass of adoption is important. Issuers of certificates will be more likely to adopt the platform if verifiers of certificates are already using it, and the converse is true. In the case of certificate issuance, some issuers have more market power (e.g., medical license issuers) than others. There are also certain consumers of certificates (e.g., license boards, federal government) that have more market power and may be able to influence adoption. Health plans and hospital chains with national presence in the United States can also help tip the market to embracing a new approach. Migration to a blockchain-based platform for verifying credentials will take a critical mass of these influential organizations to signal their intention before others in the industry follow suit. ProCredEx has assembled a strong early adopter base but has not yet achieved critical mass to tip the industry to a decentralized blockchain platform.

10.6.6 Primary source economic incentives

For issuers of certificates or 'sources of truth', economic incentives must exist for them to issue an independently verifiable certificate. Those organizations view the verification of credentials as an operational cost will need to see that the cost of establishing the infrastructure to issue digital certificates is less than the cost of verifying credentials. On the other hand, several organizations view the verification of credentials as recurring revenue, and they will be looking to replace any displaced revenue from self-verifying credentials. Many organizations that issue credentials also need to verify credentials (e.g., hospitals and license boards are both issuers and verifiers). These organizations need to realize enough cost savings in verification to offset revenue reductions. If the entire industry adopts this approach, cost savings can be realized throughout. Independent actors, however, must recognize their own return-on-investment before they will adopt. A marketplace approach like the one ProCredEx is promoting may be the right one to incentivize actors to participate in the solution, but only if the benefits of participating in the network outweigh the costs to change. Demonstrating the pricing framework to participants and transparent governance will be necessary to move forward.

10.6.7 Accreditation and regulatory acceptance

Government agencies as well as accreditation bodies such as the National Committee for Quality Assurance (NCQA), Utilization Review Accreditation Commission, and Joint Commission must recognize the validity of independently verifiable credentials signed with a private key and whose hash values are stored in a permanent and verifiable blockchain platform. NCQA has been reluctant thus far to take a public position on blockchain, and more demonstrations and popular industry support will need to occur before they take a position. Many healthcare organizations are waiting to hear the position of both government agencies and accreditation bodies before they are willing to fully embrace blockchain-based solutions.

10.7 Walmart supply chain: one non-healthcare example

10.7.1 Why are we talking about food supply chains in a healthcare book?

This non-healthcare section was included to provide background and complement Section 10.8 on the pharmaceutical supply chain. The Walmart supply chain example has widespread impact and demonstrates scale that has not yet been observed in other blockchain projects. Therefore, this example is being included to provide a model on how healthcare supply chains, including pharmaceutical, can leverage blockchain as well as how a single company with industry-wide reach can move the market towards blockchain adoption.

10.7.2 Issues with supply chain management

Supply chains have been a common early focus for blockchain-powered solutions because friction exists in the cross-company interactions. A food recall event, such as a recall of mangos, using the current technologies could span up to 2 weeks to complete. During this time, companies err towards overreaction to ensure the safety of their consumers. An audit trail is needed as mangos move from the farm to supplier to distributor to the actual storefront to support recall efforts. Stakeholders in this process are motivated to downplay their involvement to avoid liability and negative publicity. Transparency is needed within each step of the process to ensure that information is shared quickly and stakeholders can trust the accuracy of audit information regarding the 'chain of custody' of the recalled product.

Other sources of complexity in supply chains are the different combinations of interactions among supply chain participants. An ideal solution would be a unified, integrated utility across all supply chain participants that minimizes point-to-point integrations between stakeholder systems. Point-to-point integrations between multiple systems add significant friction and costs for participants to support and to maintain their connections to the supply chain. One question regarding such utility would be around ownership and trust. If a single party owned and managed the utility, can they be trusted with this competitive information such as how many mangos each store stocks or the number of mangos produced by a particular farm? If one company were to have access to all information, it may provide that company with an unfair advantage such as its ability to leverage that information for price negotiations.

10.7.3 Walmart and IBM using blockchain to address supply chain issues

Walmart has partnered with IBM to create a solution that utilizes the blockchain capabilities to address these supply chain friction points. By September 2019, Walmart's suppliers will be required to share updates for leafy green vegetables with the network so the supply chain audit trail for these products is transparent, immutable, and available in near real time [31]. Starting with leafy greens focuses on one of the most common recall targets (between 2010 and 2019, there have been nine *Escherichia coli* outbreaks in the United States caused by green lettuce or sprouts) and allows the group to learn with a limited scope prior to rolling these features out more broadly. Even though contamination is recognized as a serious issue, stakeholders in this process require additional incentive to adopt these technologies. Some farms have never experienced a recall and will need to invest in building new integration points between their systems and the supply chain. Walmart with its market power is uniquely positioned to require these stakeholders to implement these new integrations and reporting points into their process.

This solution seems straightforward; however, the details of governance, onboarding, maturity of the technology, and the concerns of supply chain participants represent potential barriers Walmart and IBM will need to overcome. The process to sort out the audit trail and inform a recall is projected to improve from 7 days to 2.2 s. These improvements are just the start of what the industry can expect as this solution evolves. IBM Food Trust is the branded name of this solution, and growers, processors, distributors, and retailers are able to utilize this product and realize the same benefits beyond the Walmart project (IBM). Food Trust product is looking to add value by improving supply efficiencies, food freshness, and sustainable sourcing. Transparency into the supply chain should allow for improved efficiencies and visibility into the freshness of the food which could be perceived as positive by the end-consumer.

10.7.4 Walmart initiative could be the first widespread non-cryptocurrency blockchain use case

An interesting by-product of this initiative may be improved public awareness of blockchain, and the capabilities offered to the public at large. A scalable production application in Walmart stores is arguably the most visible and understandable case for the technology and may represent a 'crossing the chasm' moment for blockchain. Bitcoin and blockchain are mainstream terms due to the hype of cryptocurrency speculation, but the true capabilities of the underlying technology are often misunderstood. Knowledge and hands-on experience with the Food Trust product could raise awareness for other use cases that spread well beyond the food supply chain.

10.8 Pharmaceutical supply chain management

10.8.1 What is the pharmaceutical supply chain?

The pharmaceutical supply chain is the system of manufacturers, wholesalers or distributors, and pharmacies that are required to deliver prescription medicines to patients [32]. Manufacturers are typically responsible both for the research and development and the downstream manufacturing and packaging of prescription drugs. Distributors transact with manufacturers to purchase drug products and then distribute them to pharmacies. Pharmacies purchase the product from distributors and sometimes from the manufacturers themselves and keep a local, physical inventory they can use to dispense to patients. There are different types of pharmacies, including traditional retail pharmacies, institutional (hospital or long-term care) facility-based pharmacies, and a growing number of mail-order pharmacies.

10.8.2 Issues with the pharmaceutical supply chain

About 2.5 per cent of all drugs traded globally are counterfeit [33]. Counterfeit drugs negatively impact both patient safety and the economics of the pharmaceutical industry.

There are vulnerabilities along the supply chain at all junctures, from manufacturing to distribution down to the pharmacy. These vulnerabilities can result in product theft as well as the introduction of counterfeit products. As a result, the United States enacted the DSCSA which imposed requirements on the pharmaceutical industry to establish, by 2023, traceability throughout the supply chain for all drug products sold in the United States. This includes 'chain of custody' of any product, unit-level product identifiers, and allowing downstream parties within the supply chain to trace the path of any product unit through all distribution or manufacturing nodes. Investments thus far have been made to focus on the serialization and traceability of drug product, including upstream manufacturer systems, modern packaging and palletizing technologies, and machine vision systems. Contractor packaging companies work within the supply chain and must also comply with new rules, resulting in costly investments in technology and process changes. Traditional software vendors such as IBM, Optel, and Antares are offering non-blockchain solutions to bring together data from supply chain participants.

10.8.3 How could blockchain be used to address these issues?

Internet of Things (IoT) and blockchain can be used in tandem to increase the traceability of product along the pharmaceutical supply chain [34]. IoT includes physical sensors and tags that help bridge the physical and digital worlds and would provide a secure linkage between physical assets and their digital representations on a blockchain. A blockchain-based solution would enable multiple writers, as every participant of the supply chain would need to record their transactions on the shared data infrastructure [35]. Blockchain could also address the lack of trust between participants, especially as the degrees of separation increase between downstream pharmacies and global suppliers within the pharmaceutical supply chain. With blockchain, supply chain management can be optimized by processing transactions without an intermediary. The updates are immutable which serves as a permanent record of change in 'chain of custody' of drug product and increases the reliability of audit data [34]. In addition to compliance to the DSCSA, many companies are exploring how similar approaches can be leveraged to address prescription drug abuse (opioid abuse) and to respond to drug recalls [35].

10.8.4 Early initiatives to leverage blockchain to address

The US Food and Drug Administration in February 2019 announced that it is launching pilot programmes to evaluate new technologies, including blockchain, to support the sharing of data and tracking of product between manufacturers, distributors, and pharmacies [36]. SAP announced its pharmaceutical supply chain solution built on an open blockchain and used to immutably store serial numbers for drug products [37]. MediLedger has a complementary solution that addresses organizational identity, certificates, and a directory of participants [38]. These explorations will demonstrate the possibilities of leveraging blockchain to address the growing compliance and transparency needs in the pharmaceutical supply chain.

10.8.5 Barriers to overcome to scale these solutions

The pharmaceutical supply chain use case seems to be a good fit for a blockchain-based approach, and the barriers will be common to most use cases. Getting a critical mass of pharmaceutical companies, distributors, and pharmacies aligned to participate will be a challenge; however, with consolidation in all three segments, there are relatively fewer to bring together than there were in the recent past. Establishing a robust governance framework to build and operate such utility will also be challenging and may require leveraging existing associations and alliances to incubate and provide structure to the effort. Advances in blockchain technology to ensure performant real-time transactions will also need to occur, as the pharmaceutical supply chain will not tolerate significant data-sharing lag times.

10.9 Patient identity and consent management

10.9.1 Administrative costs associated with patient identity

Understanding the identity of the patient associated with clinical or research data is a significant challenge in healthcare with both cost and privacy issues. Some estimate that the cost of patient-matching issues that result in duplicate records and repeated medical care amounts to an average of $1,950 per patient per inpatient stay and over $800 per emergency room visit [1]. Medical claims processes are also impacted with an estimated 33 per cent of all denied claims coming from inaccurate patient identification or incorrect information, resulting in $1.5M for the average hospital in 2017 and $6B for US healthcare per year [39].

10.9.2 Privacy issues related to patient identity

While patient matching is challenged in part due to the siloed nature of patient data, breaking through the silos may also begin to create vulnerabilities around a patient's privacy. The HIPAA Privacy Rule protects patient privacy, and such protections may necessitate an ability for the patient to manage how their information is shared. This affects an oft-proposed solution of simply establishing a universal patient identifier. If a universal patient identifier was implemented, and at some point, the registry of identifiers was exposed, then every dataset associated with that universal identifier is now potentially compromised because the patient associated with each data element is now known.

For example, a patient goes to the Day Clinic to treat a substance abuse issue, and the information about the visit is associated with patient identifier FN2187. Then that same patient goes to a City Pharmacy to purchase sinus medication, and that purchase is also associated with patient identifier FN2187. Should a malicious attacker obtain access to the City Pharmacy database and learn the name of the individual associated with identifier FN2187, that attacker could cross reference the Day Clinic data to identify the person who has visited the clinic to receive substance abuse treatment. As a result, most organizations operate their own siloed data source, using different identifiers and creating the patient-matching issue.

A related challenge is the consent to exchange and use patient data. Normally this type of consent is managed in a binary fashion: the company that obtains the consent can do either anything they want with the data or nothing at all. Collecting a signature for this consent is buried deep in the legal text of a clipboard-attached consent form, and few people read the text when checking in to receive treatment or enrolling in health insurance. Regulations are in place to ensure that companies use the data appropriately, but it is normally an all or nothing arrangement. Few people request data removed from databases since the United States does not have General Data Protection Regulation type regulations, and as such, the capabilities to remove data are lacking.

Revisiting the prior example, the patient could have the flexibility to manage consent around the substance abuse data differently than the sinus medication information and do so in a unified way across systems. As the regulatory environment changes in the United States and patients become more interested in stewarding their data, these capabilities will begin to emerge. With a rising number of healthcare-related breaches (15M patient records were exposed in 503 data breaches in 2018), interest and advocacy around patient privacy is increasing rapidly. Blockchain technologies provide an opportunity to add trust and transparency to both identity and consent management.

10.9.3 Blockchain solutions for patient identity issues

A blockchain-powered solution could serve a similar role to the library card catalo. Each healthcare transaction would store metadata on the blockchain, including a unique identifier for the transaction, a patient identifier for that transaction, and a pointer to where the data is stored off chain, managed, and protected by the system of record. Patients could manage their own keys for each transaction and could prove that these are associated with their identities. Once verified, the patients could then be granted access to the data held securely off-chain. Losing or deleting these keys would break the connection and could be done intentionally to remove data. Like a password reset, capabilities or protections would need to be in place to avoid doing this by accident. One way to help mitigate this risk would be for the patients to entrust a third party to store these keys, again like how password managers and key stores are used currently. Similar solutions have emerged around key management for cryptocurrency wallets, and those advancements could be leveraged for patient identity and consent management.

10.10 Electronic health record exchange

10.10.1 Current issues with medical record exchange

One persistent issue in healthcare is interoperability, and medical record exchange is ground zero for this problem. When patients receive care, they typically rely on a network of unaffiliated providers who are likely not using the same electronic health record (EHR) system. Issues emerge when the exchanges of medical records between providers within that care team are inhibited because of lack of interoperability between multiple systems. Lack of interoperability affects patient outcomes, adds to physician fatigue, and increases the cost of care.

The US federal government has taken efforts, including the HITECH Act, MACRA, and the 21st Century Cures Act, to promote EHR adoption and interoperability [40]. EHR adoption is up, with 96 per cent of hospitals and 80 per cent of provider practices having adopted and installed an EHR [41]. However, in 2015, only 12 per cent of physicians completed stage 2 of meaningful use, and only 6 per cent of healthcare providers could share medical record data with another provider using a different system [41]. Despite increased EHR adoption, data interoperability is still lacking and related issues persist.

10.10.2 Leveraging blockchain to solve medical record exchange issues

The persistent issues of EHR interoperability, combined with emerging issues of patient data security, make EHRs a likely target for blockchain entrepreneurs. Health records indeed have multiple, often unaffiliated writers, and verifiability and traceability are important. There is some evidence of lack of trust for a centralized authority as each institution, and the EHR vendors themselves desire to exert some control over medical record data. With respect to external data, many healthcare providers are distrusting of health records transmitted to them from external parties. Institutions charge fees of patients to obtain health records, and EHR vendors can charge tens of thousands of dollars to enable interoperability with third-party systems. Charging fees for health records and integration demonstrates that vendors and institutions are implicitly creating barriers to access data. Lack of trust, multiple writers, and the need for verifiability make blockchain a potential fit; however, there are open questions on the willingness of participants to collaborate and a resonance of a market-level business case.

Multiple solution concepts emerged around blockchain-based EHRs since 2016. The more modest concepts involve hashing an audit trail to an immutable ledger. Others aspire to introduce increased interoperability, clinical research recruitment, and patient-driven access control. The most ambitious strive to shift the centre of gravity of health records from institutions to the patient or individual, establishing what has remained elusive for decades: a universal, interconnected, usable, patient-managed personal health record.

10.10.3 Early start-up activity and proofs-of-concept

The earliest company to announce a solution for blockchain-based medical records was US-based Gem in partnership with Philips in 2016. However, 2 years later in 2018, the blockchain company quietly pivoted back to financial services [42]. Academic proofs-of-concept were also established, including MIT Media Lab's MedRec project which was piloted with Beth Israel Deaconess Medical Center in Boston, Massachusetts. Later start-ups in 2018 also announced notable partnerships: UK-based Medicalchain is working with Mayo Clinic [43], and

Korean-based Mediblock is working with Massachusetts General Hospital [44]. These pilot projects focused on supplementing a core EHR system with additional interoperability, audit, and patient engagement capabilities rather than entirely supplanting incumbent systems. As of the writing of this chapter, no leading EHR vendor has announced product efforts related to blockchain to solve for interoperability; however, some are conducting pilots around security and auditing.

10.10.4 Barriers to overcome to scale blockchain-based medical record solutions

While blockchain can help address these problems, there are long-standing issues that need to be addressed with the participation of incumbent players in the EHR space. Motivating vendors to embrace standards and establishing a governance structure that appeals to vendors are necessary for interoperability: blockchain or otherwise. Health Level 7, a standards organization that governs exchange of clinical data, introduced Fast Healthcare Interoperability Resources (FHIR) as a model for modern application programming interface interactions around clinical data in 2014, and it has seen steady adoption among EHR vendors seeking to expand interoperability. The US Health and Human Services Office of the National Coordinator, the federal office responsible for promoting health IT and interoperability, has recently expressed support for FHIR [45].

Universally adopted standards will be necessary for a blockchain health record platform. In terms of lack of incentives, industry coalitions such as Sequoia Project, CareQuality, and CommonWell are bringing major vendors to the table to create persistent linkages between competing solution vendors [46]. Blockchain disruptors will have to either completely disintermediate these alliances or seek to complement them in a non-competitive way. Finally, there is a sense among blockchain entrepreneurs that, at least in the early days, they should focus on solutions addressing non-sensitive data problems. Clinical data is the most sensitive, as it is governed by the HIPAA Privacy Rule, and new technologies such as blockchain are not attractive to conservative buyers such as hospitals and provider practices. Many organizations could opt to first test blockchain on less sensitive use cases.

10.11 Real-time claims adjudication

10.11.1 Costs and issues related to claims adjudication

In the United States, the primary financial mechanism used by a provider of healthcare services to obtain payment for care given to patient is a 'claim' to the health insurance company that covers the patient as part of a contracted plan. Legislation in the United States referred to as Affordable Care Act mandates all individuals who are protected by health insurance. Agreements between patient and insurance company, combined with the agreements between providers of healthcare and insurance companies, create unnecessary complexity and friction.

Healthcare spending in the United States is projected to reach $5.5 trillion by 2025 (Advisory Board), and administrative costs are estimated to account for 30 per cent of these costs [47]. A category of administrative costs referred to as BIR is estimated to account for over 60 per cent of the total administrative costs, with conservative estimates projecting $300B spent on BIR annually [3].

BIR activities include '*contracting with insurers and subcontracted providers; maintaining benefits databases; determining patient insurance and cost sharing; collecting copayments, formulary, and prior authorization; coding of services delivered; checking and submitting claims; receiving and depositing payments; appealing denials and underpayments; collecting from patients; negotiating end-of-year resolution of unsettled claims; and paying subcontracted providers*' [3]. Providers on average work with 12 or more insurance companies, which means that the provider must interact with multiple parties who have nuances and different interpretations of standards. Multiple interactions are often needed to be paid appropriately. All these interactions add incremental friction and cost to the healthcare system. There is also a significant shift in the US healthcare system to move away from 'fee for service' to more value-based, risk-sharing agreements, the latter being even more burdensome to manage. The additional burden comes from tracking on-going metrics to ensure that the services provided improve the health of the patient, incentivizing a total population health and wellness.

These complexities paired with the siloed nature of healthcare in the United States contribute to the challenges of understanding overall cost and how cost is broken down between patient and insurance company prior to services being performed. This means the vast majority of patients do not have a clear understanding of the costs incurred when healthcare services are rendered. These costs are calculated after care is provided, often taking weeks if not months to fully settle between the parties involved. Transactions are also audited by various regulatory agencies, which also occur well after the care episode. The delays in settling claims transactions could be streamlined if the industry were to collaborate on evolving current processes and platforms. Issues of ownership, governance, transparency, trust, and incentives are practical barriers that must be overcome.

10.11.2 Blockchain-based solutions for claims

A blockchain-powered utility solution could help address some of the existing challenges of ownership, trust, and transparency while also adding the incentive of removing costly intermediaries. For a medical claim to be adjudicated, there are two agreements that need to be understood and executed, one between the insurance company and provider, the other between patient and insurance company. If this logic was represented and accessible via 'smart contracts' on a shared blockchain utility, then the claim could be adjudicated in real time. A medical claim transaction normally navigates through multiple centralized silos prior to completion. An example flow may include the provider's practice management system, a third-party billing system, a clearinghouse contracted with the provider, a clearinghouse contracted with the health insurance company, and finally the health insurance company itself. Each jump incurs cost, adds complexity, and introduces another potential point of failure. The opportunity for a decentralized system is both the logic and data needed for this multi-company workflow can transition from the disparate silos to a shared blockchain. The logic can be executed without the hops between centralized system, and each of the parties needing to be involved can have transparency into the flow of the information. This utility would enable real-time adjudication and remove the need for intermediaries who are only engaged today in order to facilitate the transmission of information between systems. These capabilities would also enable solutions to equip the provider and patient with tools to more easily calculate the price and cost share prior to service. Auditing could also be improved as regulators would be able to monitor transactions in real time, spotting fraudulent and suspicious behaviour within minutes instead of months.

10.11.3 Anticipated barriers to establishing a blockchain-based claims solution

Improving medical claims is a significant challenge due to scale of incumbent claims processes, and the sheer amount of change that would need to occur to realize the aforementioned benefits. Blockchain technologies provide new capabilities; however, the challenges of governance and incentives will need to be overcome especially as it relates to incumbent organizations such as claims clearinghouses and health insurance companies. Due to the issue of rising healthcare cost in the United States and the need to efficiently manage complex contractual arrangements, there is motivation to collaborate and try new approaches. Privacy of patient data, confidentiality of these agreements, and the scalability of blockchain solutions are barriers to consider as healthcare organizations explore the adoption of decentralized technologies. Time will tell if a decentralized solution plays a key role in driving down administrative costs related to claims processing. Less complex areas of focus in healthcare, such as provider directories, will inform the approach and feasibility for more complex problem spaces such as medical claims.

10.12 Reducing of fraud, waste, and abuse in healthcare

10.12.1 Understanding fraud, waste, and abuse in healthcare

Fraud constitutes attempts to obtain money, property, or benefits from healthcare organizations through the means of misrepresenting identity, falsifying claims for payments, or other false pretences. Waste is the unnecessary utilization of healthcare-related resources. Abuse is the improper or excessive use of resources that can result in financial loss.

Fraud, waste, and abuse scenarios are diverse and can present themselves differently in various healthcare contexts. One example of fraud is when a medical practice submits two separate claims to a health plan for a single test and receives payment for both claims. Abuse was found by the US Department of Justice in a 2019 case charging 24 people, including 2 physicians, for a $1.2B Medicare telemarketing fraud scheme involving call centres targeting Medicare beneficiaries and influencing them to seek medically unnecessary braces [48]. Waste was demonstrated in the 2014 scandal within the Phoenix VA hospital where patients were waiting an average of 115 days to see a primary care physician during which as many as 40 veterans died [49]. Hospital staff then reported up to the agency-falsified logs to cover up the long wait times.

It is estimated that there are potential savings of up to $600B, if fraud, waste, and abuse are addressed at scale [50]. Some progress has been made: HHS Healthcare Fraud and Abuse Program in 2016 recaptured over $3.3B [51]. Between 2007 and 2019, the Medicare Fraud Task Force filed 1,600 cases against almost 3,500 defendants who were responsible for fraudulently billing Medicare for over $13B [52]. Commercial health plans have utilized a combination of human-driven audit efforts as well as efforts that incorporate AI and machine learning. Traditionally, human examiners would sift through mounds of claims and supporting data to manually detect patterns of fraud, waste, and abuse. Aetna, a national health insurance plan, has a special investigation unit that utilized machine learning algorithms to scale its ability to identify cases of overbilling, incorrect coding, and duplicate claims. These techniques had positive results but still represent just a small percentage of the opportunity.

10.12.2 How blockchain fits the fraud, waste, and abuse problem

The benefits of immutability and transparency a blockchain-structured decentralized database offers could help solve for many of the issues of fraud, waste, and abuse. One solution scenario involves multiple parties transacting on a tamper-proof blockchain that is tuned to detect instances of fraud, waste, and abuse [53]. Participants could transact with each other via the blockchain with the knowledge that data is tamper-proof, and transactional data can be scalably cross-referenced and monitored for fraud signatures [54]. Another example is the writing of VA wait time data onto an immutable ledger that would have increased the trustworthiness of the data and allowed the VA at the federal level to exercise more in-depth oversight of the wait time issue across all medical centres.

A blockchain-based platform could be combined with artificial intelligence and algorithms to scalably monitor for fraud among a stream of claims transactions. There are detectable signatures of probable fraud that have been used for years, and the availability and discoverability of data that blockchain affords could enhance the impact of these approaches.

10.13 Conclusion

There is an abundance of entrepreneurial activity occurring across all sectors of healthcare leveraging blockchain technologies to address a range of use cases.

Venture-backed start-ups, consortia, and academic research initiatives are all testing the feasibility, desirability, and viability of blockchain-powered solutions to compete for a share of the estimated $5.61B blockchain healthcare market in 2025 (BIS Research). The most promising use cases being targeted are those that fit specific criteria, primarily revolving around the lack of trust, and leverage blockchain's unique capabilities of immutability and decentralization.

Regulatory, economic incentive, governance, and technical barriers will need to be addressed to realize these benefits. While no initiative has yet reached scale and demonstrated sustainable returns to participants, a high degree of optimism around blockchain prevails. As the technology improves, investments increase, and the potential for critical mass in adoption also increases.

As with the Internet, it is hard to predict when growth becomes exponential for any particular use case; however, when it does, industry disruption quickly occurs and the market landscape shifts. The Internet enabled new ventures to overtake market leaders within just a decade. We see examples of this with NetFlix, AirBnB, Uber, Google, and Amazon. The new collaborative business models that blockchain may catalyse within healthcare could be equally as disruptive. Success of the early efforts described within this chapter will determine the degree and the timing around the impact of blockchain on healthcare in their respective use cases.

References

[1] Lunden I. Amazon's Share of the US e-Commerce Market is Now 49%, or 5% of All Retail Spend. TechCrunch; 2018. https://techcrunch.com/2018/07/13/amazons-share-of-the-us-e-commerce-market-is-now-49-or-5-of-all-retail-spend/ [Accessed 30 April 2019].

[2] Gordon C. A history of ATM Innovation. NCR; 2017. https://www.ncr.com/company/blogs/financial/history-atm-innovation [Accessed 30 April 2019].

[3] Institute of Medicine (US) Roundtable on Evidence-Based Medicine, Yong PL, Saunders RS, and Olsen LA, editors. The Healthcare Imperative: Lowering Costs and Improving Outcomes: Workshop Series Summary. National Center for Biotechnology Information; 2010. 25 7 2016, http://www.ncbi.nlm.nih.gov/books/NBK53942/.

[4] The Economist. The Trust Machine – The Promise of the Blockchain [online]. 2015. Available from https://www.economist.com/leaders/2015/10/31/the-trust-machine [Accessed 30 April 2019].

[5] Orcutt M. Venture Capitalists Are Still Throwing Hundreds of Millions at Blockchains [online]. MIT Technology Review; 2019. Available from https://www.technologyreview.com/s/613247/venture-capitalists-are-still-throwing-hundreds-of-millions-at-blockchains/ [Accessed 2 May 2019].

[6] McCauley A. The $100B Blockchain Proof Of Concept Hiding In Plain Sight [online]. Forbes; 2019. Available from https://www.forbes.com/sites/alisonmccauley/2019/01/09/the-100b-blockchain-proof-of-concept-hiding-in-plain-sight/#300b8ea71c8a [Accessed 2 May 2019].

[7] Kalathil M. Blockchain and Healthcare [online]. Washington, DC: Topsights; 2019. Available from https://topsights.tech/2018/07/20/blockchain-and-healthcare/ [Accessed 2 May 2019].
[8] Greenspan G. Do You Really Need a Blockchain for That? [online]. Coin Center; 2017. Available from https://coincenter.org/entry/do-you-really-need-a-blockchain-for-that [Accessed 2 May 2019].
[9] Social Security Administration. The Social Security Number Verification Service [online]. Social Security Administration. Available from: https://www.ssa.gov/employer/ssnv.htm [Accessed 2 May 2019].
[10] Centers for Medicare and Medicaid Services. NPPES NPI Registry [online]. Centers for Medicare and Medicaid Services. Available from https://npiregistry.cms.hhs.gov/ [Accessed 2 May 2019].
[11] ShortWhiteCoats.com. A Map of all Medical Schools in the United States [online]. ShortWhiteCoats.com. Available from: http://shortwhitecoats.com/2015/a-map-of-all-medical-schools-in-the-united-states [Accessed 2 May 2019].
[12] Meunier S. When Do You Need a Blockchain? Decision Models [online]. Medium; 2016. Available from https://medium.com/@sbmeunier/when-do-you-need-blockchain-decision-models-a5c40e7c9ba1 [Accessed 2 May 2019].
[13] Moukheiber Z. How Surescripts Became the Dominant Electronic Prescribing Network [online]. Forbes; 2014. Available from https://www.forbes.com/sites/zinamoukheiber/2014/04/22/how-surescripts-became-the-dominant-electronic-prescribing-network/#232369015aa0 [Accessed 2 May 2019].
[14] TradeLens [online]. TradeLens. Available from https://www.tradelens.com/ [Accessed 2 May 2019].
[15] Allison I. IBM and Maersk Struggle to Sign Partners to Shipping Blockchain [online]. CoinDesk; 2018. Available from https://www.coindesk.com/ibm-blockchain-maersk-shipping-struggling [Accessed 2 May 2019].
[16] Stanley A. Ready To Rumble: IBM Launches Food Trust Blockchain for Commercial Use [online]. Forbes; 2018. Available from https://www.forbes.com/sites/astanley/2018/10/08/ready-to-rumble-ibm-launches-food-trust-blockchain-for-commercial-use/#284f35617439 [Accessed 2 May 2019].
[17] Healthcare – Hyperledger [online]. Hyperledger. Available from https://www.hyperledger.org/resources/industries/healthcare [Accessed 2 May 2019].
[18] Hashed Health. Professional Credentials Exchange [online]. Hashed Health. Available from https://hashedhealth.com/blockchain-healthcare-solutions/professional-credentials-exchange/ [Accessed 2 May 2019].
[19] Greenspan G. Avoiding the Pointless Blockchain Project [online]. MultiChain; 2015. Available from https://www.multichain.com/blog/2015/11/avoiding-pointless-blockchain-project/ [Accessed 2 May 2019].
[20] Wust K and Gervais A. Do You Need a Blockchain? International Association of Cryptologic Research; 2018.

[21] Health IT. MACRA. Health IT.gov; 2019. https://www.healthit.gov/topic/meaningful-use-and-macra/macra [Accessed 30 April 2019].

[22] Graham J. Health Data "Interoperability": A $30 Billion Unicorn Hunt. Forbes; 2014. https://www.forbes.com/sites/theapothecary/2014/09/03/health-data-interoperability-a-30-billion-unicorn-hunt/#137725ea5a9b' [Accessed 30 April 2019].

[23] Centers for Medicare & Medicaid Services (CMS). Online Provider Directory Review Report; 2017. From cms.gov: https://www.cms.gov/Medicare/Health-Plans/ManagedCareMarketing/Downloads/Provider_Directory_Review_Industry_Report_Final_01-13-17.pdf [Retrieved 26 February 2018].

[24] CAQH. CAQH White Paper Calls for Industry Collaboration to Solve Provider Data Challenges; 2016. From https://www.caqh.org/about/press-release/caqh-white-paper-calls-industry-collaboration-solveprovider-data-challenges [Retrieved 26 February 2018].

[25] Customer Story FSMB [online]. Learning Machine. Available from https://www.learningmachine.com/customer-story-fsmb/ [Accessed 2 May 2019].

[26] Metcalf D, Bass J, Hooper M, Cahana A, and Dhilon V. Blockchain in Healthcare: Innovations That Empower Patients, Connect Professionals and Improve care. New York: CRC Press; 2019. p. 78.

[27] Grech A and Camilleri A. Blockchain in Education [online]. European Commission; 2017. Available from http://publications.jrc.ec.europa.eu/repository/bitstream/JRC108255/jrc108255_blockchain_in_education%281%29.pdf [Accessed 22 Nov 2020].

[28] Begando A. (2019 April). Phone interview with author.

[29] Bolger A. (2019 April). Phone interview with author.

[30] Kelly R. Learning Machine Update Brings Together Blockcerts and Open Badges [online]. Campus Technology; 2019. Available from https://campustechnology.com/articles/2019/01/03/learning-machine-update-brings-together-blockcerts-and-open-badges.aspx [Accessed 22 Nov 2020].

[31] Miller R. Walmart is Betting on the Blockchain to Improve Food Safety. Tech Crunch; 2018. https://techcrunch.com/2018/09/24/walmart-is-betting-on-the-blockchain-to-improve-food-safety/ [Accessed 30 April 2019].

[32] Avalere. The Kaiser Family Foundation. Follow the Pill: Understanding the U.S. Commercial Pharmaceutical Supply Chain [online]. Avalere; 2005. Available from https://avalere.com/research/docs/Follow_the_Pill.pdf [Accessed 22 Nov 2020].

[33] OECD. Global Trade in Fake Goods Worth Nearly Half a Trillion Dollars a Year [online]. OECD; 2016. Available from https://www.oecd.org/industry/global-trade-in-fake-goods-worth-nearly-half-a-trillion-dollars-a-year.htm [Accessed 2 May 2019].

[34] Deloitte. Continuous Interconnected Supply Chain Blockchain & Internet-of-Things in Supply Chain Traceability [online]. Deloitte; 2017. Available from https://www2.deloitte.com/content/dam/Deloitte/lu/Documents/technology/lu-WP-Supply-Chain-Blockchain-18102017.PDF [Accessed 2 May 2019].

[35] Clauson K. Leveraging Blockchain Technology to Enhance Supply Chain Management in Healthcare: An Exploration of Challenges and Opportunities in the Health Supply Chain [online]. Blockchain in Healthcare Today; 2018. Available from https://blockchainhealthcaretoday.com/index.php/journal/article/view/20/7 [Accessed 2 May 2019].

[36] Ledger Insights. FDA to Run Pharma Blockchain Pilots [online]. Ledger Insights; 2019. Available from https://www.ledgerinsights.com/fda-dscsa-pharma-blockchain/ [Accessed 2 May 2019].

[37] Ledger Insights. SAP's Pharmaceutical Blockchain Goes Live [online]. Ledger Insights; 2019. Available from https://www.ledgerinsights.com/saps-pharmaceutical-blockchain-goes-live/ [Accessed 2 May 2019].

[38] Ledger Insights. MediLedger: Pharmaceutical Industry's Blockchain Network [online]. Ledger Insights; 2019. Available from https://www.ledgerinsights.com/mediledger-pharmaceutical-blockchain/ [Accessed 2 May 2019].

[39] Security Magazine. Inaccurate Patient IDs Cost Hospitals $1.5M a Year. Security Solutions for Enabling and Assuring Business; 2018. https://www.securitymagazine.com/articles/88999-inaccurate-patient-ids-cost-hospitals-15m-a-year [Accessed 30 April 2019].

[40] ONC. The Office of the National Coordinator of Health Information Technology. Connecting Health and Care for the Nation a Shared Nationwide Interoperability Roadmap. ONC; 2015. Available from https://www.healthit.gov/sites/default/files/nationwide-interoperability-roadmap-draft-version-1.0.pdf [Accessed 2 May 2019].

[41] Reisman M. EHRs: The Challenge of Making Electronic Data Usable and Interoperable. *P T*. 2017;42(9):572–575. PubMed PMID: 28890644; PubMed Central PMCID: PMC5565131.

[42] Bukstel E. Why Are So Many Companies Exiting the Healthcare Blockchain Market? Medium; 2018. Available from https://medium.com/@Connected_Dots/why-are-so-many-companies-exiting-the-healthcare-blockchain-market-43cddbea4431 [Accessed 2 May 2019].

[43] Miliard M. Mayo Clinic Exploring Blockchain EHR Use Cases With UK Startup. Healthcare IT News; 2018. Available from https://www.healthcareitnews.com/news/mayo-clinic-exploring-blockchain-ehr-use-cases-uk-startup [Accessed 2 May 2019].

[44] Miliard M. Massachusetts General Hospital Piloting Blockchain Projects With Korean Startup. Healthcare IT News; 2018. Available from https://www.healthcareitnews.com/news/massachusetts-general-hospital-piloting-blockchain-projects-korean-startup [Accessed 2 May 2019].

[45] Posnack S. Heat Wave: The U.S. is Poised to Catch FHIR in 2019. Health IT Buzz; 2018. Available from https://www.healthit.gov/buzz-blog/interoperability/heat-wave-the-u-s-is-poised-to-catch-fhir-in-2019 [Accessed 2 May 2019].

[46] Dubovitskaya A, Xu Z, Ryu S, Schumacher M, and Wang F. Secure and Trustable Electronic Medical Records Sharing using Blockchain. *AMIA*

Annu Symp Proc. 2018;2017:650–659. PubMed PMID: 29854130; PubMed Central PMCID: PMC5977675.

[47] Tseng P, Kaplan RS, Barak D, Richman JD. Administrative Costs Associated With Physician Billing and Insurance-Related Activities at an Academic Health Care System. JAMA Network; 2018. https://jamanetwork.com/journals/jama/fullarticle/2673148 [Accessed 30 April 2019].

[48] Ellison A. Feds Charge 24 in $1.2B Telemedicine Fraud Scheme [online]. Becker's Hospital Review; 2019. Available from https://www.beckershospitalreview.com/legal-regulatory-issues/feds-charge-24-in-1-2b-telemedicine-fraud-scheme.html [Accessed 2 May 2019].

[49] Lopez G. The VA Scandal of 2014, Explained [online]. Vox; 2015. Available from https://www.vox.com/2014/9/26/18080592/va-scandal-explained [Accessed 2 May 2019].

[50] Sahni N, Chigurupati A, Kocher B, and Cutler D. How the U.S. Can Reduce Waste in Health Care Spending by $1 Trillion [online]. Harvard Business Review; 2015. Available from https://hbr.org/2015/10/how-the-u-s-can-reduce-waste-in-health-care-spending-by-1-trillion [Accessed 2 May 2019].

[51] US Department of Health and Human Services. Health and Human Services and the Department of Justice Return $2.6 Billion in Taxpayer Savings from Efforts to Fight Healthcare Fraud [online]. US Department of Health and Human Services. Available from https://www.hhs.gov/about/news/2018/04/06/hhs-and-department-justice-return-26-billion-taxpayer-savings-efforts-fight-healthcare-fraud.html [Accessed 2 May 2019].

[52] Nexmax. Scammers May Be Using DNA Testing to Defraud Medicare, Steal Identities [online]. Nexmax; 2019. Available from https://www.newsmax.com/finance/streettalk/scam-dna-tests-health/2019/04/17/id/912165/ [Accessed 2 May 2019].

[53] Matthews K. How Blockchain Technology Could Help Prevent Medical Fraud [online]. HIT Consultant; 2018. Available from https://hitconsultant.net/2018/07/10/blockchain-technology-medical-fraud/#.XMuysI5KiUm [Accessed 2 May 2019].

[54] ICO Spotters. 3 Ways Blockchain Technology Is Helping To Combat Healthcare Fraud [online]. ICO Spotters; 2018. Available from https://icospotters.com/blog/how-blockchain-technology-is-helping-to-combat-healthcare-fraud [Accessed 2 May 2019].

Further Reading

[55] Centers for Medicare & Medicaid Services (CMS). Online Provider Directory Review Report; 2018. From cms.gov: Centers for Medicare & Medicaid Services [Retrieved 26 February 2018].

[56] Benson E. The Challenge of Big Data and the Solution of Patient Matching. Healthcare innovation; 2018. https://www.hcinnovationgroup.com/

analytics-ai/article/13011311/the-challenge-of-big-data-and-the-solution-of-patient-matching [Accessed 30 April 2019].

[57] Advisory Board. CMS: US Health Care Spending to Reach Nearly 20% of GDP by 2025. Advisory Board; 2018. https://www.advisory.com/daily-briefing/2017/02/16/spending-growth [Accessed 30 April 2019].

[58] Beal A and Culver K. Crowdsourcing Healthcare Provider Directory Maintenance. EY; 2016. http://www.ey.com/humana [Accessed 30 April 2019].

[59] IBM. Food Trust. IBM; 2018. https://www.ibm.com/blockchain/solutions/food-trust [Accessed 30 April 2019].

[60] Viggiano L. Bitcoin and Blockchain. Bitcoin Aeon Bits. https://bitcoin.aeonbits.org/ [Accessed 30 April 2019].

[61] Federation of State Medical Boards (US). US Medical Regulatory Trends and Actions [online]. Federation of State Medical Boards; 2018. Available from https://www.fsmb.org/siteassets/advocacy/publications/us-medical-regulatory-trends-actions.pdf [Accessed 2 May 2019].

[62] Gordon WJ and Catalini C. Blockchain Technology for Healthcare: Facilitating the Transition to Patient-Driven Interoperability. *Comput Struct Biotechnol J*. 2018;16:224–230. doi: 10.1016/j.csbj.2018.06.003. PubMed PMID: 30069284; PubMed Central PMCID: PMC6068317.

[63] BIS Research. Global Blockchain in Healthcare Market: Focus on Industry Analysis and Opportunity Matrix – Analysis and Forecast, 2018-2025.

Chapter 11

A practical introduction to artificial intelligence in medicine

Kevin T. Lyman[1]

Prologue

Dr. Anthony Upton: "*The pulmonary parenchyma is unremarkable. There is no pulmonary nodule or mass, or area of consolidation. The pleural recesses are clear. Mediastinal viscera appear normal. Extensive lymph node enlargement is present within both axillae. The largest—*"

Anthony stops mid-sentence as an administrator knocks on the door and places a sheet of paper on his desk to the right of his keyboard. Without missing a beat, he gently slides his finger off of his dictation device, glances over at the paper, signs it, and returns to his study. The administrator leaves with the sheet. The entire interaction lasts under 5 s.

Dr. Anthony Upton: "*—on the right measures 4 x 2.5cm and on the left 2.8 x 1.9cm. Enlarged lymph nodes seen throughout the mediastinum, particularly in subcarinal space, prevascular and aortopulmonary windows. Enlarged posterior mediastinal node and epicardiac nodes also noted. The spleen is moderately enlarged, its—*"

Anthony stops mid-sentence as a brief but loud buzz can be heard. An intercom turns on as a voice asks him to provide a quick triage. Again, without missing a beat, Anthony stops his dictation, but this time glances up. Large screens toward the ceiling begin to display multiple series of a brain MRI quickly changing as a technologist remotely scrolls through each slice. Anthony says, "all good" and returns to his report as the voice on the intercom thanks him. The entire interaction lasts about 10 s.

Dr. Anthony Upton: "*—craniocaudal span is 18cm. Liver size and density are normal. Extensive lymph node enlargement seen throughout the mesentery, and retroperitoneum and within the pelvis and inguinal regions. This forms conglomerate lymph node masses in the upper abdomen—*"

[1]Enlitic, Inc., San Francisco, CA, USA

Anthony stops mid-sentence as the phone rings, and he places it on speaker. A referring physician asks Anthony's thoughts on a patient referred to his site a few days earlier. He immediately begins to describe the relationship between the patient's symptoms and their clinical findings with such clarity as if he can still see the entire study and his report in his mind. The two agree on a follow-up path for the patient and Anthony returns to his current report. The entire phone call lasts under 2 min.

Dr. Anthony Upton: "*—and appears to mildly obstruct the bile ducts. The kidneys, adrenals, and pancreas appear normal. There is no intra-abdominal mass or free fluid. There is no focal osseous destructive lesion. Extensive lymph node enlargement seen—*"

Anthony stops mid-sentence as the administrator returns, this time asking him to administer a contrast injection for a patient about to be scanned. He gets up and leaves the room, returning roughly 3 min later.

Dr. Anthony Upton: "*—throughout all lymph node stations in the neck and supraclavicular region. The pharyngeal mucosa, oral cavity structures, and larynx are normal. Low density lesion in the right thyroid lobe measures 1.5 cm and most likely represents a colloid nodule but can be further assessed—*"

Anthony stops mid-sentence as another radiologist, the only other one onsite today, briefly stops dictating her own report to ask Anthony for a second opinion. He quickly rolls his chair 6 ft over to her, glances at the study, and corroborates her findings. Within a minute, he is back at his desk continuing his own report.

Dr. Anthony Upton: "*—with ultrasound if clinically indicated. Large lymph node seen in the parotid glands bilaterally. Final Comment: Extensive lymph node enlargement from neck to pelvis in all lymph node groups is most compatible with stage 4 lymphoma. Splenomegaly. Ultrasound guided core biopsy of an inguinal or axillary node recommended for diagnosis. Specialist review recommended.*"

With that, Anthony finally finishes dictating his report. With a sense of accomplishment, he triumphantly returns to his work list and checks off on this study. His hopeful demeanor quickly shifts as the enormity of today's case load hits him. He takes a deep breath and jumps into the next one—number 17 of 300—all of which must be completed today.

****

The previous description is a recount of my first visit to a radiology clinic in November of 2015. I was a Forward Deployed Engineer recently hired by Enlitic, a San Francisco based start-up developing clinical applications of artificial intelligence (AI) for radiology. It was my job to shadow Anthony and other clinicians working for partners with the goal of understanding their workflow and thought processes well enough to help build them meaningful tools on the fly.

It was an eye-opening experience revealing the incredibly challenging nature of radiology—a field where one is expected to look at any part of the human body from any angle in two, three, or even four dimensions, using images constructed with fundamentally diverse physical modalities, and is on the hook to simultaneously identify potentially thousands of findings, even those which have never been seen before or are subvisual to the human eye. Despite the incredible burden they carry, we expect them to read more and more in less and less time as caseloads increase while government reimbursement rates drop. At the same time, we expect them to be infallible, despite multiple interruptions in a single report. These incredibly unrealistic expectations make imperative the true need for AI, not just in radiology, but in all of medicine.

In the 4 years since, I have had the good fortune of spending more than 2,000 h shadowing and interviewing radiologists across nearly 20 countries around the world. Today, Anthony is now Enlitic's Chief Medical Officer and I am the CEO. We have worked together every day since to bridge the gap between engineer and clinician, as we aim to change the world of diagnostics using AI to give clinicians the support they truly need.

In this brief chapter, I hope to provide further perspective on the inner workings of medical AI and the many technical, clinical, regulatory, design, market, and acceptance-related challenges that stand between research papers and clinical practice.

11.1 Why does medicine need AI and why are radiologists leading the forefront?

Nearly half a billion people will get an ultrasound, X-ray, CT, or MRI in 2020 alone [1]. Unfortunately, roughly one in five will be misdiagnosed, meaning they might receive treatment they do not even need. One in four will have their diagnosis missed all together, meaning they might never receive treatment they desperately need [2]. Perhaps even more alarming is nearly 5 billion people will lack access to these diagnostic studies altogether [3]. AI, while still in its nascency, potentially offers a means of alleviating these massive challenges among countless others in healthcare—in everything from augmenting and extending the performance of diagnosticians, to facilitating the faster and more effective development of drugs and other therapeutics, to even autonomously driving ambulances in times of emergency.

While AI will undoubtedly impact every aspect of care over time, early applications have disproportionately focused within the space of radiology for several practical reasons. Radiologists tend to be among the most forward-thinking clinicians, adopting technology long before their peers, which should stand to reason as their profession is fundamentally predicated on the existence and advancement of technology—without Wilhelm Röntgen's discovery of X-rays in 1895, radiology may not even exist [4]. That trend has persisted, with radiologists being among the first clinicians to adopt a primarily software-based workflow nearly 100 years later in the 1980s [5]. More so than simply being suggestive of a receptive mindset, these software-based workflows give AI an easier point of integration and additionally imply the potential existence of more than 30 years of already-digitized data. Importantly, radiology has become a central hub in modern diagnostics, providing a strong vertical for AI to start in with clear line of sight to additional verticals both upstream and downstream, such as cardiology, pathology, oncology, and genomics.

While primitive computer-aided diagnostic tools have been in use in radiology since the first FDA-approval of such a device in 1998, the mass-interest from radiology toward AI did not begin to pick up momentum until the mid-2010s [6]. In under a decade since, the general zeitgeist within the radiology community has shifted from fear of job loss to recognized need for useful tools to help keep up with ever-growing demands. As technology companies have dived deeper into the extreme nuances of radiology, and radiologists have been further ingrained into the world of software development, both sides have come to see that AI will enable today's critical shortage of human radiologists to serve the two-thirds of the planet currently lacking access long before it poses any substantiated risk to job security. It is unlikely AI will eliminate radiologists any time in the foreseeable future, but it is almost a certainty that it will redefine their role in diagnostics in ways that, if anything, has sparked new excitement for the field; perhaps most telling of this is that 100% of US diagnostic radiology residency positions that were filled in 2018, up from only 88% in 2014 [7].

11.2 Basics of artificial intelligence

AI is a general term referencing an entire toolbox of algorithms and methodologies that can be used to simulate intelligence. It could be argued that a simple database is a form of AI as it enables software to store information in a way that can be accessed to answer basic questions. Colloquially, when referring to AI, most people are specifically referring to machine learning (ML), a field of research into algorithms that enable software to learn and identify patterns within data.

ML, represented in Figure 11.1 as a subset of AI, is incredibly powerful, but conceptually quite simple. Given a sufficient number of completed examples of a sufficiently simple problem, a basic ML algorithm will ideally learn how to go

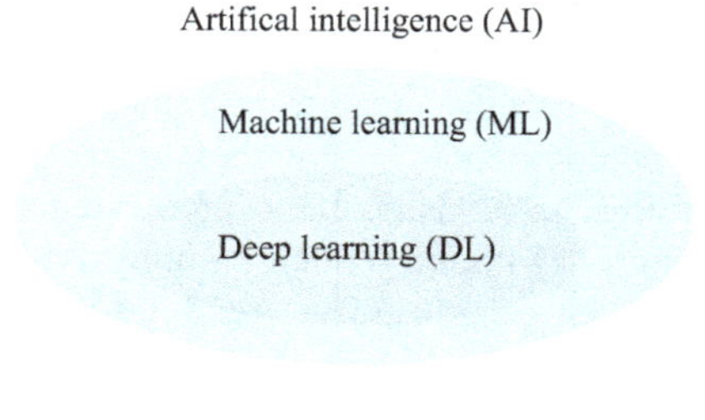

Figure 11.1 Hierarchical representation of AI buzzwords

from input to output with a reasonably high accuracy. When one knows enough about the problem at hand to clearly define what the algorithm needs to learn, this can be a very straightforward process.

One helpful example in understanding the basic workings of ML is the determination of a credit score. Most adults in the United States are assigned a number, or credit score, which can be used as a proxy for their credit worthiness. A credit score is typically between 300 and 850 and is determined by private credit bureaus using dozens of personal factors known about each individual with a credit history. Some of these factors include the number of credit lines one currently has open, the average age of their credit, and the average percentage of their available limits typically utilized. While each bureau calculates credit scores differently, with enough data and some assumptions, ML can likely be used to determine the underlying methodology.

Let us say, for example, one has access to the information in Table 11.1. The table contains each of the aforementioned factors, among many others, for a population of 1,000,000 individuals whose credit scores are known. This type of problem can be modeled as a basic series of linear equations in the form $[a_1x_1+a_2x_2+a_3x_3 = z]$, where z is the credit score, and open credit lines, average age of credit, and credit utilization are x_1, x_2, and x_3, respectively. The data in Table 11.1 can then be split randomly into three smaller datasets—70% will be used for training, 20% for testing, and 10% for validation.

A basic ML algorithm can then solve for the unknown coefficients through the process of training. During the training phase, the algorithm observes each known value of z in the training set in relation to each corresponding value of x_1, x_2, and x_3 to attempt to identify patterns suggestive of the target values for a_1, a_2, and a_3. After doing so, the algorithm then tests what it learned by attempting to solve z, for example, in the validation set. The algorithm compares its prediction for each example against the known answer and uses the difference to update its assumptions and to revisit the training set. This process is repeated until one is happy with the performance of the algorithm, at which point the training process is ended. Performance is measured one last time, this time using the test set, which is withheld from the model entirely during training to ensure an unbiased benchmark.

Table 11.1 Hypothetical example of a set of credit scores and underlying factors

ID	Credit score	Open lines	Average credit age (month)	Credit utilization (%)	...
1	750	11	88	2	...
2	620	5	60	15	...
3	800	12	120	1	...
...	...	...	...	...	...
1,000,000	510	3	18	30	...

In this simplified example,

- z is referred to as the *target output*, or the signal sought for in the noise;
- x_1, x_2, and x_3 are referred to as *features*, or the input information known to have relevance in solving for the target output;
- a_1, a_2, and a_3 are referred to as *weights*, or the amount of importance an algorithm is to place on each feature to solve for the target output.

The weights in this example are also the *learned parameters*, or the values the algorithm is trying to determine at the time of training. Once the weights are properly learned, the algorithm no longer needs to be trained. These weights can then be plugged back into the formula from which the model was built to solve for the target output in the future when only the features are known. In this example, once the weights are learned, a credit score could theoretically be calculated using only someone's number of open credit lines, the average age of their credit, and their average percentage utilization of credit.

While a naïve algorithm could also be used to solve this simplified example by randomly trying every possible combination of weights until the highest score is achieved on the validation or test set, ML algorithms tend to be much more efficient. The training process provides a closed feedback loop wherein the algorithm can essentially "search" for the right weights by monitoring the relationship between its guesses and the known answers. This efficiency might only bring marginal benefit in a basic example but has a far more substantial impact in complex problems with thousands of features, where an ML algorithm can determine in hours what may potentially take a brute force methodology thousands of years.

Some of the most interesting problems recently targeted with modern ML approaches are those with unstructured inputs where relationships to the target output are not well understood or easily expressed with a mathematical model. Consider a simple task in image interpretation such as the differentiation between pictures of cats and dogs—in this example, the expected input is an image and the target output is one of two categories. From a modeling standpoint, this is a similar problem to the previous example, but with some core differences that hugely impact the viability of traditional ML methodologies.

Unlike the credit score example where only three inputs are expected and all are known to be features with relevance in calculating the target output, the image classification example expects n inputs where n is the number of pixels in the input image. While most people could easily and reliably differentiate pictures of cats and dogs manually, very few would be able to define the math performed by their brain in making such a determination. For these sufficiently challenging problems, deep learning (DL) has become the go-to solution of choice.

DL is a form of ML largely centered around the use of artificial neural networks (ANNs), algorithms inspired by biological neural networks to efficiently learn from examples given unstructured inputs and no task-specific rules. While traditional ML methodologies are useful for identifying weights when the features are known, DL methodologies are useful for identifying both weights and features when neither are known. One can craft deep neural networks (DNNs) by stringing together several *layers* of ANNs.

DNNs are incredibly powerful algorithms, which learn by analyzing the input data hierarchically. Early layers look for features in the form of small patterns within the input data, and subsequent layers look for features in the form of patterns. In the cat/dog classification example, early layers would look for basic edges defined by adjacent pixels of different colors, subsequent layers would look for basic objects defined by those edges, and later layers would look for complex patterns defined by those objects.

DNN architectures developed for a given task tend to translate well with minimal effort to analogous tasks—a DNN developed to learn to classify cats from dogs could likely learn to classify different species of plants just as well with an appropriate training set. Most DL models developed for image interpretation use a form of DNN called a convolutional neural network and most DL models developed for sequence interpretation use a form of DNN called a recurrent neural network. The highly repurpose-able nature of DL-based architectures has enabled the research community to make massive strides in a short period of time through the shared reuse of models for different areas of application.

11.3 Problem identification

One of the many barriers to clinical adoption of AI is the nebulous and non-transparent nature of DL models—the math regarding how they learn is well understood, but the learned weights that enable future inferences do not explain well the resulting transformation in an intelligible way. While the "black box" nature of thinking this induces can often be received uncomfortably by the medical community, it forces a much simpler and more practical mental model that focuses on empirical evidence regarding the relationship between inputs and outputs. That is to say, *explaining the math is not nearly as important as proving that it works*. This is not too dissimilar from how one would train a medical student—performance is assessed by observing test results, not by issuing an FMRI (Functional Magnetic Resonance Imaging) and observing the pattern of their neurons firing as they answer a question.

While Figure 11.2 may be an oversimplification of the technical workings of a DL model, conceptually it appropriately describes the intended effect of using one as simply determining Y when given X. In the previous example, X is an image, and

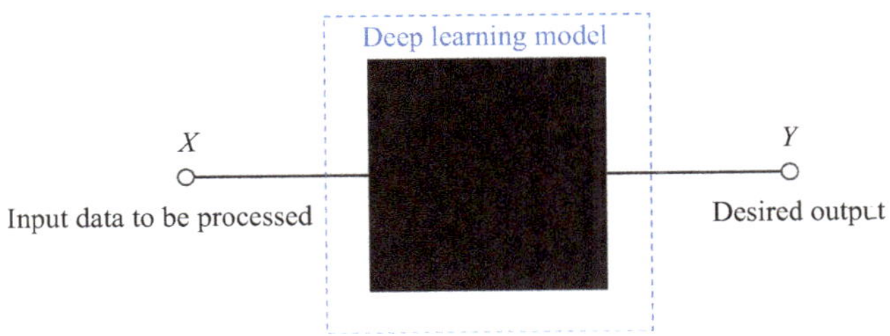

Figure 11.2 Blackbox representation of a deep learning model

Y is either "cat" or "dog." This simplification enables one to take a step back from the complex inner workings of ML/DL and properly recognize the algorithm alone is only a small piece of the puzzle. Understanding the context or system surrounding the algorithm is arguably more important than understanding the algorithm itself. This is especially true in healthcare, where most meaningful problems are incredibly nuanced and challenging for a multitude of factors.

The first step in building any AI-based application should be an assessment of the technical feasibility—*can* it even be built? Though this can be incredibly challenging to ascertain early on, there are several simple guidelines that can make the determination considerably easier. For example, the perceived complexity of a given task by a human expert can be a helpful benchmark in assuming how well an algorithm will fare in learning to do the same. As a general rule of thumb, if an expert takes only a second or fewer to determine *Y* given *X*, modern algorithms will likely be able to learn the underlying pattern reasonably well. While this means most complex problems in medicine will probably need to be broken down into a series of smaller problems, some are digestible enough to take a more naïve approach from the start. Generating an entire diagnostic radiology report from a chest X-ray may take a matter of minutes and should be seen as a complex series of smaller decisions. Most experienced radiologists, however, tend to be able to determine if an X-ray is normal or abnormal instantly upon seeing the image—unsurprisingly, DL algorithms trained to do the same have been shown to be highly performant.

Perhaps the most critical consideration in training an algorithm to go from *X* to *Y* is the consideration as to whether it is even possible to determine *Y* given only *X* under typical constraints. Chest X-rays are widely used around the world as a tool for screening—they are incredibly sensitive, meaning they contain a great deal of signal regarding a wide variety of useful clinical findings but at the same time are incredibly nonspecific, meaning they rarely contain enough information to make a decision in isolation. Tuberculosis (TB) is one of the most important diseases for which the chest X-ray is used to screen, but it is critical to keep in mind that chest X-rays are not a clinically accepted means of diagnosing TB. A radiologist interpreting a chest X-ray might confidently detect visual signs of calcified lung nodules, fluid buildup in the form of pleural effusions or consolidation, or chest deformities such as cavitation—while these signs point to TB, they also point to countless other diagnoses, and a cell-culture test would be administered to confirm. For this reason, asking DL to diagnose TB given nothing but a chest X-ray might be asking it to learn from incomplete information. Patients can have nearly every sign of TB in their chest X-ray imaginable, but unless they are coughing after a trip to a country with some prevalence of TB, the chances are slim-to-none that they themselves have it—either way, it is hard to say without access to the clinical history in addition to the X-ray.

One last critical consideration in assessing technical feasibility is, of course, whether or not one has access to a sufficient amount of representative data. There are hundreds, if not thousands, of diseases and other clinical indications that can be presented in some visual form in a chest X-ray. Further, these findings can be presented in a multitude of combinations and anatomic positions. This massive variability in visual appearances and outcomes means a fairly sizable amount of data would likely be required to learn the desired pattern in a reliable way.

Cardiomegaly, or an enlarged heart, for example, is one of the most important findings notable from a chest X-ray. It is typically indicated by measuring the cardiothoracic ratio (CTR), or the ratio of the width of the cardiac shadow over the width of the surrounding chest wall. If the CTR is 0.5 or greater, a radiologist will usually note this as enlargement of the cardiac silhouette. Existing research has shown that DL algorithms can note this finding with expert-level accuracy given thousands of training examples; but even the state-of-the-art is likely to be confounded by examples with complex circumstances, which were not sufficiently represented in the training data [8]. Congestive heart failure, which is often represented by cardiac enlargement alongside other findings, might confuse the algorithm if it has never before seen consolidation or a pacemaker. In a simpler example, dextrocardia, or an otherwise harmless anatomic variation that causes the heart to appear on the right rather than the left, might totally break the algorithm's worldview of what anatomy should even look like without having seen it.

The next step in building any AI-based application should be an assessment of the commercial feasibility—*should* it even be built? Given the nascency of both AI and the field of clinical data science, most reasonable problems are arguably worthwhile from a research perspective in the same way that space exploration is—even if there is only one person who wants to live on Mars right now. Figuring out how to make it happen today will likely result in countless scientific innovations that improve other more immediately impactful endeavors. That said, one needs to apply a much more scrutinizing lens when targeting commercial applications.

Though many prominent figureheads in AI have suggested in the past 5 years that AI will replace radiologists, most have since walked back those comments in recognition that neither the technology nor the world is ready for such a reality for a very long time. Until that time comes, if ever, no clinical executive with a checkbook cares if an algorithm reaches 99.99% accuracy on a cherry-picked dataset in a closed environment—they care if their radiologists are faster and more accurate when working alongside the algorithm, than when they are not. For that reason, any successful AI application in healthcare needs to start with an understanding of existing workflow. From there, one can determine which decisions should be augmented by AI and which should be left up to the clinician, and how an interface can be constructed to provide a seamless user experience for the two to work together side-by-side.

Further to the previous consideration as to how an algorithm can fit into workflow is the commercial understanding of whether or not the problem being solved is worth it. A hypothetical outpatient radiology center in the United States might interpret around 200 imaging studies per day. Of those, roughly 100 will be X-rays, 50 will be CTs, 40 will be MRIs, and 10 will be a mix of less common study types like fluoroscopes or DEXA scans. One might imagine based on these counts this hypothetical practice would prefer a solution that saves their radiologists 20% of their time when reading X-rays without sacrificing accuracy, because a 20% cost reduction on 50% of their studies must be a 10% overall cost reduction—in practice though, there are a number of reasons this does not even begin to hold up commercially.

First, there is no guarantee a radiologist will do 20% more work or bill for 20% fewer hours rather than using their newly freed time to play Bubble Witch Saga on their iPhone. Second, while X-rays may represent half the number of studies read daily by volume, they do not even come close to representing half of the profit generated for the practice. Radiologists in the United States are paid $401,000 per year on average [9]. Assuming 252 working days per year and 10 working hours per day, that is $159.13 per hour or $2.65 per minute. Across the 25 most common types of X-rays taken in the United States, the average government reimbursement for the interpretation of these scans is $11.30, and the average time to generate a report is 6.2 min [10].

Without even considering all of the other costs of running the practice, back-of-the-napkin math already suggests each X-ray the practice agrees to read costs them an average of $16.43 for an $11.30 return, or an overall loss of $5.13. Even in the unlikely event, a 20% time savings was fully utilized, they would still lose $1.84 per study. While this is unlikely to generate a compelling enough economic argument for most practices to make a purchasing decision, a tool that saves them 40% of their time on all of their CT and MRI studies would likely be a much easier sell, as these studies take considerably longer to read and generate a far more substantial amount of revenue and profit. While there is an incredibly valid argument that improving diagnostic accuracy or radiologist's satisfaction is a strong enough value proposition in and of itself, it is very rare purchasing decisions are made with this mindset.

One final and critical consideration in assessing commercial viability is understanding the regulatory implications and pathway for a given application. Most AI-driven healthcare applications are recognized by the US FDA as a Software-as-a-Medical-Device (SAMD). Just as with typical medical devices, SAMDs are required to be registered with the FDA. Depending on the potential risk associated with a particular SAMD, it may be classified as a Class I, II, or III medical device. Each has different associated levels of validation required prior to the FDA's allowance of marketing.

Class I medical devices are seen as the lowest risk and can be marketed immediately after being put on record with the FDA, but without needing to wait for any special designation. The introduction of AI into an SAMD will almost immediately up class it into Class II or III, but this is not necessarily true in all cases, as some basic quantitative functions can be seen as low enough risk to fall into Class I. Most AI-driven applications in radiology have historically fallen into Class II, such as those used to assist with triaging studies for urgent findings such as intracranial hemorrhages, or those used to assist with detection of common findings such as lung nodules. Though very few, if any, SAMDs using AI have been classified as Class III, this class would likely include those used to assist with the diagnosis or treatment recommendation of potentially life-threatening conditions, such as one which helps a radiologist diagnose and recommend biopsy for malignant lung cancer. Though there has been little or no discussion about applications that entirely replace a radiologist or other physician and make a standalone clinical decision, these applications would likely fall into a new class altogether, or a potential Class IV.

Regardless of class, it is important to keep in mind algorithms do not get regulatory approval—SAMDs using an algorithm in a specific context do. That is to say, two SAMDs might use the exact same underlying chest X-ray DL algorithm, one to help with triage, and the other to help with detection, but the FDA will consider these two separate devices that require independent validation. Though this is not strictly true, most Class II SAMDs seem to require a *clinical assessment*, whereas most Class III/IV SAMDs will require a *clinical trial*. The primary difference between these two terms is the methodology used to suggest the potential reward associated with the device outweighs the risk.

In a clinical assessment, one can typically use historical patient data to benchmark, either algorithm vs human performance or more likely human vs human + AI performance; in a clinical trial, one needs to create a controlled environment wherein patients are prospectively treated with or without assistance, and outcomes are studied once confirmed. This alone immediately suggests why the vast majority of approved AI-based SAMDs in the United States are triage or detection rather than diagnosis—the former can be proven cheaply and immediately on historical data, whereas the latter can potentially take years and at great expense and potential risk.

One final consideration from a regulatory standpoint is the availability of a suitable predicate device, or one already allowed by the FDA which is substantially similar enough to help with the allowance of a new one. For example, it would likely be much easier to get allowance for a device that triages chest X-rays for pneumomediastinum (a condition when air leaks into the space between the lungs and the chest wall), a time-sensitive finding, if someone has already gotten allowance for a device that triages chest X-rays for pneumothorax (a condition when air leaks into the chest cavity), another time-sensitive finding. Such devices can be submitted to the FDA through the *510(k)* program, which is reviewed on an expedited timeline and at lower cost. Devices allowed through this pathway are considered *cleared* by the FDA. For such devices without predicate, the appropriate pathway is called *de novo* and will likely require the design of a new assessment or trial—devices allowed through this program are considered *authorized* if Class II or *approved* if Class III. For those unsure which pathway or designation a given SAMD falls under, the FDA has created the *pre-submission* program, whereby one can submit a write-up petitioning their device one way or another, and the FDA will meet with them 100 days later for 1 h to discuss the appropriate way to proceed.

11.4 Data collection

Once one has identified the appropriate problem and chosen to embark upon the development of AI as a solution, the next major effort is *data collection*—the hunt for sufficient examples of *X*. Here, it is critical to consider the input data at the time of training should be representative of the input data the eventually trained model will see at the time of inference. Given that radiology involves the situational protocoling of different studies depending on clinical context, this can cause quite a challenge for algorithms exposed to a very limited subset.

Two different chest CT scans, one captured for a typical diagnostic setting, and the other captured in a screening setting, are likely to have completely different protocols. One is likely to have a much greater slice thickness, or the depth of anatomy pictured in a single image, and the other may have a higher dose of radiation, or a potentially sharper image. One may have contrast, or the administration of a radiopaque agent to highlight certain properties, whereas the other likely will not. To a lay person, these will likely appear reasonably similar, but to a radiologist or an AI trained to simulate one, these are completely different inputs.

These differences are persistent in a multitude of unique ways for every modality. X-ray images can be captured to view the anatomy from a variety of different angles, and the image itself can be captured digitally or in an analog fashion and digitized after the fact. MRI scans are perhaps the most complex in this regard, as a technologist is given several dozen parameters whereby both the visual appearance and the physical meaning of a given study can be changed entirely. None of this is to suggest that AI cannot overcome these hurdles, but rather the onus is on the one training the algorithm to expose it to enough examples of every scenario it will be expected to perform once released into the world.

The collection of training data poses a massive challenge in a variety of ways. First and foremost is finding and accessing the data, which is typically stored in antiquated systems deliberately designed to keep others out and safeguarded by people who do not understand these systems but have been charged with keeping them safe. Within radiology, there are three main systems of interest—the PACS, or picture archiving and communication system, the RIS, or radiology information system, and the EMR/EHR, or electronic medical/health record. For the most part, the PACS stores the images, the RIS stores the reports, and the EMR/EHR stores the patient histories and associated billing data.

Unfortunately, all three systems are typically produced by different companies that have never communicated with one another nor even contemplated the idea of providing some reasonable means of external integration by a third party. Further, all three are highly fragmented markets, meaning a multitude of completely different vendors providing slightly different solutions, despite everything really just being an SQL (Structured Query Language) table under the hood. While this is likely to create some frustration for engineers, who need to interface with said systems to extract data, not all hope is lost, as most of these systems do need to abide by some common standards to ensure they work in a real-world environment.

Most PACS store medical data in DICOM, or digital image communication format, which essentially wraps the pixel data associated with a given medical image with a series of potentially hundreds of other headers containing information about the patient and the study itself. Most PACS can be interfaced with over a network using a common protocol of simple commands, CFIND, CSTORE, and

CMOVE, to find, store, and move/copy studies to/from the PACS respectively. Most RIS and EMR systems store data in structured tables and can be communicated with through a bus-based bar-delimited protocol called *HL7*. Though the principle behind HL7 is roughly the same in most contexts, it is important to keep in mind different clinics and practices have probably configured their HL7 messages to look and operate differently.

Extracting data from the PACS, RIS, and EMR can each be long and challenging endeavors depending on the age of the system, the level of access granted, the hardware that system sits on, and the approach taken to extraction—in some cases, it may even require working with the vendor who implemented the system at the request of the clinical organization. Especially with PACS, it is unlikely one would be extracting less than a terabyte of data, and much more likely to be in excess of hundreds of terabytes or even petabytes of data—meaning a difference of approach can be the difference between 3 years and 3 months for a comprehensive data pull. Regardless, the next challenge once all the relevant data has been pulled from each system is linking it together, as the images and reports tend not to be very useful unless one can join them. This is typically done using an *accession number*, which is often found in the header of a given DICOM image, but may require some mapping to other figures such as a report ID in the RIS or EMR.

Of course, beyond the technical challenges of data collection, there are the considerable associated privacy and security constraints that vary from country to country and from site to site. As with all things clinical, patient safety must be the top consideration, and privacy is an important subset. As of 1996, the Unites States mandated compliance with HIPAA, the Health Insurance Portability and Accountability Act, which sets rules and regulations around the storage and sharing of protected health information (PHI). There are currently two recognized methods of remaining compliant with HIPAA, one of which is called *Safe Harbor*, a protocol which outlines which specific types of information are considered PHI and how to handle them. The other is referred to as the rule of "expert determination," whereby each healthcare organization can appoint their own internal expert to verify no two pieces of information exist in a given dataset such that one could reasonably be expected to be able to reidentify a given patient [11]. Unfortunately, the latter approach is far more common, and no one in an organization wants to take on the responsibility or risk of being the appointed expert. This creates a need for highly customizable approaches to the deidentification or anonymization of patient data in a number of different ways.

Deidentification should always occur onsite, using a server or virtual machine physically located at the site the PHI is stored. Deidentification of structured patient fields, such as those stored in DICOM headers, or in an RIS or EMR, tends to be a trivial implementation of situational rules. For example, one knows the patient's name is stored in the "PatientName" field, so one can simply throw this value away. One also knows that the patient's ID or Medical Record Number (MRN) is stored in the "PatientID" or "MRN" field, so one can simply replace this with a new artificial ID that cannot be linked back to the original. One important consideration: one should not necessarily throw away all dates, times, and unique patient numbers but rather replace these values with new ones that maintain the associated nature of different studies from the same patient and the delta in time between them. For example, it is not important for development that an AI know a patient had a pelvic X-ray on September 20, 2012, but it may very well be important for the AI to know that same patient had a prostate MRI 16 days later. Patient age is also likely to be highly relevant to algorithm development, but one must consider this within limits—for example, knowing a patient is 72 at the time of their prostate MRI is unlikely to help a bad actor track them down, but it would be a completely different story if the patient was 112 as there are not very many super-centenarians out there. For that reason, Safe Harbor recommends changing any patient age 90 or above to the value 89, and otherwise keeping it.

The greatest challenge by far in deidentification is the piece least considered—dealing with unstructured data. What happens when a patient gets X-rayed wearing a dog tag with their name engraved on it? How about when the clinical notes, handwritten or digital text, mention the patient by name? How about when someone reconstructs a patient's face from a high-resolution brain MRI and then runs it against a database of pictures pulled from Facebook to figure out their name? While unlikely, these scenarios are distinct and provable possibilities, which should not stand in the way of AI development but should force those working with PHI to develop sophisticated solutions to minimize risk and highly scrutinize said work prior to copying data externally.

11.5 Data labeling

Once one has collected sufficient examples of *X*, the next great challenge is *data labeling*—the hunt for sufficient examples of *Y*. Labeling can be done in a variety of different ways, and the correct approach always depends entirely on the circumstance. Regardless, labeling ultimately always comes down to application of some tag to an input indicating the corresponding outcome of interest. More likely than naught, labeling will require some form of human expert interaction with many examples of *X*, but this is not always the case. Either way, labeling strategy should start with an understanding of what *Y* one wants an algorithm to output when presented with *X*—as a rule of thumb, the *Y* used to train an algorithm should look exactly like the algorithm's desired output. That is to say, if one wants the algorithm to output a yes/no answer, one should train the algorithm with *Y* in the form of yes/no answers. If one would rather an algorithm output a segmentation mask around a region of interest (ROI), one should train the algorithm with *Y* in the form of segmentation masks around said ROIs.

To provide a few examples of fundamentally different tasks in radiology and the general shape of the corresponding label, consider the differences among the tasks of triage, detection, measurement, characterization, and co-registration.

Triage is the task of classifying a study as containing the presence or absence of a given finding, primarily for the sake of prioritization. If one is triaging head CT scans for intracranial hemorrhages, or brain bleeds, the input *X* is a head CT scan,

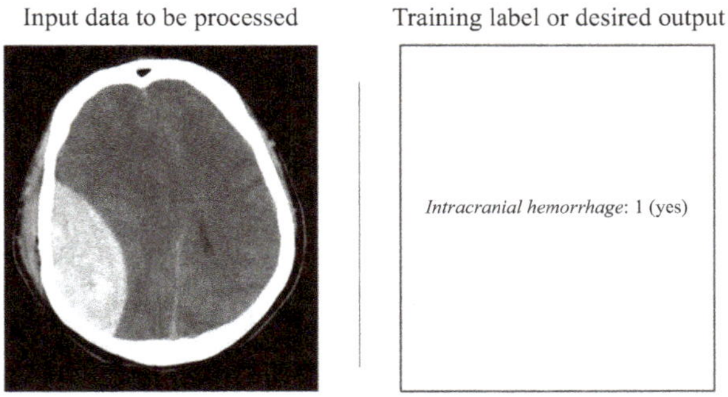

Figure 11.3 Example input and training label for a triage task. The input image features one axial slice of a head CT scan containing an intracranial hemorrhage [12]. The training label is 1 to affirm the indication

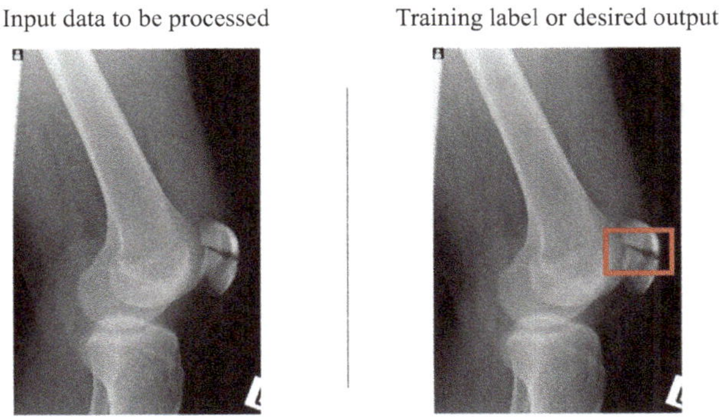

Figure 11.4 Example input and training label for a detection task. The input image features an X-ray of the knee containing a transverse fracture through the mid portion of the patella. The training label is a bounding box centered on the finding. Image and label provided by Enlitic

and both the desired training label and the output *Y* are 1 if a hemorrhage is present and 0 otherwise (Figure 11.3).

Detection is the task of producing a nondescript ROI, such as a circle or a bounding box, to indicate the visual location of given finding in a study. If one is detecting fractures in X-rays of the extremities, the input *X* is an extremity X-ray, and both the desired training label and output *Y* are bounding boxes or circles around each fracture (Figure 11.4).

Measurement is the task of finely segmenting the boundaries of a finding for the sake of indicating the linear axis measurements, the area, or the volume. If one is measuring lung nodules in a chest CT, the input *X* is a chest CT scan, and both the

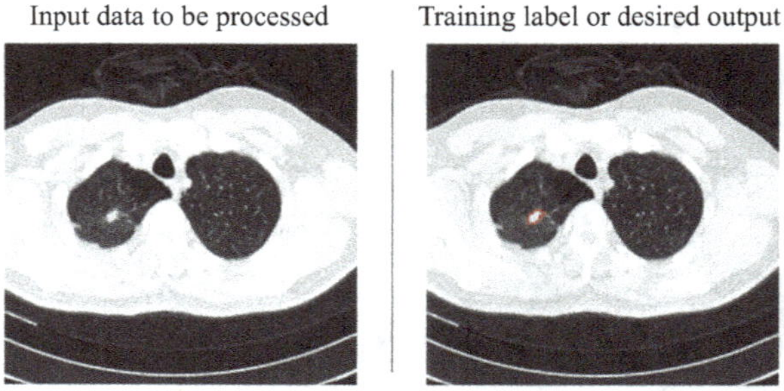

Figure 11.5 Example input and training label for a measurement task. The input image features a CT of the chest containing a lung nodule. The training label is an ROI tightly contouring the finding. Image and label provided by Enlitic

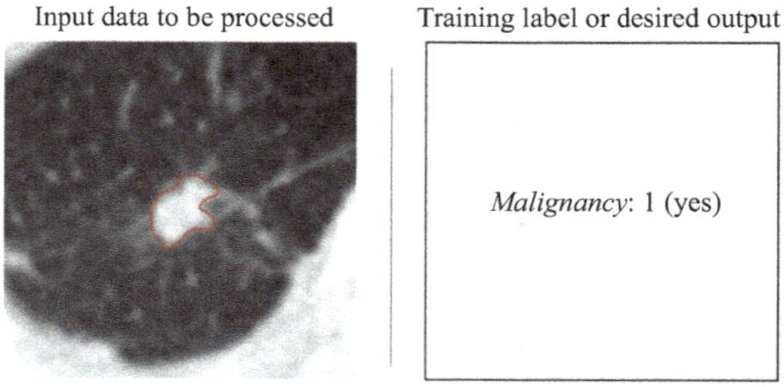

Figure 11.6 Example input and training label for a characterization task. The input is an ROI within a CT of the chest segmenting a lung nodule. The training label is 1 to affirm the characteristic. Image provided by Enlitic

desired training label and output Y are tightly contoured ROIs cleanly hugging the margins of each lung nodule (Figure 11.5).

Characterization is the task of further classifying a given finding within a study, typically for the sake of diagnosis or the determination of other descriptive features. If one is characterizing lung nodules in a chest CT as being benign or malignant, the input X is an ROI around a given lung nodule, and both the desired training label and output Y are a "1" if the nodule is malignant and a "0" otherwise (Figure 11.6).

Co-registration is the task of locating a given finding within a study when given the location of that same finding in a different study, typically for the sake of determining change over time. If one is co-registering lung nodules between two chest

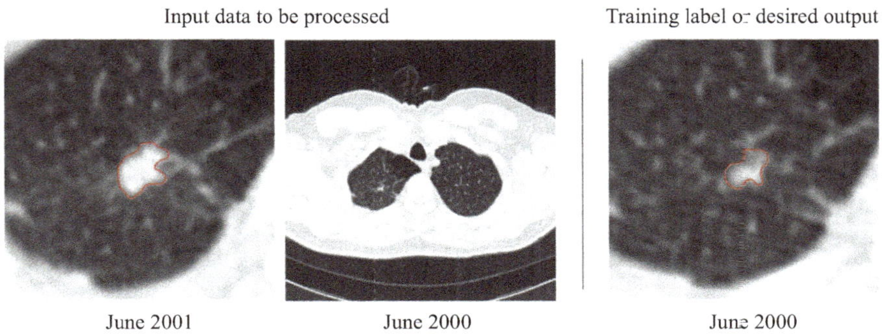

Figure 11.7 Example input and training label for a co-registration task. There are two inputs, an ROI segmenting a lung nodule in a chest CT from June 2001, and an entire chest CT from 1 year earlier. The training label is an ROI segmenting the nodule, but in the CT from June 2000. Image and labels provided by Enlitic

CT scans from the same patient, the input X is an ROI around a given lung nodule in the first scan, and both the desired training label and output Y are an ROI around that same nodule in the other scan (Figure 11.7).

It is important to note that in this context some labels are more useful than others, but usefulness tends to scale directly with cost to acquire. Co-registration data with fine contours around every nodule in two different scans is very expensive to collect but can be used to train algorithms for co-registration, measurement, detection, and triage all at the same time. A triage label on the other hand would not contain enough information to properly train any other types of algorithms without other techniques that might introduce unintended consequences.

For some of the previous problems, training labels can be bootstrapped, or determined using semiautomated methodologies much faster and more cost-effective than manual annotation by human experts. Triage labels, for example, can often be determined through the use of natural language processing (NLP). To explain this example, consider a different problem from those discussed earlier—one where the input X is a radiology report, and both the training label and output Y are a set of tags corresponding to each clinical finding indicated in the report. This algorithm would be substantially cheaper to train than most imaging models because many professionals can read radiology reports, such as medical transcriptionists, nurses, medical coders, and technologists, and not just the most expensive radiologists. The resulting algorithm can be used to analyze millions of historical radiology reports, distilling each down to yes/no answers across a series of findings. These yes/no answers can then be applied as triage labels to the image study about which each report was originally written, thus enabling the creation of millions of image triage training labels in a matter of hours (Figure 11.8).

Another example would be in the space of detection and measurement, borrowing from annotations historically applied to images for clinical purposes. In an

Chest X-ray

Clinical history:
Right pleural effusion with known aortic dissection.

Findings:
There is mild cardiomegaly with a cardiothoracic ratio of 175/335. sternotomy sutures are seen. there is no evidence to suggest pulmonary edema. a moderate right-sided pleural effusion is noted. the visualized lungs appear clear with no suggestion of any nodule or mass. surgical clips are seen in the right axilla.

Cardinomegaly: 1 (yes)
Medical device: 1 (yes)
Pleural effusion: 1 (yes)
Edema: 0 (no)
Nodule or mass: 0 (no)
Fracture: 0 (no)
Consolidation: 0 (no)
Pneumothorax: 0 (no)

...
...
...

Figure 11.8 Example input and training label for an NLP task. The input is a clinical radiology report describing a chest X-ray study. The training labels are "1" to affirm each positive finding and "0" to negate any number of negative or unmentioned findings. Report provided by Enlitic

oncology setting, for example, countless hours by radiologists and technologists are spent painstakingly segmenting cancerous lesions and other surrounding anatomy for the sake of progression tracking and treatment planning. Simple scripts can easily be written to ingest these historical annotations to extract segmentation ROIs for the sake of bootstrapping detection and measurement image labels. While bootstrapping and other semi-supervised learning techniques are invaluable tools for building strong algorithms, they should never be trusted as the sole source of training data in clinical applications where the potential risk of error is quite high.

The most valuable training data in building any clinical AI is likely to come from human annotation of studies by experts. When this is the case, one will likely need access to some tool for *crowdsourcing* these labels, or enabling labeling by a large pool of distributed individuals. This introduces a great deal of interesting new challenges which clearly highlight the development of good radiology AI is much more akin to the development of a clinical radiology quality improvement program than the development of traditional software. It is true that labeling is both an art and science of standardizing inputs, ensuring that every radiologist is providing answers in a consistent format, and with high accuracy, even in recognition that training labeling and clinical interpretation are similar but different tasks. This means radiologists need to be tested prior to being able to label—some people read brain MRIs much better than chest X-rays and vice versa, while some struggle to do either because it feels so different from clinical reporting. Even once labeling, radiologists need to be tested on an ongoing basis to ensure quality never dips. This can be facilitated much more easily by ensuring that some number of studies are the same across all labelers, monitoring the resulting agreement rates.

Even with an army of the world's best radiologists labeling around the clock, one might wonder how an AI could ever hope to exceed expert-level performance. The solution to this is actually quite straightforward—by giving the radiologists far more context when labeling than they would typically have at the time of clinical interpretation. For example, false positive rates (FPRs) are notoriously high when radiologists recommend lung nodules for biopsy in a screening setting, but this is only because it is better to be safe than sorry when the downside is untreatable malignancy. If at the time of labeling a historical study, a radiologist is given access to the biopsy which eventually followed the said study, the radiologist can label the study with proven knowledge of the future rather than an educated guess. Further, research consistently suggests studies are read more accurately when seen by more radiologists. While this might be too cost prohibitive in an everyday clinical setting, it is a helpful means of ensuring high-quality training data when cost is not an issue.

11.6 Validation

There is only so much utility in collecting a massive supply of high-quality training data if one ultimately has no idea how well the resulting algorithm is performing. For that reason, good clinical algorithm development is contingent on the definition and understanding of *ground truth*. Ground truth is meant to represent the factual physical answer key to a given problem, which exists beyond human opinion and can differ wildly for different problems and in different clinical contexts. For the most part, the ideal ground truth is some form of proven follow-up that can confirm an outcome with much greater certainty than the data provided at the time of inference.

Borrowing a previously aforementioned example, the ground truth used to benchmark performance at the task of lung cancer diagnosis from a chest CT should not be human opinion, but rather the results of a biopsy following that scan to definitively indicate the state of that nodule with much greater confidence than could be discerned from a CT scan alone. In the task of fracture detection from a foot X-ray, the ground truth for subtle fractures should be determined from a follow-up CT or MRI that can show the finding in much greater detail. In the event a definitive ground truth is not available, then the best one can do is typically to rely on the joint opinion of several experts, with the more asked resulting in higher confidence. In the task of lung nodule detection from a chest CT, the best ground truth one can rely on is probably a panel of experts, as it is incredibly unlikely one has a sizable dataset wherein every single lung nodule in a set of patients was removed to prove it was not in fact a blood vessel.

Once one has an understanding of ground truth for the problem of interest, the next important activity is the development of a gold standard validation set, or a dataset with ground truth for a sufficient number of examples of each endpoint targeted by the algorithm. Consider an algorithm trained to triage chest X-rays for

14 simultaneous findings—one cannot have confidence the algorithm is performing sufficiently well on each of these findings unless one has gold standard validation data with enough examples of each finding, as well as an overall equivalent number of "normal" examples.

Further, it is important to ensure that these findings exist in roughly similar proportions to validate the algorithm that is not simply generalizing to the contextual probability of any given finding. That is to say, one wants to ensure an algorithm does not learn to just always say "no" to pneumothorax because it was trained on outpatient data, where pneumothoraces are far rarer than in an ICU, and "no" would probably be the correct answer 99.99% of the time in that setting. It is also important to ensure sufficient diversity of the presentation of each abnormality and in different combinations in the gold standard validation set. For example, it is important to ensure that an algorithm says "yes" to pneumothorax only when it properly sees one, and not just when it sees a chest tube—this can be a problem given the vast majority of pneumothorax training cases will come from an ICU where it is already being treated by the administration of a chest tube. In the same validation set, one will want examples of patients who are upright, or standing up, as well as supine, or laying down, as both are common settings wherein chest X-rays are taken, and they can have drastic differences in the deformity of anatomy and the appearance of a finding. Further, one will want examples of pneumothoraces of all sizes.

Gold standard validation sets are incredibly challenging to prepare correctly but are a critical step in any algorithmic development. The determination of the size of a gold standard validation set, as well as the sub-characteristic distribution, should be done through a power calculation based on the target accuracy and the statistical confidence one desires in the resulting answer.

Accuracy is a loaded term, as most clinical contexts call for far more meaningful performance metrics. For example, consider a test wherein 1,000 patients are being screened for breast cancer, and only one has a malignant lesion. A radiologist, or an algorithm for that matter, could simply answer "benign" to every study without looking, and either party would be 99.9% accurate. This simple example immediately highlights why accuracy is the wrong metric—arguably, it would have been better to incorrectly biopsy 20 of the 1,000 patients if it meant the one with breast cancer did not go untreated.

Different clinical tasks are properly benchmarked differently, and in many cases these benchmarks can be challenging to interpret. Triage tasks, for example, are typically measured in terms of *sensitivity*, or true positive rate (TPR), the percentage of positives correctly classified as such, and *specificity*, or the percentage of negatives correctly classified as such, which can be calculated as one minus the FPR. Triage algorithms do not actually output a "0" or a "1," but rather a decimal value in between, which can be converted into a yes/no value by comparison against some preset threshold value. By changing the definition of this threshold to each possible value between 0 and 1, and recording the corresponding TPR and FPR at each step, it is possible to draw a curve of all possible *operating points*, or achievable trade-offs of TPR and FPR. This curve is called the receiving operating characteristic (ROC) curve.

The area under the ROC curve, or AUC, is probably the most popularly reported metric for triage algorithm performance in a research setting, as it is sort of a holistic measure that can be indicated in a single number between 0 and 1, where "0" is always wrong, "1" is perfect, and "0.5" roughly mimics a coin flip. The issue with AUC as a measure for practical purposes, however, is most real-life applications that must be shipped with a fixed threshold as per regulations, meaning an AUC is relatively meaningless compared to the fixed operating point at which the algorithm is required to stay. That said, the ability to shift this threshold would potentially be quite useful, as many clinical contexts may very well trade TPR for a lower FPR and vice versa.

Detection algorithms are considerably more difficult to benchmark, largely because detection is a task of locating one or potentially many of a finding which may or may not even be present, and determining a hit or a miss cannot be done by simple comparison of yes/no answers. This hit/miss determination can be done on a finding-by-finding basis through the use of a metric called intersection over union (IOU), which essentially measures the ratio of the area a guess and an answer overlap divided by the area jointly covered by both the guess and the answer. The IOU is then compared against some preset threshold, typically 0.5, to convert it to a hit or a miss. This analysis can be done across all findings in a study or set of studies to produce a curve that reports the average sensitivity against the number of false positives per scan.

Fortunately, some clinical tasks do properly call for a simple accuracy metric. Measurement, for example, is often an intuitive comparison of guess vs answer. An algorithm that reports the volume of a 1,000 mm^3 mass as 950 mm^3 is 95% accurate. The challenge here will be making sure there is a proper comparison—clinical radiologists will typically report the volume of a mass through the use of the protocol known as RECIST, or response evaluation criteria in solid tumors, whereas an algorithm is going to attempt to interpolate area on each 2D slice across the full range of 3D space much akin to a Riemann sum. Given that RECIST provides a crude estimate of volume by taking a single linear axis measurement and plugging it into the formula for the volume of a sphere, $[V = (4/3)\pi r^3]$, the algorithm may be marked as wildly inaccurate despite using a far more sound methodology and arriving at a more accurate answer.

One additional critical consideration when validating is whether to validate against human performance or alongside it. There is only so much value in measuring the performance of a detection algorithm against a panel of human experts if the intended use of the resulting product is to help human experts achieve more accurate results in a shorter amount of time. If that is the case, a proper validation would have a panel of expert radiologists reading each of some number of studies at two different points in time, once with help from the product, and once without, and with enough separation in time between the two points, or a *wash-out period*, for each to forget the studies they saw the first time. One would then compare the results of each radiologist against the ground truth for each of the two reads on each study and look for a statistically significant improvement in TPR, FPR, or speed.

Regardless of the task at hand or the method of validation, it is important to note validation must be performed for every intended setting and population for which the resulting product is intended for use. Every patient population has different incidences of abnormalities and anatomical variations, technical imaging protocols and definitions of follow-up, and imaging vendors and equipment. Without testing a product in each of these settings, or validating the underlying algorithm on representative data, it is impossible to know with confidence whether or not it will perform as intended.

11.7 Deployment and integration

There is little utility in product no one trusts or that which worsens human performance, even if it is powered by the world's most highly performant algorithm. Perhaps the most difficult part about developing clinical applications of AI is making them useful. This requires a deep understanding of the modern condition in radiology, from the needs that drive radiologist adoption, to the bar one needs to pass to get there. One particularly challenging question is "when is an algorithm good enough?" A naïve response might be when the algorithm meets or exceeds human performance—but if the goal is to improve human performance, then why does solitary algorithm performance matter?

Consider the example of an algorithm that triages chest X-rays for several different findings simultaneously—is the algorithm with 0.95 AUC for cardiomegaly and 0.80 for nodules better than the one with 0.80 for cardiomegaly and 0.95 for nodules? If one is planning to deploy the resulting product in the United States, the correct answer is probably neither, unless either somehow has a substantially positive impact on human performance. If one is planning to deploy in the developing world, the correct answer is probably either, because both will probably substantially elevate the performance of technologists who have to read scans in isolation without an expert radiologist for miles. In essence, the answer to "when is good enough" is entirely driven by the context of one's application and the validation metrics one has set to prove that it sufficiently solves a real market need at the time of testing.

Once rigorous internal validation has provided confidence that an algorithm meets or exceeds expectations, the next major step is deployment; or its release in a way made accessible to the outside world. For this phase, it is highly recommended to surround one's algorithm with the necessary infrastructure to provide it as an API, or abstracted program interface. APIs are common constructs frequently used throughout software engineering to simplify the interface between multiple potentially large or complex code bases by representing distinct functions or sets of functions as separable callable services that return the expected output when provided the expected input.

Google Translate is a convenient example of why APIs are important—it is an enormously complex system likely comprising tens of millions of lines of code, and yet it is a critical component of their service offering used to translate Google searches, web pages in Chrome, and countless applications for their partners and subsidiaries. To manually integrate each of these lines of code into each of the hundreds of other programs that use it would be a nightmarish, if not impossible undertaking. Google has instead simplified this process with good software engineering principles by hosting their translation software as an API. Any service, including those developed by third parties, can now benefit from the value of Google Translate by simply sending the API a body of text and a target output language, and the API will return the body of text in the desired language.

The API model is conceptually an excellent fit with the input/output black box model of DL, and more importantly, enables the development of complex pipelines of models, or *ensembles*, with relative ease. For example, say one were aiming to develop a comprehensive solution for the analysis of brain tumors in MRI, simultaneously providing the core functions of detection, measurement, tracking, and characterization. Given the complexity of this overall task, it is highly unlikely a single algorithm would do particularly well end-to-end. One logical approach would be to train four algorithms, one for each function, and tie them together in an ensemble.

For example, a detection algorithm is sent a brain MRI and returns an ROI corresponding to a bounding box around a suspected tumor. The ROI, as well as the MRI, and any historical MRIs, are then sent to a tracking algorithm which returns ROIs corresponding to bounding boxes around the same detected tumor but in the historical MRIs. Each set of ROIs is then sent to a measurement algorithm, which returns a new set of ROIs with much tighter contours around the tumor as well as volumes at each point in time, and a characterization model, which returns the prognosis.

This approach provides substantial benefits by enabling each component to be validated and reused independently and for different purposes. Without the use of APIs, such an ensemble could be incredibly challenging to build as each algorithm could likely be anywhere between 100 and 10,000 lines of code. By abstracting each algorithm as an API, however, each function can be tied together with only a few extra lines of code in the way conceptually laid out in Figure 11.9. This has the added benefit of drastically simplifying integration into external systems as well.

One final but substantial consideration is the user experience of the application. This, even more so than the accuracy of the underlying algorithm, will

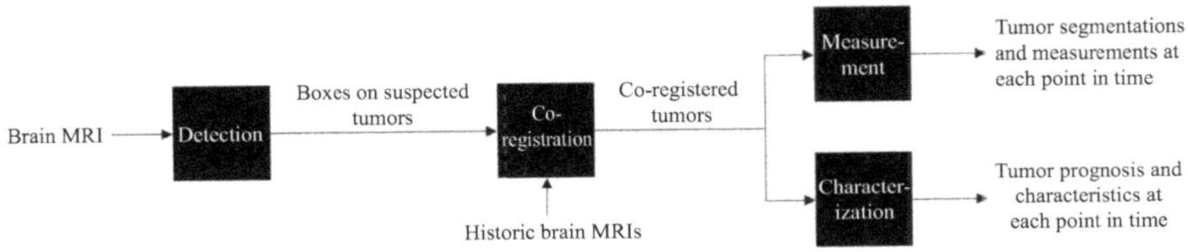

Figure 11.9 Example ensemble tying together DL models for detection, co-registration, measurement, and characterization to perform end-to-end brain tumor analysis in MRIs

ultimately make or break the market's view of the application. Unless one's application enables a fundamentally new function, preferably one that opens previously inaccessible streams of revenue, it is critical that the application feels seamless, familiar, and overall, as if it solves more problems than it creates. This is an especially challenging prospect in radiology, as most radiologists are experts in diagnostic image interpretation and not in the adoption of new software.

Most radiologists use their RIS, PACS, advanced image viewers, and other clinical and administrative software as a means to an end, more out of necessity than desire. Most hospital software is installed with multi-year multi-million-dollar contracts that are challenging and expensive to break. For that reason, most radiologists simply learn whatever software was purchased by their employer, who intends to keep using it for at least a decade at a time. Riddled with bugs and confusing interfaces, radiologists tend to dislike whatever software they use on a daily basis, but at least they know it; they tend to be skeptical of yet-another-screen-or-program to look at and will need to be eased into the modern world of pragmatic and intuitive software. While it is clear the modern radiological workflow can be fundamentally reworked for major improvement leveraging modern technology, jumping straight to something completely new will likely cause more harm than good. Early applications should plan to be minimally invasive, likely confined to a simple augmentation of a radiologist's existing interfaces, and only get more complex and differentiated from current practice as users build confidence and comfort with the system. Above all, successful developers of clinical AI products must value human centric design as one of the most important considerations.

References

[1] "Medical/Diagnostic Imaging Market – Global Opportunity Analysis and Industry Forecast, 2015 – 2022." Allied Market Research.

[2] "Overview of Imaging Market." Bain & Company.

[3] "Essential Diagnostic Imaging." World Health Organization, Department of Essential Health Technologies, http://www.who.int/eht/en/DiagnosticImaging.pdf.

[4] "History of Radiology." CME Science, https://cmescience.com/history-of-radiology/.

[5] Oosterwijk, Herman. "PACS Fundamentals." Aubrey: OTech Inc, 2004. ISBN 978-0-9718867-3-5.

[6] Doi, Kunio. "Computer-aided diagnosis in medical imaging: historical review, current status and future potential." Computerized Medical Imaging and Graphics. 31 (4): 198–211. doi:10.1016/j.compmedimag.2007.02.002. PMC 1955762. PMID 17349778.

[7] Casey, Brian. "New Data From Match 2018 Underscore Radiology's Rebound." Aunt Minnie, 16 March 2018, https://www.auntminnie.com/index.aspx?sec=log&itemID=120257.

[8] Yao, Li. "Learning to Diagnose From Scratch by Exploiting Dependencies Among Labels." Enlitic, Inc., 2018, https://arxiv.org/pdf/1710.10501.pdf.
[9] "Physician Compensation Survey 2019." Medscape.
[10] "Time & Revenue Analysis of Top 25 X-ray CPT Codes." Fahrenbach and Associates of Chicago.
[11] "Guidance Regarding Methods for De-identification of Protected Health Information in Accordance With the Health Insurance Portability and Accountability Act (HIPAA) Privacy Rule." U.S. Department of Health and Human Services, https://www.hhs.gov/hipaa/for-professionals/privacy/special-topics/de-identification/index.html.
[12] Bell, Daniel. "Intracranial Hemorrhage." Radiopaedia, https://radiopaedia.org/articles/intracranial-haemorrhage?lang=us.

Chapter 12

Under the hood: developing the engine that drives personalized medicine

Edward Kiruluta[1], Björn Stade[2] and Rona Margaret Relova, M.D.[3,4]

12.1 Introduction

One of the greatest achievements in human history was the completion of the DNA sequence for the human genome in 2001 [1]. Since then, many individuals have been sequenced, and as expected, the genetic material is more than 99% identical. Variations in the genome explain traits, such as eye color, skin and hair color. However, variants also cause genetic diseases, predispose us to certain diseases like cancer, or compromise the effectiveness of drugs. The correct interpretation of the effect of variants in a genome can be used to create an individual's personalized diagnosis for health conditions.

Personalized Medicine (PM) moves away from a "one size fits all" approach to the treatment and care of individuals. PM has a powerful impact in management of disease risks [2], in therapeutic treatments accounting for individual drug efficacy [3], and as the focus of this chapter, in treatment for hereditary genetic diseases. This approach is transforming medicine by providing an individual's genetic profile that guides decision-making in prevention, diagnosis, and treatment of diseases. This approach also maximizes health benefits and minimizes the risks of disease progression by enabling diagnostic and prognostic information based on genetic profile not previously available. PM not only has the potential for extricating the underlying cause of a disease, but also discovering better treatments that usher improved health outcomes.

Over 850 genes have been linked to epileptic seizures. We now have the capability of pinpointing defects in those genes. Instead of prescribing generic drugs, genes can be specifically targeted. Ninety of those 850 genes have effective treatments, thus can profoundly change the course of the disease and patients'

[1]Calgene, Summit, NJ, USA
[2]Fabric Genomics, Oakland, CA, USA
[3]VA Palo Alto Health Care System, Stanford University, Palo Alto, CA, USA
[4]National Institutes of Health, Bethesda, MD, USA

clinical outcomes. For example, defects in the metabolic gene ALDH7A1 not only cause seizures in newborns but can also lead to lifelong cognitive impairment. Instead of prescribing generic seizure drugs, patients with this gene mutation can be treated with a simple change in diet which prevents the seizures and the concomitant decline of cognitive brain function (PMID 30930802, PMID 30671974). In the case of ENPP1 and ABCC6 mutations, instead of heart transplant intervention for the newborn or more frequently, acceptance of mortality within 6 months due to a calcified heart, targeted bisphosphonate treatments may save the patient's life (PMID 30206659).

To benefit from the genomic medicine in improving patient care, clinicians need to gain better understanding of inheritance pattern of diseases, confirmation process of clinical diagnoses with genetic tests, and inclusion of novel gene-based therapies in medical armamentarium. Genomic techniques that allow molecular-level analyses as a standard in investigating a patient's diagnosis and determining therapeutic interventions may be the imminent breakthrough in patient care. However, there are hindrances to overcome; like translating next-generation sequencing (NGS) results for routine clinical care would entail management and interpretation of such an enormous amount of information produced by genomic techniques. There are also the challenges of identification of disease etiologies for genetic conditions with substantial genetic heterogeneity and ethical issues related to this novel method [4]. The technologies are explained in the following sections.

12.2 Sequencing

To discover DNA variants, the individual's DNA needs to be sequenced. Understanding human variant analysis and its pitfalls requires some basic knowledge of this technology. Depending on the clinical needs, either the whole genome, the exome (the coding regions that form the functional proteins), or specific, targeted, genes can be sequenced.

The major innovation called NGS or second-generation sequencing has served as the impetus for PM. NGS generates many millions of nucleotide short reads in parallel in a much shorter time than Sanger sequencing, which was used to sequence the first human genomes. Sequencing of the first human genome cost $2.7 million and the duration to complete the sequencing took 10 years. But already in 2008, the cost decreased to $100,000 [5] and in 2015 went further down to $1,500. Today, the sequencing of a whole genome is already available for less than $1,000 [5].

NGS parallelizes the sequencing process, producing millions of sequences concurrently at high speed and low cost. The advent of inexpensive high-throughput sequencing has paved the way to exponential discoveries of causes of genetic diseases, new underlying pathways, and identification of novel mutations that has extensively expanded genotype–phenotype relationships.

NGS refers to multiple deep, high-throughput, in-parallel DNA-sequencing technologies. Generally, DNA is extracted with a chemical process from tissue samples, most commonly from easily obtainable blood. For whole-genome sequencing, the workflow for the most widely applied NGS platforms starts with the fragmentation of the DNA into smaller segments (shotgun sequencing). For exome or targeted gene sequencing, protein coding parts of the DNA are selectively amplified with polymerase chain reaction. The nucleotide sequence of these fragments is then determined by in vitro synthesis or ligation with individual nucleotides that were modified to emit a light signal indicating the identity of the base. An image-capturing device records the light signals produced along the growing second strand. The synthesis or ligation at a single strand of DNA is not enough for emitting sufficiently strong light signals. Consequently, the single fragments are first amplified and fixed on a medium to form colonies prior to the synthesis or ligation step. Light signals emitted by these colonies can now be recorded by image-capturing devices and analyzed for determining the nucleotide sequence. In principle, the available platforms differ in the way the colonies are formed and amplified and also how the nucleotide sequence is determined in the end [6,7]. The read types generated by NGS are digital and therefore enable direct quantitative comparisons [8]. Raw sequencing signals produced by the manufacturer's sequencing machine or system are converted into nucleotide bases of short-read data (base calling) with base quality scoring into the FASTQ format (this is a text-based file used for storing both as biological sequence and its corresponding scores), or the more compact Sequence Alignment Map format and its compressed Binary Alignment Map (BAM).

While extremely powerful, NGS introduces several problems affecting the interpretation of the DNA sequence. Instead of getting a single strand of DNA comprising the chromosomes, NGS yields small fragments that need to be reassembled or aligned to a known genome to reconstitute the original sequence. The underlying process depends on in vitro chemistry, which, unlike biological systems, is not accurate. Not every DNA fragment will be represented in equal quantities. For this reason, much more DNA is sequenced than required for reconstituting the genome. This DNA overrepresentation is usually referred to as 1×, 10×, or even 100× sequencing, resulting into 1- to 100-fold quantities of DNA fragments. Having multiple DNA fragments not only allows for error correction, but also increases the computational complexity for reconstituting the individual's sequence.

12.3 Secondary analysis

Comparing the DNA sequences of two individuals reveals differences in the individual DNA sequences. At a certain DNA position, a cytosine nucleotide corresponds to a thymine nucleotide in another person. Computational processing of NGS fragments to such variants is called secondary analysis. The goal of this process is to generate a file with positions that differ to a known reference genome. Since genomes are largely identical, representing an individual's genome with differences will result into a more compact and easily maintainable file.

The most common reference for the human genome is defined and updated by the Genome Reference Consortium [9], an international collective of academic and research institutes with expertise in genome mapping, sequencing, and informatics.

This standard genome is based on the historical first genome sequence, input from various individuals, and ongoing improvements of the assembly. All past and current technologies are based on sequencing small fragments. The genome has many repetitive and nonunique regions, which render reconstituting a genome from such fragments a computationally challenging problem. There are ongoing improvements, both in the sequencing and computational technologies, resulting into multiple, progressively more complete assemblies. The newest reference is called GRCh38 (Genome Reference Consortium—human build 38), first published in 2013, the latest updated version was released in 2017. Due to inertia and the substantial scientific community using the human genome, the most commonly used assembly is still GRCh37. However, GRCh37 has not been updated for several years and is ultimately expected to be replaced by the current 38 release. National Institutes of Health (NIH) also published its own reference genome, called RefSeq [10].

The first step is aligning the sequences of the NGS fragments to the reference genome. This is not only complicated by the aforementioned NGS problems, but also by the fact that the individual's sequence will not be identical to the reference.

A difference between base pairs is referred to as a single-nucleotide variation (SNV) or point mutation. Of course, variations can be bigger than one single nucleotide. They can also be small deletions or insertions (inDels) of a few nucleotides or changes in large regions, called structural variations. Single-nucleotide changes are easy to describe without ambiguity, but others allow for multiple descriptions depending on the choice of start and end of the nucleotide stretch and its replacement. Such variability can have a profound impact on matching the variation to known data predictors. Therefore, variants need to be normalized to a standard representation. Complex rules have been developed and implemented either in proprietary pipelines or public tools (e.g., VT tools [11]). The latter has become a quasi-standard and increasingly widely used for this process.

One now speaks of a mutation when an individual has a variation compared to the described reference. Compared to an individual, the reference has only one set of chromosomes. For typing a variant, both chromosome strands of an individual are always used. If an individual has the same base on both strands, but they are different from the reference, this is called a homozygous SNV. If the bases of an individual differ in the same place, this is called a heterozygous SNV. In this context, the expression of a single-nucleotide polymorphism (SNP) is also called a genotype. For example, an individual has an A/C genotype at a particular location with alleles A and C if they have a heterozygous SNP at that location. Depending on where in the DNA and with which genotype a variant occurs, it may interfere with protein production and, thus, influence the phenotype (external characteristics) of an individual. During translation, an altered amino acid is formed from the SNP-containing codon. This process is also called amino acid substitution. If a variant alters the stop codon of a gene, the protein formed can mutate to become harmful to the body.

12.3.1 False-positive filtering

Filtering is an essential step in reducing the number of false-positive SNP calls. Typically applied, filters check for deviations from the Hardy–Weinberg equilibrium, minimum and maximum read depth, adjacency to inDels, strand bias, etc. While filtering might also remove real variants from the candidate list, it is an important tool for minimizing variant calling artifacts.

Most variant calling tools have the option to generate the data in the variant call format (VCF) [12]. The VCF files contain a tabular description of the variations of the probing individual to this standardized genome. Each line contains one continuous variation on the DNA sequence with additional information, such as a quality assessment from the preceding laboratory process, copy number variation, and the variant's zygosity (i.e., if the individual is homo- or heterozygous for a given variant). This file allows for a more compact description of the individual's genome because it encompasses only the differences. Usually, the file for a whole genome contains between 4 and 10 million lines or variants. Optionally, this file can contain multiple samples, e.g., for the proband and both parents, allowing for an even more compact format for a case.

While VCF is a standardized defined file format, in practice, various details are not particularly well described and therefore, individual genome submissions contain many derivations. For an annotation pipeline, having a robust parsing and standardization is a quintessential feature. A vigorous pipeline must be able to deal with simple problems such as premature line or file endings, differences to expected number or samples as well as more complex issues. For example, the initial step should conduct a sanity check with the reference genome to inspect if the reported file fits to the genome assembly. In this initial step, the pipeline must also decide if the VCF file is salvageable or needs to be flagged and reported as incomprehensible.

12.4 Tertiary analysis

The tertiary analysis encompasses annotation of variants with prior knowledge or predictions. Variants are placed in context to the protein coding and noncoding regions of the genome, associated with any known data and scored with probabilistic prediction tools. These associations allow for clinical analysis and provide input to computational prioritization tools: Exomes/Genomes.

12.4.1 Variant annotation

The variant calling process on the whole-exome data generated about 20,000 variants, based on the stringency of the former false-positive filter. A whole genome has 4–9 million variants. Thus, following up on each variant manually is clearly out of scope, even more so for whole-genome re-sequencing studies. The purpose of the variant annotation is to document the consequences of a variant on the amino acid sequence. This requires linking the chromosome location to a previously annotated protein and computing the change of the amino acid caused by this variant, if any.

Types of amino acid consequences can be derived and classified as the following:

- Nonsense variants: A codon in the gene is changed so that a stop codon is formed, and the transcription is prematurely terminated.

- Read-through variants: The SNV modifies the stop codon of a gene so that transcription continues beyond the actual gene.
- Start-lost variants: The start codon of a gene is changed, and the transcription starts at a later time.
- Synonymous variants: The variant causes an amino acid substitution but has no further effects on transcription.

Variants occurring in a coding region of a gene but causing no substitution are called synonymous SNVs. A human being has about 3–5 million SNVs of which about 1% occur in coding areas.

There are various tools to annotate the nucleotide changes against a reference and compute the amino acid change. Examples are the ENSEMBL variant effect prediction and ANNOVAR. Both toolsets also query other databases to deliver further information to a variant, like its allele frequency or prediction score.

12.4.2 Variant categorization

Simplified PM is based on detecting the disease-causing variants in the patient's genome. The human genome has about 6 million variants, and its exome has about 20,000. Most of them are benign, or even if they are causing a malfunction of the protein, the human body itself is very often able to repair this damage [13].

The challenge in the variant categorization is to detect those variants that are most likely to cause diseases. In general, there are the following two types of variant categorizations:

- On variant base level, only the position of the variant is important. An example is the frequency of a variant based on the population.
- On protein/transcript level, the influence of a variant of the transcripted protein is important, for example, how much a variant disturbs its function.

Many databases that detail the deleterious variants and many tools that predict the adverse effects of a variant were published in recent years. Some of these variants will be introduced next.

1. Categorize based on frequency

   Perhaps, one of the most important pieces of information about a variant is its allele or genotype frequency. The frequency describes how often the allele or genotype of a variant is observed in the human population. Simplified, if a variant is observed often in the population, it is most likely benign. For Mendelian diseases, causative variants are non-existing or very rare in populations. Thus, frequently occurring variants can be easily discarded as injurious, whereas novel or very rare variants are key candidates. However, frequencies require a large number of sequenced individuals and a statistically representative sample of the population. The first usable frequency resource was derived from the Thousand Genomes Project [14], a major undertaking at its time but ultimately hugely important. More recently, the Gnomad [15]

Project from the Broad Institute [16] expanded to a larger number of individuals, thus characterizing many more variants.

2. Categorize based on evidence

   Previous characterizations of variants are increasingly frequent and have become a critical annotation. If an identical variant or amino acid change has been previously shown to cause the disease, it will instantly become the prime candidate. Numerous databases have assembled literature information of submitted variants. Efforts include Online Mendelian Inheritance in Man (OMIM) [17], Human Gene Mutation Database (HGMD) [18], and NIH's ClinVar [19]. ClinVar has increasingly become a primary source for collecting literature variants and for clinical laboratory submissions. At the beginning of 2019, the number of variants submitted in the ClinVar database was 778,673. HGMD has 248,700 submissions, but with the manual curation of every entry in the database, it is known to be very trustworthy.

12.4.3 Prediction scores

Computational tools provide the means to predict the deleteriousness of the annotated variants. Generally, these tools fall into one of three categories:

1. Primary scores

   These scores use various features and the known variant effect with supervised learning algorithms to compute a probabilistic effect. Features include conservation, known variant frequencies, and effects of amino acid changes on secondary amino acid structure. This feature dataset is used with various machine-learning algorithms with known pathogenic and benign variants to learn a probabilistic score for variants.
2. Composite scores

   Various primary scores have different strengths and weaknesses. The composite scores act as a "mixture of experts." These scores use machine learning to find the optimal combination of primary scores to find a better prediction. Omicia score [20] was one of the first scores, showing remarkable improvements over the primary scores. Most recent scores, such as REVEL [21] or ClinPred [22], take advantage of this conceptual idea and include both primary features and more recent training datasets to high prediction accuracy.
3. Frequency and conservation

   Frequency and conservation are powerful tools to predict the pathogenicity of a variant. The most common conservation score is PhyloP [23]. To detect a conservation area, it compares the human genome with the genomes of other mammals like the ape or zebra. Genetic areas that are equal must be inherited from ancestral species and are known as very robust against diseases.

Also, the Variant Annotation, Analysis and Search Tool [24] (VAAST) is a probabilistic search tool for identifying damaged genes and their disease-causing variants.

VAAST 2 builds upon existing phylogenetic conservation, amino acid substitution, and aggregative approaches to variant prioritization, combining elements of all into a single unified likelihood framework that allows users to identify damaged genes and deleterious variants with greater accuracy, and in an easy-to-use fashion. VAAST 2 can score both coding (SNV, InDel, and splice site) and noncoding variants (SNV), evaluating the cumulative impact of both types of variants simultaneously. VAAST 2 can identify variants causing rare genetic diseases, and it can also use both common and rare variants to identify genes responsible for common diseases. VAAST 2 has a much greater scope of use than any existing methodology to prioritize candidate disease genes in sets of unrelated affected genome sequences.

Another prediction tool is called VAAST Variant Prioritizer [25] (VVP). It computes a likelihood prediction for a variant without a training dataset. VVP provides rapid and scalable scores and prioritizes any sequence variant.

List of evidence databases and tools

Name	**Description**
ClinPred [22]	ClinPred is a prediction tool used to identify disease-relevant nonsynonymous SNVs
ClinVar [19]	ClinVar is a public archive of reports of the relationships among human variations and phenotypes, with supporting evidence
COSMIC	COSMIC, the Catalogue of Somatic Mutations In Cancer, is the world's largest and most comprehensive resource for exploring the impact of somatic mutations in human cancer
GWAS	GWAS (genome-wide association study) is an observational study of a genome-wide set of genetic variants in different individuals to see if any variant is associated with a trait
HGMD [18]	The Human Gene Mutation Database (HGMD) represents an attempt to collate all known (published) gene lesions responsible for human-inherited disease
LR	Composite score based on ten component scores and the maximum frequency observed in the 1,000 genomes populations
LRT	Likelihood-ratio test using an alignment of 32 vertebrate species' genomes
MutationAssessor	Uses multiple sequence alignments of homologous proteins to assess the deleteriousness of a mutation
MutationTaster	MutationTaster employs a Bayes classifier to predict the disease potential of an alteration. The prediction of disease-causing polymorphism is either from the Bayesian model or based on external data, which is noted in the classification
OMIM [17]	OMIM (Online Mendelian Inheritance in Man) is a comprehensive, authoritative compendium of human genes and genetic phenotypes
phyloP [23]	phyloP computes conservation or evolutionary acceleration *p*-values based on an alignment and model of neutral evolution
Polyphen-2 [26]	Polyphen-2 predicts possible impact of an amino acid substitution on the structure and function of a human protein using straightforward physical and comparative considerations

(Continues)

(*Continued*)

List of evidence databases and tools	
Name	**Description**
RadialSVM	Composite score based on ten component scores and the maximum frequency observed in the 1,000 genomes populations
REVEL [21]	REVEL is an ensemble method for predicting the pathogenicity of rare missense variants
SIFT [27]	SIFT predicts whether an amino acid substitution affects protein function, by aligning homologous protein sequences using PSI-BLAST
VVP	The VAAST Variant Prioritization (VVP) provides a variant-specific VAAST score that incorporates allele frequency, amino acid substitution severity, and phylogenetic conservation into a unified score that is normalized to a given feature such as a gene or genomic bin

12.4.4 Variant prioritization

The categorization of variants narrows the disease-causing candidates, but which is the one variant that causes a specific disease is still unknown. The next step is to prioritize the variants, which of those are the most likely disease-causing variants.

A common way is to assess which of the variants have the most evidence in disease causation. For example, the candidates have disease-causing prediction scores as listed in ClinVar, or the containing genes in OMIM are associated with the patient's disease. This step requires substantial effort in curation by a geneticist. To reduce this effort, a periodization tool called Phevor was developed [28]. Phevor integrates phenotype, gene function, and disease information with personal genomic data in order to identify disease-causing variants. It uses an algorithm that propagates information across and between phenotype and genotype ontologies.

12.4.5 Further filter options

1. Filtering based on pedigree

   Another way to find disease-causing candidate variants is to compare the patient's genome/exome with that of the parents or other close relatives. For example, if one parent has the same disease as the patient, it is very likely (at least for monogenetic diseases) that the patient has the same disease-causing mutation. We differ between two kinds of inheritance modes, autosomal dominant and autosomal recessive.

   (i) Autosomal dominant inheritance

   An autosomal dominant disease can be transmitted from both parents to their children. If a parent has a heterozygous pathogenic variant in a gene that is associated with a disease, the probability is 50% for the parent to pass on the disease-causing allele to a child.

If a parent is homozygous, it is expected that all the children will inherit the disease. An example of this inheritance is aniridia (missing iris). Autosomal dominant inheritance can be recognized by the following criteria [29]:

(a) Both sexes are equally affected by the disease (cross-family tree).
(b) The disease occurs in every generation of a family.
(c) If a person is affected by the disease, at least one parent is also affected.
(d) About half of the children of a person affected will also have the disease.

(ii) Autosomal recessive inheritance

In the case of autosomal recessive inheritance, affected patients have mostly unaffected parents. In contrast to autosomal dominant inheritance, the disease gets inherited always from both parents. If the disease-causing gene site is heterozygous in both parents, the child inherits the corresponding, then homozygous, disease alleles with a probability of 25%.

Well-known examples of autosomal recessive diseases are lactose intolerance (in adults) [30] and cystic fibrosis. Autosomal recessive inheritance can be recognized by the following criteria [29]:

(a) Both sexes are equally affected by the disease.
(b) The disease does not occur in every generation of the family. (Often the parents of an affected person are not ill.)
(c) Both parents have, as described earlier, a heterozygous allele expression at the disease-causing locus, the child has a homozygous.
(d) Often the parents of a person are related, for example, cousin/cousin.

If monogenic diseases are caused by variants in the gonosomes, this is referred to as X-linked dominant or pseudoautosomal recessive diseases.

2. Filtering based on cases/controls

In case control studies, as many sample genomes with the same phenotype as possible are collected and analyzed. It is determined which variants the samples have in common. The results are compared with healthy control genomes to filter candidate variants.

12.5 Technical implementation

12.5.1 Scalability and parallelization

As sequencing costs for genomes and exomes drop constantly, and PM gains more significance in modern diagnostics and therapeutics, the amount of genomic data that has to be analyzed has increased dramatically [5]. To process this huge amount of data, researchers and geneticists may require weeks or months if they utilize their own workstations. Parallelism techniques can be applied to reduce the total processing time and to ease the management, and analyses of this data.

The pipeline can be installed in high-performance environments such as Cloud or Spark systems [31]. The different database queries and runs of the prediction tools during the evaluation step are highly parallelizable. Analysis pipelines must scale with respect to the resources on a single compute node, to the number of nodes on a cluster, and to cost performance [32].

A relatively new state-of-the-art parallel and scalable computing platform is Apache's Spark system. It is a fast, in-memory, iterative computing framework for large-scale data processing and high scalability by introducing the resilient distributed dataset abstraction. In terms of performance, Spark system can be up to 100 times faster in terms of memory access and 10 times faster in terms of disk access than a conventional system [33].

12.5.2 Handling big data

Big data refers to large, complex datasets that are beyond the capabilities of traditional data management systems to store, manage and process in a timely and economical manner. Often in petabytes, structured, semi-structured, and unstructured big data creates impediment in data capture, transfer, encryption, storage, analysis and visualization [34].

Managing big data is to take care of the three Vs of data: volume, velocity, and variety [35]. It is not only important to store a big amount of data, its quick access is also mandatory to enable a fast analysis and interpretation. It is imperative to oversee the various source databases, for example, confidential patients' medical records including their genomic profiles.

1. Data volume

   The large amount of data to be stored, to be kept available for the customers for years, and to be backed up has increased exponentially. Modern data centers maintain multiple storage systems, each designed for a particular use case or workload.

   An insight of the immense data sizes involved in analyzing the human genome is provided as follows [36]:

   (i) The raw data (FASTQ files) coming from a sequencer for a single human genome has a size from approximately 300 to 250 GB.
   (ii) After aligning to the reference, the produced binary files (BAM) have a size from approximately 75 to 100 GB.
   (iii) After the variant calling is finished, the resulting VCF file has a size from approximately 100 MB to 1 GB.

2. Data velocity

   With the growth of stored data, it gets more overriding to guarantee a fast access to the data. Initially, companies analyzed data using a batch process. One takes a chunk of data, submits a job to the server, and waits for delivery of the result. This scheme works when the incoming data rate is slower than the batch processing rate and when the result is useful despite the delay [37].

12.5.3 Validation

Data validation is one of the most cardinal parts in every PM pipeline. Nothing is worse than incorrect evidence scores getting displayed and a physician making a misguided decision based on the incorrect scores. Though all data must be validated regularly, the process occurs at distinct levels:

1. Regression test

   The regression test is the most important validation test. This test ensures a change or addition to the pipeline code or to the computer system itself has not broken any existing functionality of the pipeline. The regression test must pass on a regular basis, at least with every code or data source change, or within a system update.

   The test for an annotation pipeline includes the annotation of selected variants. To pass the test, all scores and other annotation data must be exactly the same as before the changes were implemented. In the case of a database update or a bug fix, all differences must be expected and justifiable.
2. Proof of the data

   With every update of a data source, the new scores or data must be proven to be accurate. The displayed scores in the pipeline, for example, must be the same as that on the data source homepage. If possible, an automated test system compares the pipeline data with the original data source after every data update. If an automatization is not possible, the data must be spot-checked manually. This is very time consuming but quite necessary.

12.6 Challenges

12.6.1 Managing updates of published clinical data

Most of the published clinical data is updated on a regular basis, biannually, monthly, or even daily. Reasons for the updates are discovery of new diseases-causing variants and the algorithm to calculate an evidence score has improved. These updates must be implemented into the annotation pipeline as well regularly. The update process itself of the data source is easily automated. It always follows the same steps: download the new data, reformat data to work with the pipeline, store the data, and run the validation process.

12.6.2 Managing changes to data and algorithms

It is important to emphasize that analyzed genomes are risky to compare between different update builds. The evidence of a variant to be disease causing or not may have changed, or prediction scores may have ranked a variant differently. It is critical that all genomes of a study are analyzed with the same data build that includes the previously annotated genomes. All genomes must run through the pipeline again if the annotation pipeline does not offer older data builds to analyze a genome.

12.7 How this engine will redefine healthcare

In a Journal of American Medical Association (October 2019) article, Shrank *et al.* published that the United States spends more on healthcare than any other country, with costs approaching 18% of the gross domestic product (GDP). Prior studies estimated approximately 30% of healthcare spending may be considered waste. The cost of waste in the US health-care system ranged from $760 to $935 billion [38]. A deeper dive in multiple publications attributes wasteful spending to a constellation of factors such as unnecessary services, missed prevention opportunities, inefficient delivery of care (undertreatment), and overprescribing unnecessary medications and costly tests (overtreatment). Could PM furnish the holy grail that reduces the continued increases in US health-care expenditures?

Personalized Medicine (now more popularly referred to as Precision Medicine) is a multidimensional perspective on the patient that is not just one data modality. It is integrating information of an individual's genomic profile, health records, and personal lifestyle variables for a well-rounded view of the patient. This enables tailoring of diagnostic intervention, therapeutic decision-making, and predictive prognosis.

This chapter spotlights the technological driver of genomic information. To underscore what was discussed in the introduction of this chapter, DNA sequencing has now become cheaper and faster than it used to be. In addition, it has also exponentially produced better quality results. Rapid, low-cost, large-scale throughput of genomic data is defining the trajectory of DNA-based hyper-individualized approach into mainstream medicine. Could this be the watershed moment when disparate practices, genetic discovery, clinical care, advanced informatics coalesce to make achievable the quest for Precision Medicine?

Medical informatics and bioinformatics (use of computer science in medicine and life science) are the ecosystems that fuel acceleration of Precision Medicine. The capability of the algorithms to sift through humongous volumes of data search is of the essence, a feat unmatched by human cognitive faculties.

1. Precision prevention: Genomics can identify various gene alterations that can suggest susceptibility to a specific condition. With this information, an individual may now take preemptive action to delay or even eliminate the possibility of the disease state from progressing.

   One example of disease interception is when women, who have BRCA1 or BRCA2 genetic mutations that put them at high risk of developing breast cancer, opt for elective prophylactic mastectomy (surgical removal of breasts).
2. Precision diagnosis: Comprehensive databases of genetic biomarkers can be instrumental in accurate and definitive diagnosis of a disease. In the United States, The Cancer Genome Atlas (TCGA) [39] has mapped the key genomic alterations of 33 types of malignancies. TCGA has produced a rich dataset of immeasurable value for precision diagnosis. TCGA is a trusted reference that will be mined for many years.

3. Precision treatment: Genomics facilitates a critical element of Precision Medicine through pharmacogenomics (study of how genes affect a person's response to drugs). An individual's gene may influence a very different reaction to a standard medication in the same dose that is well tolerated by another. Identification of gene variations or polymorphisms enables alternative treatments that will optimally deliver similar effectiveness.

The uniqueness of one's genetics determines one's therapeutics. A shift to gene-based prescription that minimizes side effects (also referred to as targeted treatment) is reshaping current drug discovery.

Precision Medicine holds both promise and peril alike. This ambitious innovation may indeed deliver tailored care, thereby eliminating "trial and error." This may then improve clinical outcomes and reduce wasteful therapeutic costs. However, the proponents should remain acutely cognizant of the potential technical vulnerabilities of Precision Medicine platforms and databases. There remain mostly uncharted questions. The cautious design of platforms and the use of diverse databases may assiduously minimize inadvertent glitches in the algorithms and inaccuracies of interpreted results.

It may be amiss not to mention the emerging field of gene editing or gene manipulation in the offing. Would not it be intriguing to be able to pinpoint a precise segment of a malfunctioning DNA, cut it out, and replace it with a good DNA? The medical applications and concomitant societal consequences and ramifications of genome engineering are quite immense.

May the thought leaders, active implementers, and passive advocates of Precision Medicine carry on until potential breakthroughs come to full fruition; yet remain mindful and responsible to eschew the health seeker's endangerment.

References

[1] Lander ES, Linton LM, Birren B, *et al.* Initial sequencing and analysis of the human genome. *Nature*. 2001;409(6822):860–921. doi:10.1038/35057062.

[2] NHS. Personalised medicine. https://www.england.nhs.uk/healthcare-science/personalisedmedicine/. 2018.

[3] Vogenberg FR, Barash CI, and Pursel M. Personalized medicine, Part 1: Evolution and development into theranostics. *P T*. 2010;35(10). https://www.ncbi.nlm.nih.gov/pmc/articles/PMC2957753/pdf/ptj35_10p560.pdf.

[4] Haghighi A. Next generation sequencing in personalized medicine: Advances, translational impact, and future directions. *J Pharmacogenomics Pharmacoproteomics*. 2014. doi:10.4172/2153-0645.S1.004.

[5] Black Friday for Genome Sequencing – IEEE Future Directions. http://sites.ieee.org/futuredirections/2018/11/21/black-friday-for-genome-sequencing/. Accessed March 14, 2019.

[6] Altmann A, Weber P, Bader D, Preuss M, Binder EB, and Müller-Myhsok B. A beginner's guide to SNP calling from high-throughput DNA-sequencing data. *Hum Genet*. 2012;131(10):1541–1554. doi:10.1007/s00439-012-1213-z.

[7] Metzker ML. Sequencing technologies — the next generation. *Nat Rev Genet*. 2010;11(1):31–46. doi:10.1038/nrg2626.

[8] Kulski JK. Next-Generation Sequencing — An Overview of the History, Tools, and "Omic" Applications. *Next Generation Sequencing – Advances, Applications and Challenges*. Jerzy K Kulski, IntechOpen; 2016. doi:10.5772/61964.

[9] Genome Reference Consortium. https://www.ncbi.nlm.nih.gov/grc. Accessed March 15, 2019.

[10] Pruitt KD, Tatusova T, and Maglott DR. NCBI reference sequence (RefSeq): a curated non-redundant sequence database of genomes, transcripts and proteins. *Nucleic Acids Res*. 2005;33(Database issue):D501–D504. doi:10.1093/nar/gki025.

[11] Tan A, Abecasis GR, and Kang HM. Unified representation of genetic variants. *Bioinformatics*. 2015;31(13):2202–2204. https://doi.org/10.1093/bioinformatics/btv112.

[12] Danecek P, Auton A, Abecasis G, *et al*. The variant call format and VCFtools. *Bioinformatics*. 2011;27(15):2156–2158. doi:10.1093/bioinformatics/btr330.

[13] Sanca A. DNA repair in humans. *Annu Rev Genet*. 1995;29:69–105. https://www.annualreviews.org/doi/pdf/10.1146/annurev.ge.29.120195.000441.

[14] The 1000 Genomes Project Consortium. A map of human genome variation from population-scale sequencing. *Nature*. 2010;467(7319):1061–1073. doi:10.1038/nature09534.

[15] Kruglyak L, Daly MJ, Reeve-Daly MP, and Lander ES. Parametric and nonparametric linkage analysis: a unified multipoint approach. *Am J Hum Genet*. 1996;58(6):1347–1363. http://www.pubmedcentral.nih.gov/articlerender.fcgi?artid=1915045&tool=pmcentrez&rendertype=abstract.

[16] Lek M, Karczewski KJ, Minikel EV, *et al*. Analysis of protein-coding genetic variation in 60,706 humans. *Nature*. 2016;536(7616):285–291. doi:10.1038/nature19057.

[17] Amberger JS, Bocchini CA, Schiettecatte F, Scott AF, and Hamosh A. OMIM.org: Online Mendelian Inheritance in Man (OMIM®), an online catalog of human genes and genetic disorders. *Nucleic Acids Res*. 2015;43(D1):D789–D798. doi:10.1093/nar/gku1205.

[18] Stenson PD, Mort M, Ball EV, Shaw K, Phillips AD, and Cooper DN. The Human Gene Mutation Database: building a comprehensive mutation repository for clinical and molecular genetics, diagnostic testing and personalized genomic medicine. *Hum Genet*. 2013. doi:10.1007/s00439-013-1358-4.

[19] Landrum MJ, Lee JM, Benson M, *et al*. ClinVar: public archive of interpretations of clinically relevant variants. *Nucleic Acids Res*. 2016;44(D1):D862–D868. doi:10.1093/nar/gkv1222.

[20] Coonrod EM, Margraf RL, Russell A, Voelkerding KV, and Reese MG. Clinical analysis of genome next-generation sequencing data using the Omicia platform. *Expert Rev Mol Diagn*. 2013;13(6):529–540. doi:10.1586/14737159.2013.811907.

[21] Ioannidis NM, Rothstein JH, Pejaver V, *et al.* REVEL: an ensemble method for predicting the pathogenicity of rare missense variants. *Am J Hum Genet.* 2016;99(4):877–885. doi: 10.1016/j.ajhg.2016.08.016.

[22] Alirezaie N, Kernohan KD, Hartley T, Majewski J, and Hocking TD. ClinPred: prediction tool to identify disease-relevant nonsynonymous single-nucleotide variants. *Am J Hum Genet*. 2018;103(4):474–483. doi: 10.1016/j.ajhg.2018.08.005.

[23] Pollard KS, Hubisz MJ, Rosenbloom KR, and Siepel A. Detection of non-neutral substitution rates on mammalian phylogenies. *Genome Res*. 2010;20(1):110–121. doi:10.1101/gr.097857.109.

[24] Yandell M, Huff C, Hu H, *et al.* A probabilistic disease-gene finder for personal genomes. *Genome Res*. 2011;21(9):1529–1542. doi:10.1101/gr.123158.111.

[25] Flygare S, Hernandez EJ, Phan L, *et al.* The VAAST Variant Prioritizer (VVP): ultrafast, easy to use whole genome variant prioritization tool. *BMC Bioinformatics*. 2018;19(1):1–13. doi:10.1186/s12859-018-2056-y.

[26] Ramensky V, Bork P, and Sunyaev S. Human non-synonymous SNPs: server and survey. *Nucleic Acids Res*. 2002;30(17):3894–3900.

[27] Ng PC. SIFT: predicting amino acid changes that affect protein function. *Nucleic Acids Res*. 2003;31(13):3812–3814. doi:10.1093/nar/gkg509.

[28] Singleton MV, Guthery SL, Voelkerding KV, *et al.* Phevor combines multiple biomedical ontologies for accurate identification of disease-causing alleles in single individuals and small nuclear families. *Am J Hum Genet.* 2014;94(4):599–610. doi: 10.1016/j.ajhg.2014.03.010.

[29] Ziegler A and König I. *A Statistical Approach to Genetic Epidemiology.* Wiley-VCH; 1 edition; 2010. http://www.amazon.com/Statistical-Approach-Genetic-Epidemiology–learning/dp/3527323899/ref=sr_1_1?s=books&ie=UTF8&qid=1321015660&sr=1-1. Accessed November 11, 2011.

[30] Torniainen S, Parker MI, Holmberg V, Lahtela E, Dandara C, and Jarvela I. Screening of variants for lactase persistence/non-persistence in populations from South Africa and Ghana. *BMC Genet.* 2009;10(1):31. doi:10.1186/1471-2156-10-31.

[31] Ocaña K and de Oliveira D. Parallel computing in genomic research: advances and applications. *Adv Appl Bioinform Chem.* 2015; 8:23–35. doi:10.2147/AABC.S64482.

[32] Fjukstad B and Bongo LA. A review of scalable bioinformatics pipelines. *Data Sci Eng.* 2017;2(3):245–251. doi:10.1007/s41019-017-0047-z.

[33] Guo R, Zhao Y, Zou Q, Fang X, and Peng S. Bioinformatics applications on Apache Spark. *GigaScience*. 2018;7(8). doi:10.1093/gigascience/giy098.

[34] Nambiar R, Bhardwaj R, Sethi A, and Vargheese R. A look at challenges and opportunities of Big Data analytics in healthcare. *Proc – 2013 IEEE Int Conf Big Data, Big Data 2013*. 2013:17–22. doi:10.1109/BigData.2013.6691753.

[35] Estrada R. From big data to fast data – O'Reilly Media. https://www.oreilly.com/ideas/from-big-data-to-fast-data. Accessed March 16, 2019.

[36] He KY, Ge D, and He MM. Big data analytics for genomic medicine. *Int J Mol Sci*. 2017;18(2):412. https://doi.org/10.3390/ijms18020412.
[37] The 3Vs that define Big Data – Data Science Central. https://www.datasciencecentral.com/forum/topics/the-3vs-that-define-big-data. Accessed March 16, 2019.
[38] Shrank WH, Rogstad TL, and Parekh N. Waste in the US Health Care System: Estimated costs and potential for savings. JAMA. 2019;322 (15):1501–1509. doi:10.1001/jama.2019.13978.
[39] The Cancer Genome Atlas Program https://www.cancer.gov/about-nci/organization/ccg/research/structural-genomics/tcga.
[40] Schwarze K, Buchanan J, Taylor JC, and Wordsworth S. Are whole-exome and whole-genome sequencing approaches cost-effective? A systematic review of the literature. *Genet Med*. 2018;20(10):1122–1130. doi:10.1038/gim.2017.247.

Afterword

The impacts of novel and emerging technologies on a pandemic

Rona Margaret Relova, M.D.[1,2] *and*
Leonard Goldschmidt, M.D., Ph.D.[1]

Around December 2019, the emergence of a cluster of pneumonia of unknown etiology started appearing in Wuhan City, Hubei Province of China. Subsequent virus isolation from patients and genetic analysis showed that the pathogen was a new coronavirus (CoV) [1].

On January 13, 2020, the first case outside China was reported in Thailand [1]. This marked the swift expansion and spread of the virus within hospitals (nosocomial infection) and by family transmission (close-contact spread), exacerbated by travel. Already by January 23, six foreign countries had confirmed cases [1]. By January 30, the World Health Organization (WHO) declared this outbreak a public health emergency of international concern [2].

On February 11, 2020, WHO announced "COVID-19" as the name of the new disease; and the International Committee on Taxonomy of Viruses designated SARS-CoV-2 "Severe Acute Respiratory Syndrome Coronavirus 2" as the name of the new coronavirus [3]. By March 11, COVID-19 was declared a pandemic [4,5].

As of November 2020, the number of confirmed cases globally was over 62 million, with mortality reported well over 1.4 million in 191 afflicted countries [6]. With no antiviral drugs nor vaccines, and with the presence of asymptomatic carriers (people who do not manifest symptoms), traditional public health intervention measures struggle to combat the high transmissibility of COVID-19. Efforts across the globe on containment and mitigation (physical distancing, masking, shelter in place, lockdown) have demonstrated varying degrees of success. These measures have precipitated ramifications on most societies, inevitably wreaking havoc on health systems and economies on a scale not seen in more than 100 years, specifically since the 1918 Influenza pandemic.

[1]VA Palo Alto Health Care System, Stanford University, School of Medicine, Palo Alto, CA, USA
[2]National Institutes of Health, Bethesda, MD, USA

How could digital healthcare technologies alleviate the deleterious impacts of this public health crisis or facilitate strategies geared at quashing this pandemic? Digital healthcare technologies have been adopted by many countries in the management of COVID-19 pandemic. Applications of novel and emerging technologies have been implemented in various facets of the response, such as surveillance, testing, contact tracing, quarantine, drug and vaccine development, clinical management, continuity of care, logistics and personnel training.

A.1 Pivot to telemedicine and telehealth

Mandatory shelter in place orders and lockdowns necessitated the shift to remote health-related services in hyperdrive. Services include online monitoring, advice, consultation and education between doctors and patients over a secure connection. According to J.D. Power's US Telehealth Study data, only 10% of healthcare consumers were using virtual care platforms in 2019 [7]. This may have attributed to the lackluster development of the infrastructure prior to the current situation. This pandemic brought telemedicine and telehealth into a new light as health organizations turn to alternative solutions to deliver care while curbing the disease's spread.

At Lucile Packard Children's Hospital Stanford, prior to pandemic the organization was conducting approximately 20 telehealth visits per day in ambulatory setting. When shelter-in-place was ordered, the health system increased to 800 telehealth visits per day [8].

Many outpatient services and elective procedures were paused due to capacity issues or safety concerns. With a healthcare system stretched too thinly to operate as usual, patients with treatable chronic conditions have suffered disproportionately [8]. Prompt transition to remote health services has become the norm during this period for many institutions, businesses and individuals. Convenience, efficiency and necessity have all contributed to this changeover. Because COVID-19 pandemic is unlikely to be the last global public health crisis, this event may be the impetus to promulgate and extend the widespread adoption of remote health-related services (such as video visits) as an integral part of a healthcare system.

A.2 Logistics and supply chain optimization

Personal protective equipment (PPE) is used every day by healthcare workers (HCW) to protect themselves, the patients and others when providing care. PPE supply chains have been acutely disrupted by the pandemic, producing long lead times and unreliable deliveries. The use of machine learning technologies can ensure that inventory meets the facility's current or anticipated utilization rate. Secure centralized platforms that estimate how long the remaining supply of PPE will last, based on the average consumption rate also referred to as burn rate, can then facilitate order projections for future needs. This replaces the traditional purchasing systems in which each service is tasked to hunt for its own supplies, at times even competing with each other to fulfill the demand.

Another strategy worth spotlighting is the technology of 3D-printing. Some facilities have creatively resorted to 3D-printing of swabs for screening tests, as prompted by the shortage during the surge.

As for supply distribution, by deploying self-driving robots and drones to deliver supplies (PPE, linens, medications, test kits), many facilities have effectively eliminated human-to-human contact.

A.3 Tracking, screening, contact tracing and quarantine

The Internet of Things (IoT) is the interconnection via the Internet of computing devices embedded in everyday objects, enabling them to send and receive data. The data generated can then be analyzed and used to predict or create desired outcomes.

Data dashboards, migration maps, real-time monitoring gadgets, smartphone apps, wearable technology (tracking temperature or heart rate), global positioning systems, thermal cameras—these digital tools allow visible depiction of viral upticks, highlight area restrictions (hot spots) and inform forecasts.

The Center for Systems Science and Engineering at Johns Hopkins University developed an online dashboard to visually track the reported cases and mortality rates on a daily timescale [5]. This is intended to provide the public with an understanding of the outbreak situation as it unfolds, using transparent data sources.

Another relevant technology in this public health crisis is artificial intelligence (AI), also referred to as deep learning, smart algorithms, augmented intelligence or cognitive computing. AI, which was deemed a futuristic aspiration until very recently, has become the reference point for expeditious data integration and analyses that human cognitive capabilities cannot match. Several countries now use AI to gather information on disease prevalence and pathology, and to identify individuals for testing, contact tracing and isolation or quarantine [9]. AI also facilitates infection control and supports point-of-care clinical decision-making, fast-evolving diagnostics and risk prediction by aggregating and analyzing massive data at scale.

Mount Sinai researchers used AI combined with imaging and clinical data to analyze patients with COVID-19. The proof of concept study, published in Nature Medicine on May 2020, demonstrated the high sensitivity of the AI model that can provide a "second opinion" to physicians in cases where computed tomography scan is either negative (in the early course of infection) or shows nonspecific findings [10].

A.4 Virtual education and dissemination of information

The pandemic has invigorated the paradigm shift from conventional, in-person learning to remote, interactive education and collaboration. Virtual education models render requisite trainings to healthcare personnel; and digital tools (like chatbot and web bot) support bidirectional mass communications for COVID-19 notifications and public health advisories.

A.5 "Social distancing" out, "distant socializing" in

According to Aristotle, man is by nature a social animal. This means human beings will naturally seek the companionship of others as essential to their well-being. This foundational human dynamic includes cultivating relationships, mostly through face-to-face interactions. During these onerous circumstances, chronic stress may lead to long-term mental and physical health conditions. Isolation and loneliness may increase sleeplessness, depression, as well as immune and cardiovascular problems.

Dr. Jamil Zaki, Director of the Stanford Social Neuroscience Laboratory, encourages the practice of "distant socializing" [11]. Experiments show that the support of loved ones softens our response to stress and even our brains' response to painful electric shocks [11]. People can remain together even while being apart. Applications with multiparty video-chatting functionality can host virtual coffee breaks, play dates, concerts and memorial services. These tools enable sustained connectedness and social support network with far-reaching benefits on one's wellness.

A.6 COVID-19 therapeutics, drug and vaccine development

Clinical trials are an extension of clinical care. SARS-CoV-2 is a novel strain of coronavirus without any existing evidence-based armamentarium. Therapeutic and prophylactic interventions against COVID-19 are urgently needed. The pathogen's gene sequencing, made possible by advanced technology, provides an accelerated trajectory to discovering drug therapies and vaccines.

The medical and scientific communities could hardly keep pace with the colossal torrent of scholarly publications about SARS-CoV-2. COVID-19 Open Research Dataset (CORD-19) aims to facilitate research work by being an easily accessible resource for clinicians and scientists. CORD-19 allows machine learning algorithms to mine for pertinent knowledge that can aid crucial research in antiviral agent and vaccine development [12]. This dataset is intended to mobilize researchers to apply recent advances in natural language processing and generate new insights in support of the fight against this infectious disease.

Classical vaccine platforms have contributed to past major public health breakthroughs: whole inactivated virus (polio), live attenuated virus (measles, mumps, and rubella), protein subunit (seasonal flu) and virus-like particle (human papillomavirus). The next-generation vaccine platforms include viral vector (modified adenovirus), DNA, RNA, and antigen-presenting cells. The main advantage of next-generation vaccines is the capability to develop them based on sequence information alone. This makes these platforms highly adaptable and agile, speeding up vaccine development considerably [13].

The integration of computational immunology, bioengineering and robotics has also enabled the rapidity with which antiviral monoclonal antibodies can be isolated and engineered. This technology offers an alternative option for passive

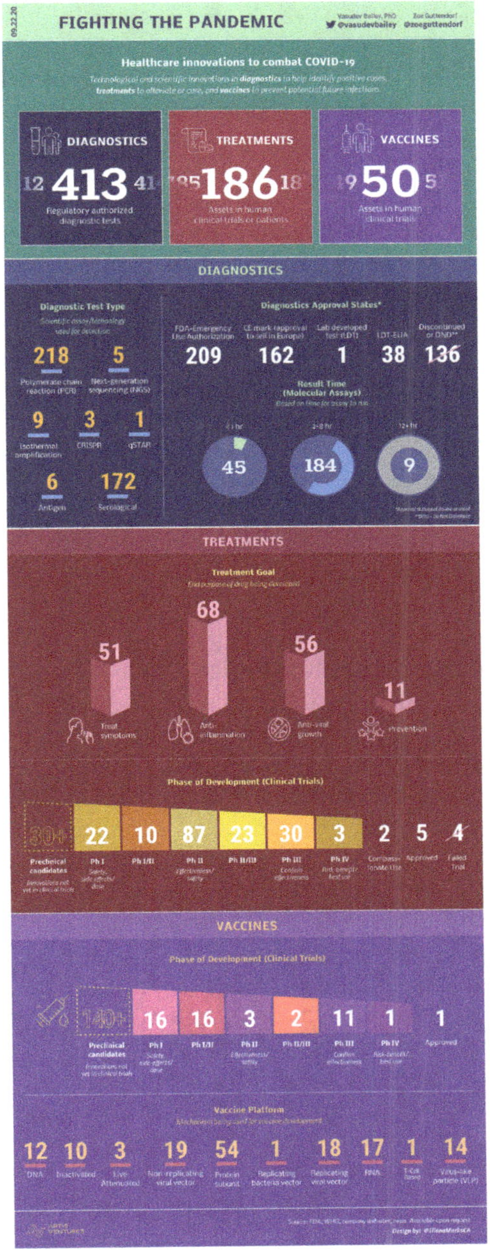

Acknowledgment: Artis Ventures, San Francisco, CA, USA https://www.av.co/covid

immunization against SARS-CoV-2. Monoclonal antibodies can be produced quickly, safely, and in large volumes with current techniques [14]. Establishing the therapeutic or prophylactic efficacy and safety (considered as the "holy grail") of vaccines and monoclonal antibodies will be decisive in suppressing and mitigating the COVID-19 pandemic.

On June 16, 2020, the United States initiated the Operation Warp Speed (OWS) that aims to deliver 300 million doses of a safe, effective vaccine for COVID-19 by January 2021 [15]. OWS is part of a broader strategy to accelerate the development, manufacturing and distribution of COVID-19 vaccines, therapeutics and diagnostics; collectively known as "medical countermeasures" [15]. Ongoing COVID-19 vaccine clinical trials involving next-generation platforms have been implemented within months of the first outbreak; a process that typically takes 5–10 years to launch under usual circumstances.

In collaboration with OWS, Accelerating COVID-19 Therapeutic Interventions and Vaccines (ACTIV) led by the National Institutes of Health (NIH) aims to develop a research strategy for prioritizing and speeding the development of the most promising COVID-19 vaccines and treatments [16]. ACTIV government and biopharmaceutical industry partners will provide infrastructure, subject matter expertise, technology and innovation ecosystem to address this global health crisis.

A.7 Caveats of digital technologies

The digital transformation of healthcare presents both promise and peril.

Digital health interventions, specifically applications intended for surveillance, can infringe on privacy and threaten civil liberties. It is sensible to be vigilant about the risks that come with the use of technologies during this unprecedented time.

Digital health initiatives involve internet, smartphones and wearable technology. This can amplify the digital divide in diverse socioeconomic populations. Technologies may end up benefitting only the more affluent groups. The IoT has been disproportionally more commonplace in high-income than in low- and middle-income areas; 82% in Europe vs. 28% in Africa [17].

Data is the lifeblood of machine learning systems. It is then critical to have robust, heterogeneous datasets, which can produce predictive models that will be beneficial to diverse populations with least possible biases.

This pandemic presents an opportunity to reduce healthcare disparities even as it underscores the gaps and unmet needs of mostly minority communities. The imperative goal is for digital health technologies to be nondiscriminatory and equitably accessible for everyone; thus fostering inclusive, just and fair societies.

A.8 Path forward

Countries that deployed digital health technologies in their pandemic response remain front-runners in containment, mitigation and the management of disease burden. Ongoing and future progress in digital healthcare technology will undeniably redefine medicine and human health, well beyond the COVID-19 pandemic. This public health crisis has fueled major advancements in the biomedical space. The threat of harm or death led to a sense of urgency that galvanized a common resolve to stimulate technologies that could defeat, or at least arrest such a lethal virus.

But how to balance enthusiasm with caution at this inflection point? Uncertainties around technological maturity, scalability, accessibility, governance, data security and impact on health outcomes call for significant prudence on our part. Being mindful that human-to-human interface remains to be the bedrock of practice of medicine should serve as the beacon while navigating the digital revolution.

The readers, authors and editors of this book (an implicit yardstick of shared curiosity and interest) are collectively charting the course of healthcare's patient-centered novel and emerging technologies.

A.9 Glossary of pandemic terms [18]

Contact tracing	the process of identifying people who might have come into contact with an infected person
Containment	the use of available tools to restrict the spread of infection
Lockdown	the active restriction and control of the movement of people by governments
Incidence	the number of individuals who develop a *condition* during a particular time period
Mitigation	the action of reducing the severity of the *pandemic*
Per-capita mortality	a measure of deaths in a particular population, scaled to the size of that population
Quarantine	the process of isolating and restricting the movement of potentially exposed or infected people
Screening:	assessing for signs of disease in an apparently asymptomatic population
Testing:	using medical procedures to confirm a diagnosis in individuals suspected of having a disease
Tracking:	monitoring the spread of infection across locations

References

[1] Sun J, He WT, Wang L, *et al.* COVID-19: Epidemiology, evolution, and cross-disciplinary perspectives. Trends Mol. Med. 2020;26(5):P483–P495. Published online March 21, 2020. DOI: https://doi.org/10.1016/j.molmed.2020.02.008.

[2] WHO. COVID-19 Public Health Emergency of International Concern (PHEIC). 2020. https://www.who.int/publications/m/item/covid-19-public-health-emergency-of-international-concern-(pheic)-global-research-and-innovation-forum (Accessed August 6, 2020).

[3] WHO. https://www.who.int/emergencies/diseases/novel-coronavirus-2019/technical-guidance/naming-the-coronavirus-disease-(covid-2019)-and-the-virus-that-causes-it (Accessed August 6, 2020).
[4] New ICD-10-CM Code for the 2019 Novel Coronavirus (COVID-19). April 1, 2020. https://www.cdc.gov/nchs/data/icd/Announcement-New-ICD-code-for-coronavirus-3-18-2020.pdf (Accessed August 6, 2020).
[5] STAT. WHO Declares Coronavirus Outbreak a Global Health Emergency. 2020. https://www.statnews.com/2020/01/30/who-declares-coronavirus-outbreak-a-global-health-emergency/ (Accessed August 6, 2020).
[6] Johns Hopkins University & Medicine. Coronavirus Resource Center. https://coronavirus.jhu.edu/map.html (Accessed August 6, 2020).
[7] Power JD. 2019. https://www.jdpower.com/business/press-releases/2019-us-telehealth-satisfaction-study (Accessed August 6, 2020).
[8] Healthcare Innovation. 2020. https://www.hcinnovationgroup.com/population-health-management/telehealth/article/21147065/the-telehealth-tidal-wave-has-arrived-will-it-come-crashing-down (Accessed August 6, 2020).
[9] Medical Express. 2020. https://medicalxpress.com/news/2020-05-hospital-artificial-intelligence-covid-patients.html (Accessed August 6, 2020).
[10] Mei X, Lee H, Diao K, *et al.* Artificial intelligence–enabled rapid diagnosis of patients with COVID-19. Nat Med. 2020. https://doi.org/10.1038/s41591-020-0931-3.
[11] Stanford News. 2020. https://news.stanford.edu/2020/03/19/try-distant-socializing-instead/ (Accessed August 6, 2020).
[12] Lu Wang L, Lo K, Chandrasekhar Y, *et al.* CORD-19: The COVID-19 Open Research Dataset. Preprint. ArXiv. 2020;arXiv:2004.10706v2. Published 2020 Apr 22.
[13] Van Riel D and de Wit E. Next generation vaccine platforms for COVID-19. Nat. Mater. 2020;19:810–812. Published 23 July 2020. DOI: https://doi.org/10.1038/s41563-020-0746-0.
[14] Marovich M, Mascola JR, and Cohen MS. Monoclonal antibodies for prevention and treatment of COVID-19. JAMA. 2020;324(2):131–132. doi:10.1001/jama.2020.10245.
[15] HHS. Fact Sheet: Explaining Operation Warp Speed. 2020. https://www.hhs.gov/about/news/2020/06/16/fact-sheet-explaining-operation-warp-speed.html.
[16] NIH. Accelerating COVID-19 Therapeutic Interventions and Vaccines (ACTIV). https://www.nih.gov/research-training/medical-research-initiatives/activ (Accessed August 6, 2020).
[17] GSMA. The State of Mobile Internet Connectivity. https://www.gsma.com/mobilefordevelopment/wp-content/uploads/2019/07/GSMA-State-of-Mobile-Internet-Connectivity-Report-2019.pdf (Accessed August 6, 2020).
[18] Whitelaw S, Mamas M, Topol E, *et al.* Applications of digital technology in COVID-19 pandemic planning and response. Lancet Digital Health. 2020;2(8): E435–E440. Published online June 29, 2020. DOI: https://doi.org/10.1016/S2589-7500(20)30142-4.

Index